ON SCHIZOPHRENIA, PHOBIAS, DEPRESSION, PSYCHOTHERAPY AND THE FARTHER SHORES OF PSYCHIATRY

On Schizophrenia, Phobias, Depression, Psychotherapy and the Farther Shores of Psychiatry

Selected Papers of

SILVANO ARIETI, M.D.

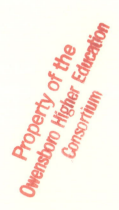

BRUNNER/MAZEL, *Publishers* • New York

Library of Congress Cataloging in Publication Data

Arieti, Silvano.
    On schizophrenia, phobias, depression, psychotherapy, and the farther shores of psychiatry.

    Bibliography: p.
    1. Psychiatry—Addresses, essays, lectures.
II. Title.

RC458.A73   616.8'9   77-25333
ISBN 0-87630-161-8

Copyright © 1978 by SILVANO ARIETI

Published by
BRUNNER/MAZEL, INC.
19 Union Square West
New York, New York 10003

MANUFACTURED IN THE UNITED STATES OF AMERICA

Contents

NOV 7 9

Part III: COGNITION AND ITS RELATION TO PSYCHODYNAMICS

Part IV: RELATED FIELDS

Introduction

When Brunner/Mazel invited me to publish a selection of my papers, I found the suggestion exciting and to be taken very seriously. This publisher, when it was named Robert Brunner, was the firm which published the first edition of my book *Interpretation of Schizophrenia* in 1955. But although a sentimental attachment is undeniable, it was not this feeling that made me react so positively to the suggestion. It was the opportunity to reevaluate most of my work, to retrace the steps of its development, and to decide what I think can be offered again to the professional reader.

Although some of my writings have appeared in book form, the articles published in professional journals have prepared the ground for them and have often contained material which, for one reason or another, could not be included in the books. I believe it is appropriate to make that material available again.

To select 30 papers out of over 100 that I had written by the end of 1977 was not easy. It is not certain that an author is the best judge of his own work. But he is generally called upon to make the selection, and must adopt some criteria which at times do not coincide with his wishes. Some papers which are very dear to the author have to be omitted to avoid repetition or copyright infringements. The order of presentation may also present some problems.

Part One of this collection consists of eleven papers on the subject to which I have devoted most of my activities, schizophrenia. It starts with an overview of the predominantly psychological approach to schizophrenia, followed by a series of papers ranging from practical and therapeutic procedures to theoretical issues.

Part Two presents a number of papers which deal with subjects other than schizophrenia. Depression, phobias, and psychopathic personality are among the subjects studied psychodynamically, therapeutically, or theoretically.

Part Three deals with cognitive studies, which differ from those generally reported by psychologists. Their main objective resides in determining how and to what extent cognitive constructs constitute the inner reality of the human being and have a psychodynamic influence in health and mental disease.

Part Four deals with issues related to psychiatry and especially with the creative process.

Each article is preceded by an introductory note which explains the significance of the paper at the time of publication and, in the cases in which it is pertinent, what change in its significance has occurred since then.

It may be of some interest to the reader to know some details of the author's personal and professional development. When I left Italy in 1939 to escape Fascist persecution and came to this country, I was a young doctor not yet 25 years old. I had graduated from the medical school of Pisa and finished the equivalent of a rotating internship. I had written my thesis, required by European medical schools for graduation, on a neuropsychiatric subject, under the direction of Professor Giuseppe Ayala, Chief of the Institute of Psychiatry and Neurology of the University.

I arrived in the United States with a good preparation in neurology, learned from Professor Ayala, who was an excellent neurologist. However, his psychiatry, which he considered secondary to neurology, left much to be desired. It was exclusively Kraepelinian and followed the major trends of the German psychiatry of that time. Nevertheless, I had studied Freud on my own, as well as other psychoanalysts, a translation of the famous German textbook by Bunke, and the first edition of the French textbook of psychology by Dumas.

When I left Italy, Professor Ayala gave me a letter of introduction for Dr. Armando Ferraro, who was chief of the department of neuropathology of the New York State Psychiatric Institute. Dr. Ferraro was very helpful and encouraging and willing to take me on as a research fellow in neuropathology if I could obtain a fellowship from some foundation. I applied to the Dazian Foundation, which granted me a fellowship of $100 a month for a year to do research work in neuropathology. That fellowship was later renewed for a second year, and I supported myself on that amount. Although at that time, too, my main interest was in clinical psychiatry, working in the department of neuropathology of the Psychiatric Institute gave me wonderful and welcome opportunities.

First of all, when I arrived in this country, I knew many languages, but not a word of English. Thus it would have been impossible for me to work with patients. However, I started to learn the language by myself; soon I could follow the lectures and clinical presentations which were given at the Psychiatric Institute.

At that time the Institute was probably in one of the most glorious periods of its existence. Under the direction of Dr. Nolan Lewis the Institute flourished in many ways. Dr. Lewis was and still is a very liberal and open-minded person who made available the facilities of the Psychiatric Institute to many psychiatrists, innovators, and celebrities who had escaped from Europe. Among those who were there, and whose influence I came under during my stay, were Paul Hoch, Lothar Kalinowsky, who did the first studies of ECT in the United States, Zygmund Piotrowsky, an authority on the Rorschach test, Franz Kallman, an authority on the genetics of mental illness, Hans Strauss, one of the first authorities on the electroencephalogram, and George Jervis and Leon Roizin in neuropathology, in addition to the already mentioned Armando Ferraro. But whereas all the Europeans I have mentioned came to this country already prepared, and many of them introduced a new field or area of research into the United States, I was a youngster with nothing to offer; I had much to learn and to receive.

I was to some extent influenced by all those whom I have mentioned, and of course by the American staff, which included such people as Nolan Lewis, Philip Polatin, Carney Landis, Joseph Zubin, Leslie Hinsie, and William Horwitz. My research was confined, howeved, to neuropathology. What I learned then enabled me even later on to continue some neuropathological work and to publish some ten papers on neuropathological subjects, all of which have been excluded from the present collection. At this point I want to state parenthetically that if there is no paper in this collection which deals with what is generally called biological or organic psychiatry, this omission is not due to the fact that I consider such studies unimportant. On the contrary, I believe that, whenever possible, an attempt should be made to integrate the biological with the psychological (see Chapter 11). I consider the years spent first with Dr. Ayala and then with Dr. Ferraro very important. They have provided me with a biological foundation which I have never forgotten. Even today I am very much interested in the physiology of the central nervous system. If no purely biological study is included in this collection, it is because I had to recognize that my other papers were more appropriate for this book. Although I am convinced that every function (or dysfunction) of the brain is mediated by a biochemical change, I have always found myself drawn more toward inquiries into the psychological factors which bring about suffering or dysfunction, or are powerful enough to change what is only a biological predisposition into clinical actualization.

When I left the Psychiatric Institute, I obtained a residency at Pilgrim State Hospital starting November 1, 1941. That hospital was the largest psychiatric hospital in the world, with a population of over 10,000 patients. There was abundant case material of every kind, an infinite possibility for study, research, and treatment. I had been there just a little more than a month when, on December 7, the Japanese attacked Pearl Harbor and the United States entered the Second World War. The medical staff, nurses, and attendants were reduced to a minimum. We did the best we could under those circumstances. There I found in Dr. Newton Bigelow and Dr. Henry Brill two excellent teachers with extraordinary diagnostic skill. I learned a great deal from them. But because wartime conditions did not permit special facilities and because the general climate of the hospital was not oriented toward research, I continued to pursue my project alone.

In Pilgrim State Hospital I became interested in the longitudinal study of schizophrenia from the earliest to the most advanced stages. I felt that many writings on this psychosis had failed to offer a detailed description and interpretation of the gradual progression of the illness. In this type of research I was very much helped by my readings of the book on comparative development psychology by Heinz Werner, which I discovered shortly after my arrival in America. I felt that I could make an effort to combine and coordinate the basic notions of Heinz Werner, the principles of dissolution of Hughling Jackson, and the theories of regression of Sigmund Freud, and reach an understanding of schizophrenic regression in the various stages of the psychosis (see Chapters 9 and 10).

In addition, I developed two other important fields of interest during my stay at Pilgrim State Hospital (November 1941 to February 1946), first as a resident and later as a staff psychiatrist. The first concerns thought disorders in schizophrenia. Actually, the origin of my interest in this area is much more remote in time than my reading of Eugene Bleuler's and Heinz Werner's writings. It goes back to my studies of the eighteenth-century philosopher Giambattista Vico while I was in college. Vico's study of the cognitive ways in which the ancients, the primitives, children, and poets conceive of the world and respond to it fascinated me. In my opinion, Vichian conceptions were among the best preparation for understanding the schizophrenic reality and the schizophrenic experience (see Chapter 29). In Pilgrim State Hospital I made many observations which were the foundations of my subsequent studies on schizophrenic cognition.

The second field of interest deals with psychotherapy of the psychotic, which I first attempted in a rudimentary way. I had discovered that a few patients who resided in back buildings and had been considered hopeless would apparently recover or improve enough to be discharged, at times after many years of hospitalization. At that time these were considered cases of "spontaneous recovery." I was not satisfied with this explanation and looked more deeply into the matter. I soon discovered that these so-called spontaneous recoveries were not spontaneous at all, but the result of a relationship which had been established between the patient and an attendant or a nurse. I made these observations only in services of female patients, but I assumed that the same situation could take place in male services. The relationship went through two stages. In the first stage, by giving the patient special consideration and care, the nurse or the attendant had met some of her needs, no matter how primitive they were. The patient had improved somewhat and the nurse had developed attachment and deep involvement with her. The patient soon would become the pet of the nurse. In a second stage, the patient had become able to help the nurse with the work on the ward. In those war years, with acute scarcity of personnel, any help was very welcome. The patient would then be praised, and an exchange of approval, affection, and reliability was established. In this climate of exchange of warmth and concern the patient had improved to the point of being suitable for discharge. Much to my regret, however, I almost invariably observed that these formerly regressed patients would soon relapse and be readmitted to the hospital. Outside they were not able to "make it."

Nevertheless, I was impressed by the fact that even an advanced schizophrenic process had proved to be reversible or capable of being favorably influenced by a human contact. These were quite unusual notions at that time. I thought that perhaps methods could be devised by which we could help the patient maintain, increase, strengthen the achieved amelioration, even outside of the hospital environment. But of course I had no idea of how to do it. I had nevertheless learned that whatever benefit the patient could receive, had to come from his bonds with at least another human being. It was something that neither Vico, nor Bleuler, nor Werner could teach me. It seemed to be so difficult to establish a human bond with the schizophrenic, at a professional level; and Freud, whom I read extensively, did not seem much interested in the subject.

That is why, when I left Pilgrim State Hospital, I applied to become a candidate at the William Alanson White Institute, where I knew it was possible to receive what I wanted—that interpersonal approach which I had already understood was so important even for the schizophrenic. And at the White Institute were the people about whom I had heard so much, whose writings I had admired, and whom I was eager to meet in person. I refer to Harry Stack Sullivan, Clara Thompson, Erich Fromm, and many others. At the White Institute I learned that one becomes a person by virtue of relations with other human beings and not because of inborn instinctual drives. I have not yet mentioned Frieda Fromm-Reichmann, and yet it was particularly her teaching that I was searching for. She was the one from whom I had to learn those modalities which would maintain in a state of remission the patients whose temporary improvement I had seen at Pilgrim State Hospital.

The teaching of Frieda Fromm-Reichmann was very fruitful. Fromm-Reichmann was indeed among the first to emphasize that the schizophrenic is not only alone in his world, but also lonely. His loneliness has a long and sad history. Contrary to what many psychiatrists used to believe, the patient is not happy with his withdrawal but is ready to resume interpersonal relations, provided that he finds a person who is capable of removing the suspiciousness and distrust that originated with the first interpersonal relations and made him follow a solitary path. From Fromm-Reichmann I learned that there is a part of the patient that has retained an adult life and would resent being treated in a babyish way. Fromm-Reichmann tried to explain to the patient that his symptoms are ways of remodeling his life experience in consequence of, or in accordance with, his thwarted past or present interpersonal relations. She wanted the patient to become aware of the losses he sustained early in life, but he must become aware of them on a realistic level. That is, he must not distort or transform symbolically these losses, but must accept the fact that they can never be made up and that he is nevertheless capable of becoming integrated with the interpersonal world.

Not only from Frieda Fromm-Reichmann, but from the whole faculty of the White Institute I learned that a characteristic unique to the human race—prolonged childhood with consequent extended dependency on adults and need of lasting and solid interpersonal relations—is the basis of the psychodynamics of schizophrenia. What occurs at any subsequent age is also relevant and may bring about the decisive turns of events that trigger the psychosis. The childhood situation, however, provides preparatory factors that have a fundamental role inasmuch as they narrow the range of choices of life directions, thwart the possibility of compensation, determine basic orientations, and facilitate abnormal sequences of events.

In summary, my training at the White Institute taught me to study the world which the child meets and the child's way of experiencing that world, especially in its interpersonal aspects. It also taught me what people can do to one another. I was able thus to attempt some formulations of the psychodynamics of schizophrenia. I was gradually filling the numerous gaps and doubts that my original observations at Pilgrim State Hospital had left in me.

All this for the good. But soon other doubts started to creep in, and I saw different types of gaps. By stressing the interpersonal, Sullivan and the interpersonal school did not intend to subtract the intrapsychic, but in practice many Sullivanians did so. They focused on the individual as if he were a tabula rasa molded passively by the interpersonal events of his life. Although by no stretch of the imagination should interpersonal theories be confused with behaviorism, the stress was on the relation with the external world, and on the response to such relation. The inner self was neglected, at least in theoretical conceptions.

Yet no influence is received from the environment like a direct and immutable message. Multiple processes involving interpersonal and intrapsychic dimensions go back and forth and undergo a continuous integration. I thought that I could find the clue to this integrative activity in cognition, an area of psychology which was looked upon with great suspicion in the late 40s and early 50s, when either behaviorism, instinctual Freudianism, or interpersonalism prevailed. I not only went back then to my Giambattista Vico and Heinz Werner, but immersed myself also in Hughlings Jackson, Kurt Goldstein, Jean Piaget, Susanne Langer, Kasanin, Von Domarus, and the Russian Vygotsky. My approach aimed at finding structural forms for a psychodynamic content. This approach, which I called structural or psychostructural, was developed independently and along different lines from the studies of Lévi-Strauss, and preceded Chomsky's application of structuralism to other fields of inquiry. The topic on which I focused my research was thought disorder in schizophrenia.

At that time only a few people knew what I was talking about. One of them was David Rioch, who, in 1948, accepted enthusiastically my paper on the special logic of schizophrenia for publication in the journal *Psychiatry* (see Chapter 2). That paper opened to me the possibility of writing a book, and in 1955 the first edition of *Interpretation of Schizophrenia* appeared. In that book I tried to formulate a psychodynamics of schizophrenia, to lay the basis for a psychotherapy of schizophrenia, and to integrate such formulations with my cognitive-structural studies.

After the publication of the first edition of *Interpretation of Schizophrenia*, I became involved with the editorship of the *American Handbook of Psychiatry*, which was published in 1959. In the preparation of the *Handbook*, especially in the six volumes of the second edition, which appeared in 1974 and 1975, I endeavored, with the help of co-editors, to bring together several hundred authors, specialists in the various fields. We all worked together in an effort to prepare a worthy representation of American psychiatry. Many works on cognition and feelings became integrated in my book *The Intrapsychic Self*, which appeared in 1967. My research on volition, inspired originally by my work on the catatonic type of schizophrenia, was integrated with sociological studies and reported in the book *The Will to Be Human* (1972). In the meantime I devised several psychotherapeutic procedures for the treatment of schizophrenia (see Chapters 3 and 4) and drastically revised my conceptions on the psychodynamics of the disorder (see Chapters 1 and 5), so that a new edition of *Interpretation* could appear in 1974, expanded and almost entirely rewritten.

The readers of this collection of papers will soon recognize that schizophrenia has not been my only field of inquiry. From the beginning of my psychiatric studies I had a strong interest in phobias (Chapters 13 and 14), and in the last few years I have been applying myself more and more to the study and therapy of depression (Chapters 15 and 16)

However, I must repeat here what I have had the opportunity to write elsewhere, that the study of schizophrenia not only transcends schizophrenia, it transcends the whole field of psychiatry. The readers of this book will easily understand how the study of this major psychosis led me to make direct inquiries into fields which seem completely unrelated, for instance, the creative process (see Chapters 25 and 26).

In conclusion, although this collection is only a small sample of the work of a psychiatrist who follows a predominantly psychological approach, I hope it is sufficient to stimulate others to pursue the possibilities of depth and of multiple expansions offered by this approach.

SILVANO ARIETI, M.D.

Part I
SCHIZOPHRENIA

1

An Overview of Schizophrenia from a Predominantly Psychological Approach

This article was written at the invitation of the Editor of the American Journal of Psychiatry. *Published in 1974, it is an overview of a predominantly psychological approach to the study and treatment of schizophrenia as developed over a period of 30 years. It reviews psychodynamics, psychological structures and mechanisms, and psychotherapy. I also discuss the areas in which changes of position or emphasis are called for, particularly the formation of the maternal image and the self-image, and present a critique of the new conceptions of schizophrenia that view it as simply a variety of human existence rather than as a disease. Many of the issues which are briefly reviewed in this paper in the large context of the psychology of schizophrenia receive a more elaborate presentation in the papers which follow.*

IN VIEW OF THE INCREASED INTEREST in the genetic and biochemical studies of schizophrenia, it is pertinent to reevaluate the position of a predominantly psychological approach to this major psychosis.

In my opinion, a predominantly psychological orientation in the study and treatment of this psychosis is a fundamental one and will remain so in the foreseeable future. However, certain positions assumed in the past have to be reconsidered, and cognizance has to be taken of changes in emphasis and even of some perspectives.

The psychological approach includes all methods that study the psychogenesis, psychodynamics, psychological structures and mechanisms, and psychotherapy of the psychosis. In a broader sense, within the psychological approach we must also include sociocultural studies. It is apparent that in most instances sociocultural factors affect the individual through the intermediary action of psychological processes. For example, it is not enough to find out that poverty, immigration, being a member of a minority, or living in slum areas increases the incidence of the disorder. We must also be able to translate these statistical data in terms of human suffering. For instance, we may investigate whether or not these social factors become pathogenetic by decreasing among a certain group of people the possibility that they will either become good parents or receive good parenthood.

It is important to stress in these introductory remarks that the majority of authors (including myself) who focus on the psychological aspect of schizophrenia do not deny a nonpsychological, most probably hereditary, component. It is true that no Mendelian law acting in families of schizophrenics has been found; it is true that nothing resembling the distribution of such hereditary diseases as Huntington's chorea, hemophilia, or muscular dystrophy has been observed in schizophrenia. It is also true that the genetic claims made by such people as Rüdin and Kallman have not passed the test of time. On the other hand, certain situations that seem to prove a less definite but nevertheless existing genetic component have been recognized. The incidence of schizophrenia in the general population is calculated to be 0.85 percent. But if we take a population of monozygotic twins, in which one member of each pair has or had schizophrenia, in 25-38 percent of the cases the other monozygotic twin also is or was suffering from schizophrenia (1). Authors differ as to the exact concordance rate in monozygotic twins, but there seems to be little doubt, according to the reported studies, that the incidence is approximately 36 times greater than one would expect in the general population.

This finding is certainly impressive, but, in my opinion, even more impressive is the fact that in 64 percent of pairs of monozygotic twins, one twin is not suffering and is not going to suffer from schizophrenia.

If it is true that monozygotic twins are genetically equivalent, as the geneticists tell us (2), differences between them must be the result of nongenetic factors. And the difference or discordance in relation to schizophrenia in identical twins is approximately twice as frequent as the concordance. If schizophrenia were a purely genetic condition, the concordance would have to be 100 percent. It is thus fair to assume that nongenetic factors "are influencing the phenotype, either by enhancing expression of the illness in the affected twin or by retarding it in the nonaffected twin" (2). In other words, the genetic factor provides a potentiality, but other factors are necessary to change the potentiality into a clinical entity. The potentiality may be a psychobiological vulnerability or a purely biochemical one.

Those authors, including myself, who have studied cases of schizophrenia intensely and psychodynamically have found not even a single case that did not come from a very disturbed environment and that did not present a very revealing psychodynamic history. Now, it could very well be that the same psychodynamic disturbances of environmental origin would not have been enough in themselves to unchain the disorder. As a matter of fact, we find similar factors among nonschizophrenics. However, if the hereditary vulnerability pre-existed, the psychodynamic disturbances might have been able to change potentiality into a clinical disorder. I do not know whether the genetic potentiality could be labeled pathological per se. It could be that in other circumstances it would actualize itself in constructive or desirable ways. Similarly the environmental disturbance, in different contingencies, genetic or otherwise, could even help the individual to transcend the environment and become a creative person, an innovator, a reformer. However, the combination or the casual encounter of the genetic and environmental factors, or the absence of compensatory opportunities, may have determined the disorder.

Since at the present time we cannot change the genetic code of people, it seems much more promising to change the psychological factors. The organicists may think that if we cannot change the genetic code, we can try to change the effects of the anomalous genetic code by biochemical means. For instance, even when diabetes has a hereditary or familial basis, we treat it with insulin. The fact remains that the biochemical mechanisms inherent in the genetic potentiality have not yet been detected, and their existence has not been proved. The function attributed by some authors to serotonin has been denied by other authors, and the existence of such components as taraxein has not been confirmed.

The basic premise of the psychiatrist who adopts a predominantly psychological approach is that, if schizophrenia is the result of a set of etiologic organic and psychological factors, it will be enough to remove one of the two types of components of the set to disrupt the set and to prevent the occurrence of the disorder. If the disorder has already appeared, it is plausible that by removing or altering one of the two components a condition will come about in which schizophrenia will no longer be possible, or if possible, will be ameliorated. It is thus very important to study the psychodynamics, the psychological structure, and the psychotherapy of schizophrenia and to review the major changes that have occurred in these fields recently. Space limitation requires brevity and a selection of topics that may be arbitrary.

Although the individual psychotherapy of schizophrenia has received no adequate representation in the recent psychiatric literature, or a representation comparable to that of a few years ago, the involvement of practicing psychiatrists with it has not diminished. I think we can surely affirm that no psychiatrist can ignore the psychotherapy of schizophrenia, nor can he escape practicing psychotherapy with schizophrenics even if he is determined to do so. Even a psychiatrist whose practice consists predominantly of administering phenothiazines cannot help inquiring about the dynamics of the patient's anguish and conflict, cannot help observing and interpreting what happens between the patient and himself. He may not apply all the insights that people who have devoted themselves to the psychotherapy of schizophrenia have communicated, but some of them have rubbed off on every psychiatrist. What Frieda Fromm-Reichmann, other pioneers, and we, their followers, have tried to do has not been ignored but assimilated, even if at times in very diluted forms.

PSYCHODYNAMICS OF FAMILY INTERRELATIONS

Most psychodynamically oriented authors believe that most psychogenic traumas occur in childhood. From the first period of life the future schizophrenic finds himself in a family that is not able to offer him a modicum of security or basic trust. The world he meets in childhood consists of interpersonal relations characterized by intense anxiety or hostility, by false detachment, or by a combination of these feelings. Some authors have attributed great psychogenetic importance to the abnormality of the family as a whole; others have focused on the unhappy marriage of the parents or on the personality of the father or on the interaction with the siblings. The personality and attitude of the mother remain, in the opinion of many, the most important psychogenic factors.

I reported similar findings in the first edition of my book *Interpretation of Schizophrenia,* which appeared in 1955 (3). However, in these intervening years I have become aware of many other factors that have compelled me to rewrite my book almost completely (4). I have become increasingly convinced that, among many other things, we have not taken into sufficient consideration what is happening intrapsychically to the child. During childhood, and also later, the future patient not only has to sustain the impact of intense negative emotions, such as tension, fear, anxiety, hostility, and detachment; he also has to contend with the alterations in his development that are consequent to such exposure and, perhaps, with some of his own intrinsic qualities that make him less capable of coping with adverse circumstances. Certainly it is very important to study what kind of interpersonal world the patient met early in life. That is the first item on our list of inquiries, but only the first. It is also of crucial importance to determine how the child experienced this world, how he internalized it, and how such internalization affected the subsequent events of his life, which in their turn acted as feedback mechanisms.

To illustrate this point of view I must repeat here what I have reported in recent writings (4, 5) and reconsider the concept of the "schizophrenogenic mother." The mother of the schizophrenic has been described as a malevolent creature, deprived of maternal feeling. John Rosen (6) spoke of her perverse sense of motherhood. She has been called a monstrous human being. At times, it is indeed difficult not to make these negative appraisals in some cases that stand out for these very negative qualities and that therefore seem typical. Quite often, however, a generalization is made that seems to me no longer warranted.

First of all, in the largest majority of cases the mother is not a monster or an evildoer but a person who has been overcome by the difficulties of living. These difficulties have become enormous not only because of her unhappy marriage but, most of all, because of her neurosis and the neurotic defenses she built up in interacting with her children. There is another important point that has been neglected in the literature. These studies of the patient's mother, starting from those of Frieda Fromm-Reichmann (7) and John Rosen (8), were made at a time during which drastic changes in the sociological role of women were in a state of incubation. It was a period that immediately preceded the women's liberation era. It was the beginning of a time when a woman had to contend fully but tacitly with her newly emerged need to assert equality. She could no longer accept submission, yet she strove to fulfill her traditional role. These social factors entered into the intimacy of family life and complicated the parental roles of both mothers and fathers.

I wish to add that this was the time when the "nuclear family," an invention of urban industrial society, came into its full existence. The nuclear family is destructive not only for the children but also for the parents, and especially for the woman of the house. The home is often greatly deprived of educational, vocational, and religious values. It consists of a small number of people who live in little space, compete for room and for material and emotional possession, and are ridden by hostility and rivalry.

A few years after the publication of *Interpretation of Schizophrenia* in 1955 I started to compile some private statistics and, although personal biases cannot be excluded and the overall figures are too small to be of definite value, I have reached the tentative conclusion that only about 25 percent of the mothers of schizophrenics fit the image of the schizophrenogenic mother; 75 percent do not fit. We must then ask ourselves why so many authors, including Sullivan (9), Rosen (6, 8), Hill (10), Lidz and associates (11), Laing (12), and (alas!) myself (3), have portrayed these mothers in this intensely negative, judgmental way. Of course somebody could say that I have been led to error, that I have not been able to uncover the hidden perverse qualities of these mothers. However, in fairness to myself I cannot believe that I have grown so insensitive in many years of practicing psychoanalysis and psychotherapy as to become less aware now than in the past of the real personality of these mothers.

Study of the subject and repeated observations have led me to different conclusions. Schizophrenics who are at a relatively advanced stage of psychoanalytically oriented psychotherapy often describe their parents, especially the mother, in these negative terms, the terms used in the psychiatric literature. We therapists have believed what our patients have told us. Inasmuch as approximately 25 percent of the mothers have proved to be that way, it was easier for us to make an unwarranted generalization that included all the mothers of the schizophrenics. We have made a mistake reminiscent of the one made by Freud when he came to believe that his neurotic patients had been assaulted sexually by their parents. Later Freud realized that what he had believed to be true was, in by far the majority of cases, only the product of the patient's fantasy. The comparison is not quite apt, however, because in possibly 25 percent of the cases the mothers of schizophrenic patients have really been nonmaternal, and we do not know what percentage of mothers of nonschizophrenics have been nonmaternal.

The Transformation of the Parental Image

If my interpretation is correct, we must find out why many patients have transformed the image of the mother or of both parents into one that is much worse than the real one. In my opinion what happens in the majority of cases is the following: the mother has definite negative characteristics—excessive anxiety, hostility, or detachment. The future patient becomes particularly sensitized to these characteristics. He becomes aware only of them because they are the parts of his mother that hurt, and to which he responds deeply. He ignores the others. His use of primary process cognition makes possible and perpetuates this partial awareness—this original part-object relationship, if one wants to use Melanie Klein's terminology. The patient who responds mainly to the negative parts of his mother will try to make a whole out of these negative parts, and the resulting whole will be a monstrous transformation of the mother.

In later stages this negative image may attract other negative aspects of the other members of the family or of the family constellation, so that her image will be intensified in her negative aspect. This vision of the mother is somewhat understood by the mother, who responds to the child with more anxiety and hostility. A vicious circle is thus organized that produces progressive and intense distortions and maladaptations. Two tendencies thus develop. One is to repress from consciousness the reality of the mother-patient relationship, but this is not a task that can be fully achieved. The other tendency is to displace or project to some parts of the external world this state of affairs. But this tendency also is not actualizable unless a psychosis occurs, and for the time being it remains only a potentiality. What I have said in relation to the mother could, in a smaller number of patients, be more appropriately said in reference to the father. In the majority of cases, the full extent of the negative image of the mother (and/or father) is repressed. It reappears in psychotherapy when defenses and protections are eliminated.

Why do schizophrenic patients who, in the course of treatment, become aware of the negative image of their parents continue during a long stage of psychotherapy to see them in a negative way? Why in childhood did they focus on the negative aspects? We can give only hypothetical answers to this problem. The genetic vulnerability that I have referred to, or other particular contingencies occurring in early life, make the future patient experience more intensely a phenomenon that occurs to some degree in every living animal organism. Inasmuch as painful characteristics or negative parts of complex stimuli generally hinder adaptation, they are as a rule more dangerous from the point of view of survival. Evolution has thus probably favored a stronger response to them. We react more vigorously to pain than to pleasure, and to sorrow than to joy. Psychotherapy must help to put back the previous components in their proper proportion. The psychological hurt that the patient has so strongly experienced, and is still experiencing, is mainly hostility, to which I shall return later.

The therapist's knowledge that the patient transforms his experiences drastically is very important in psychotherapy. Until recently the therapist and the patient established a so-called therapeutic alliance based mainly on recrimination for what the parents have allegedly done in engendering the patient's misery. Certainly the parents have played a role, but to magnify that role is also to alter the truth and to hinder the progress of psychotherapy beyond the initial stages.

The Self and the Others

Whatever I have said about the parental image could be repeated, with the proper modifications, about the self-image of the future schizophrenic. The self, although it is related to parental appraisals, is not a reproduction of them but a grotesque representation. Space limitations prevent me from dealing with this very important subject; the reader is referred to other writings of mine (4, 13).

From a general point of view we can conclude that a large part of the psychiatric literature of psychodynamic orientation has made the error of seeing not only the child but also the adolescent and young adult as completely molded by circumstances, a passive agent at the mercy of others, either parents or society. Although these environmental forces are of crucial importance, we should not forget other factors. The person, even at a young age, is not a tabula rasa, or a sponge that absorbs whatever is given him without his adding an element of individuality and creativity to what he receives and thus contributing to his own transformation. The individual, whether he will be a psychiatric patient or not, will never reproduce the experiences of childhood as an historian would; he always transforms and recreates, in favorable or unfavorable ways. Some of the authors who study the effect of the family and of the environment on the schizophrenic patient do so in a crude way, as if they were describing a rapport of simple linear causality. It would be like studying the intake of food but not the function of the digestive system and the metabolic process of the body.

Authors like Lidz (14), Wynne and Singer (15, 16), Jackson (17, 18), and Bateson and others (19) have enlarged greatly our understanding of schizophrenia by showing the ways in which the family affects the patient. However, they have not illustrated how the environmental forces have passed through and been transformed by intrapsychic agencies. Lidz spoke of the transmission of irrationality directly from parents to children. In an article published in 1969 (20) and again in his recent book (21), he quoted the case of a girl whose mother wished her to become a good writer like Virginia Woolf, even if that would imply committing suicide. Eventually the patient did commit suicide. How could irrationality be more clearly transmitted, Lidz seemed to ask. This case is very dramatic, but it is not the typical case of schizophrenia. As a matter of fact, I dare say that this patient committed suicide *not because* she was schizophrenic, but *in spite of* her being schizophrenic. The direct execution of an order, as originally (or presumably) received from parents, is more typical of other states than of schizophrenia.

Between the conflict, originated in the parents, and the carrying out of psychotic orders and overt unusual or bizarre behavior, many intermediary displacements and transformations—affective, cognitive, and conative—take place. More typical are cases like the following: the patient who believes he is Jesus Christ and wants to act and to be treated as if he were Jesus Christ; the patient who believes that people put poison in his food; the patient who receives messages from other planets; the patient who thinks he is powerful enough to control the world, to have the human race exterminated and replaced by a population of dogs. It is hard to believe that the parents transmitted literally these irrationalities to the patients. Had they done that, they too would have been schizophrenics.

The schizophrenic irrationality is not transmitted directly, as a language is. However, a fine distinction is to be made: the schizophrenic irrationality is certainly related to the influence of others, especially parents, but in a much more subtle way. Let us take the example of the patient who thinks he is Jesus Christ. His parents probably were not able to promote his self-esteem; with their attitude they discouraged him and did not instill in him belief in the promise of life. Because of his own distortions and magnifications he saw the attitude of his parents as proof that he would be defeated in every attempt to assert himself, that there was no hope for him; he would not "make it." When the inner turmoil became very intense and he decompensated, he adopted a way of thinking that permitted him to have the greatest possible image of himself and nourish the hope that he would redeem his fellow human beings from similar predicaments. The important thing is that he would not have been able to transform his anxieties and conflicts into a particular delusion if he had not adopted a special type of thinking. And that type of thinking, from a structural point of view, did not originate from his parents (see the section on Schizophrenic Cognition).

Let us consider another one of the mentioned examples, the patient who believed that he could control the world, make the human race perish, and have it replaced by a population of dogs. This patient lost his mother at the age of three. He was brought up by two much older sisters, who resented having to take care of him, and by a father who was a perfectionist. Because of his own frustrations, the father was unhappy and hard to please. In order to stimulate the patient toward constant improvement the father provoked great anxiety in his son, who came to believe he would never succeed in anything he tried. When the father remarried, the patient saw the stepmother as a caring person at first, but as hostile later and as a source of sexual stimulation from which he could not escape. The poor communication, the inability to properly ventilate the problems, and the resulting anxiety predisposed the patient to think that his father would always find fault with him and would never love him. And yet love from his father was what the patient wanted most; nothing could be more precious or more difficult to attain. Was there in the world a creature toward whom his father was lenient and not demanding, and on whom he bestowed love? Yes, the dog of the family, or rather the series of dogs that succeeded one another.

Only the adoption of a different type of thinking made the patient change from a state of hopelessness and worthlessness into a position from which he felt he had the power to control or transform the world. The new world would be populated not by people, who withdraw from love, but by those who could obtain love—the dogs. When the acute phase of the episode was over and the patient was able to give a detailed personal history, he was easily helped to trace back the origin of his delusions. It was also explained to him that his original relations with his father, although unhappy and unhealthy, were already unrealistically transformed in childhood and made worse by poor communication, inability to see the totality of the picture, difficulty in finding compensations, and especially by the tendency to experience the rapport with his father in a restricted and unfavorable way. As we have already mentioned, the patient's relationship with his stepmother proved to be a difficult one and in its turn made the relationship with his father even more complicated because of a new and rather late oedipal situation.

PSYCHODYNAMIC DEVELOPMENT OF SCHIZOPHRENIA

Space limitations prevent presenting in detail the sequence of events that unfold in the life of the patient from birth to the onset of the psychosis. I shall only attempt to offer here a brief and incomplete outline. Although great variations are possible, I have been able to differentiate in the majority of cases four periods (4, part II). It is in the first period (early childhood) that, for a variety of reasons, the future patient cannot accept entirely the "Thou," the other person, generally the mother, who is necessary for the formation of the child's "I" or self. This is the beginning of the schizophrenic cleavage. The other comes to be perceived as a *malevolent Thou* and the I as a *bad me*. In most cases this cleavage is patched up and the psychological status is protected by deacquisition of a schizoid personality that blunts feelings or a stormy fenses. In the second period (late childhood), either because of the personality that is capable of a variety of responses, the Thou tends to be transformed and experienced as a *distressing other* and the bad me is transformed into the *weak, inadequate me*. The child will see himself as a weakling in a world of strong and distressing adults.

The third period, which generally starts at puberty, is characterized not only by sexual urges but most of all by conceptual life. What may prove most pathogenetic are not instinctual impulses or instinctual deprivations, but ideas—the cognitive part of man, which has been neglected in psychoanalysis as well as in general psychiatry (13, 22). From now on the self-image will consist predominantly of such concepts as personal significance, one's role in life, and self-esteem. The defenses that the person had adopted in the previous two periods and that were adequate for the little world of the family become less reliable now that the patient is extending his relations with the big social world. He does not feel prepared for what he experiences as perennial challenge. The characteristics of the nuclear family, to which I have already referred, sharpen the contrast between the home and the world. The patient comes to believe that the future has no hope, the promise of life will not be fulfilled. He feels unaccepted and unacceptable, unfit, alone.

He may undergo a prepsychotic panic that is caused by a strange emotional resonance between something that is very clear (like the devastating self-image brought about by the expansion of conceptual life) and the unrepressed experiences of the first period of life, when he sensed with great intensity the threat of the world. The concordance and unification of the experiences of the first and third periods complete and magnify the horrendous vision of the self. In the totality of his human existence, and through the depth of all his feelings, the individual sees himself as totally defeated, without any worth or possibility of redemption.

In most cases only one solution, one defense, is still available to the psyche: to dissolve or alter his cognitive functions, the thought processes that have brought about conceptual disaster and that have acquired an ominous resonance with the original and preconceptual understanding of the self. It is at this stage that the fourth, or psychotic, period begins. Whereas during the period of panic everything "inside" the patient appeared to be in a state of turbulent change, in the fourth period the external reality seems difficult and strange.

In the paranoid type of schizophrenia, the patient projects to the external world the evaluation of the self that he had previously accepted. No longer will he accuse himself. The accusation now comes from the external world.

SCHIZOPHRENIC COGNITION

At the onset of the psychotic period the patient adopts a different type of cognition, which to a large extent is responsible for his manifest symptomatology and alters his ways of relating to the world and to himself. The new ways are neither learned nor based on imitation. It would be incorrect to think that they are learned or transmitted from the other members of the family. They constitute special structures of thought and language that are available to every person, irrespective of the culture, historical time, or family to which he belongs. If we adopt a Freudian frame of reference, we can say that the primary process, which in normal persons does not prevail in most activities of the mind, acquires supremacy over the secondary process.

Since 1948 (23) I have illustrated the characteristics of this less differentiated or paleologic type of cognition and the ways by which it becomes connected psychodynamically with the content of the patient's thought and language. I put a new and different stress on Bleuler's cardinal concept that it is chiefly through the thought disorder that this psychosis unfolds. Since 1948 many studies of schizophrenic thought and language have been published by many authors. The interpretations have been quite different. Many authors have seen the thought disorder as predominantly a disorder of attention (24, 25). It is true that attention is disturbed in the majority of patients, but to me it seems impossible to attribute the complexity of schizophrenic phenomena to the secondary symptom of disturbed attention. It will be hard to demonstrate that it is because of a disturbance in attention that a patient "hears messages from other planets."

Some other authors have attempted to find in the parents of the patient the same thought disorder that the patient presents. They have described the parents' thoughts as diffused and fragmented (15, 16). Of course, some parents, relatives, and even friends of patients, as well as reputedly normal persons, may present occasional thought anomalies and a diffuse or fragmented chain of thoughts, but not in typically schizophrenic modalities.

Another group of authors (26-28) has given importance to another characteristic of schizophrenic thought—"overinclusiveness," described long ago by Cameron (29). For instance, when a schizophrenic patient was asked to continue this list of names: dogs, cats, horses, elephants, donkeys, etc., he added "spiders, parrots, snakes." Another patient added "stones, galaxy, infinity."

In his recent book Lidz (21) gave more consideration to schizophrenic thinking, which now holds an important place in his revised theory of schizophrenia. I mention Lidz again at this point because he fundamentally accepts Cameron's concept of overinclusiveness, but adds that this overinclusiveness is egocentric. The parents of the patient are egocentric since they are unable to recognize that the other person has different feelings, needs, and ways of experiencing. In order to adapt to the parents' needs, the patient becomes egocentric by being parent-centered: "His feelings of being central to his parents' lives lead to feelings of being central and important to everyone, including God" (21). This egocentricity of the patient leads him to "cognitive regression," specifically to "an intercategorical realm" of thinking. In other words, the patient becomes particularly preoccupied with material that lies between categories.

It is not very clear how Lidz puts together egocentricity and overinclusiveness. The "overinclusiveness" that leads the patient to believe that many events refer particularly to him may be egocentric, but that is quite different from the overinclusiveness that makes him believe, for instance, that pencil and shoe belong to one category because they both "leave traces" (30). It seems to me that overinclusiveness is the manifestation of a more basic problem.

Vygotsky (31) and Goldstein (32), using special tests, have very well demonstrated that the patient's inability to form acceptable categories appears in attempts to solve problems that require abstract thinking and is not necessarily associated with egocentricity. In the examples mentioned above, the first patient, in spite of his education, was not able to abstract the class "mammal," and the second patient was not able to abstract the class "animal." The second patient probably conceptualized more in terms of space and thought that animals are in the country, which is part of a galaxy, which in its turn is part of infinity. Contrary to what some authors believe, not only is there no increase in capacity for abstraction, but there is a severe impairment in the capacity for abstraction. The occasional use of abstract words has a different significance (4, chapter 16). This impairment of the capacity for abstraction is not permanent and is probably psychogenic in origin. It disappears in patients who recover, just as primitive types of thinking that occur in dreams disappear when the dreamer awakes. The schizophrenic retains the potentiality to abstract.

Elsewhere (4, part III) I have reported my interpretation of schizophrenic thought and language disorders and have synthesized the work originally published in more than 30 publications. I wish to indicate here, however, that in my opinion schizophrenic cognition is based on: 1) concretization (or perceptualization) of the concept, 2) identification based upon similarity (the principle of Von Domarus [33]), and 3) a changed relationship between connotation and verbalization. In other words, the usual semantic value of the word is altered and what acquires special value is the word itself, with diminished or ignored relation to its original meaning.

Lack of space does not permit me to discuss here the biological origin of this type of cognition, nor can I give examples of the varieties of forms under which this type of cognition manifests itself (4, part III). However, I would like to stress the following points:

1. My interpretation of schizophrenic cognition applies to all forms of thinking in which the primary process prevails. For instance, it is also related to what occurs in dreams and neuroses.

2. Schizophrenic cognition is based on psychological structures that are inherent in every human being in health or disease. As a matter of fact, primary process cognition with the characteristics that I have mentioned above occurs also in the process of creativity (although it is blended or harmoniously matched with other forms of cognition [34]).

3. In schizophrenia, primary process cognition is used to fit psychodynamic necessities or tendencies.

4. It is not the psychodynamic component that gives to the disorder its schizophrenic essence, but the primary process organization that the psychodynamic component undergoes in a predominant way.

SCHIZOPHRENIA AND SOCIETY

In the larger context of the psychology of the psychosis, it is important to evaluate those recent conceptions that consider schizophrenia not a disease but an imposition or creation of society, or a strategy with which one can face society, or even something good for society. Prominent among these conceptions are those of Szasz (35), Laing (36), and Siirala (37, 38). Most of these approaches have been labeled "antipsychiatry." They have to be distinguished from those approaches, like that of Goffman (39), that limit themselves to pointing out the bad aspects of institutional psychiatry.

Again the topic is too vast to be treated here adequately. Whether schizophrenia is a disease or not depends on what we call disease. Certainly the concepts of Virchow and a medical model that was conceived exclusively in relation to physical illness are not applicable to mental illnesses. In my opinion the medical model was too narrowly conceived at a time when psychiatry had not yet gained full consideration as a science. To adhere to a medical model that followed Virchow's tenets would be like following in physics a Euclidian-Newtonian system after Einstein and Heisenberg had conceived a more inclusive one. If in the concept of disease we include a dysfunction of psychological mechanisms, then schizophrenia is certainly a disease (or syndrome or pathological condition). With a few exceptions, schizophrenia causes a great deal of suffering to the patient; it is inimical to the patient's self-fulfillment and in serious forms it does not permit survival without help from others. Thus schizophrenia cannot be called a variety of human existence, like blue eyes or left-handedness. It may be based, however, on a variety, perhaps an organic variety, that later, with the participation of environmental components, becomes a pathological condition.

For Laing (12) the schizophrenic psychosis is a normal reaction to an abnormal situation. It is not a disease but a broken-down relationship. The environment of the patient is so bad that he has to invent special strategies in order "to live in this unlivable situation." The psychotic does not want to do any more denying. He unmasks himself; he unmasks others. The psychosis thus appears as madness only to us ordinary human beings who have a vision limited by hypocrisies and ingrained habits.

In my opinion schizophrenia is an *abnormal* and *specific* way of dealing with an abnormal situation. The previous situation may have been unlivable, but the rebellion is abnormal and also hardly livable. If the patient had to rebel or reject the previous situation, he could have become a revolutionary, a dissenter, a hermit, a poet, a writer, or a politician, but instead only a pathological possibility was available to him; he became a schizophrenic. We must help him to lose the pathology and, if he finds meaning in life through dissent, we must help him to find other, nonpathological media for his dissent. Unlike Laing (36), I do not believe that the term "schizophrenia" is a political label, or at least no more than any other medical term is political. This is not to deny, of course, that society has a great deal to do with provoking human suffering and that human suffering, in indirect but certain ways, promotes mental illness.

Siirala (37, 38) saw the patient as a victim and as a prophet to whom nobody listens. He saw the therapist as a person who has the duty to reveal to society the prophecies of these patients. These prophecies would consist of insights into our collective sickness, into the murders that we have committed for many generations and that we have buried so that they will not be noticed. He felt that schizophrenia emerges out of a common sort of sickness, a sickness shared by others, the healthy.

For several years I have been quite intolerant to Siirala's views, but recently I believe I understand him better and some of his ideas seem to me partially acceptable. Why has Siirala called the schizophrenic a prophet? I am not sure, but it seems to me that perhaps we can find some similarity (certainly not identity) between many schizophrenics and the prophets of the Old Testament. The Biblical prophets were people extremely sensitive to evil or to surrounding hostility. They were also extremely sensitive to society's callousness to evil. The schizophrenic, especially the paranoid, in both his prepsychotic and psychotic stages, behaves and thinks as if he had a psychological radar that enabled him to detect and register the world's hostility much more than the average person can. Must we assess this characteristic as a positive value that we can share or as the manifestation of illness? Although hostility exists in the world, the psychotic's version of it is pathological. Although the hostility is related etiologically to the psychosis, other predisposing factors enable it to become related. Although the hostility is a very active psychodynamic factor, other important psychodynamic factors are involved.

The point I am trying to make, however, is that, even if the patient—in both his prepsychotic and psychotic stages—responds abnormally to the world or misinterprets the world, we should not see only the negative part of his position. By trying to understand him fully we can become aware that normality (or what we call normality) may require mental mechanisms and attitudes that are not so healthy. At times what is demanded of us is callousness to the noxious stimuli. We protect ourselves by denying them, hiding them, becoming insensitive, or finding a thousand ways of rationalizing them or adjusting to them. We become a silent majority. By being so vulnerable and so sensitive the patient may teach us to counteract our callousness. By spending so much energy in adapting, we survive and live to the best of our ability, but we pay a big price, which may result in the impoverishment of a part of our personality. This impoverishment of the personality is particularly pronounced, not always but often enough, in the nonpsychotic members of the patient's family. As I have indicated elsewhere (40), if we try to separate the patient's insights and positive values from the more conspicuous psychotic picture, it will be easier to reach the patient, to become his peer, and to help him greatly with psychotherapy.

PSYCHOTHERAPY

Since the early efforts of Federn, Sullivan, Fromm-Reichmann, and Rosen, the psychotherapy of schizophrenia has continued to make many advances, which I cannot possibly even enumerate in this paper. Particularly noteworthy are the efforts of Sechehaye (41) and Benedetti (42) in Switzerland, and of Rosenfeld (43), Bion (44), and the Kleinian school in general. Inspired at first by Fromm-Reichmann, Lewis Hill (10), Harold Searles (45), and Otto Will (46, 47) have made many psychodynamic contributions in which the relation between parent and child was particularly studied.

In the second edition of *Interpretation of Schizophrenia*, I have illustrated in detail my technique as it has developed in the course of many years (4, part VII). It aims at reestablishing the bond of human relatedness with the patient, attacking psychotic symptoms with specific techniques, understanding the psychodynamic history, especially in the misinterpreted relations with the family, and helping the patient to unfold toward new, nonpsychotic patterns of living. Thus, although the psychotherapy of schizophrenia retains the interpretative technique and the uncovering of the repressed, as in the original Freudian psychoanalytic therapy, it expands in many directions. It is just as nourishing as it is interpretative. Although it helps the patient to reacquire communication, concern, and love for the other, it promotes autonomy, individuality, and self-assertion. Although at first the therapist assumes a parental role, he gradually becomes a peer of the patient.

Although I have obtained the best results with patients who did not receive drug therapy, I am not against its use. As a matter of fact, I consider it a useful adjunct in many cases. However, whereas drug therapy removes only the symptoms, psychotherapy aims at changing the patient's self-image and his attitude toward himself, others, and life in general. It aims at undoing part of the past and at changing one's attitude toward the present and the future. Whereas physical therapies in psychiatry as well as in other medical fields aim at a *restitutio quo ante* (return to a premorbid condition), the psychotherapist does not consider this a desirable goal for the psychotic. In fact, the premorbid condition was already morbid, although in a different way. A return to a prepsychotic condition would mean to settle for the retention not only of a biological vulnerability but also of a psychological one. The potentiality for the psychosis would thus persist.

To summarize, with many patients who receive intensive and prolonged psychotherapy we reach levels of integration and self-fulfillment that are far superior to those prevailing before the patient became psychotic. As I have said elsewhere (4, chapter 39), this does not mean that all the troubles of the patient will be over, even after successful psychotherapy. We must repeat once again the famous words of Frieda Fromm-Reichmann that we cannot promise a rose garden. It would be utopian to believe that the promise of life is a life comparable to a rose garden, utopian for the patient and utopian for us, who want to be his peers. But I think it is not utopian to promise to the patient what we promise to ourselves, his peers, sooner or later in life: to have our own little garden.

REFERENCES

1. KRINGLEN, E.: New studies on the genetics of schizophrenia. In *The World Biennial of Psychiatry and Psychotherapy*. Edited by S. Arieti. New York: Basic Books, 1970, pp. 476-504.
2. ROSENTHAL, D.: *Genetic Theory and Abnormal Behavior*. New York: McGraw-Hill, 1970.
3. ARIETI, S.: *Interpretation of Schizophrenia*. New York: Brunner, 1955.
4. ARIETI, S.: *Interpretation of Schizophrenia*, 2nd ed. New York: Basic Books, 1974.
5. ARIETI, S.: The psychodynamics of schizophrenia: A reconsideration. *Amer. J. Psychotherapy*, 22:366-381, 1968.
6. ROSEN, J.: *The Concept of Early Maternal Environment in Direct Psychoanalysis*. Doylestown, Pa.: Doylestown Foundation, 1963.
7. FROMM-REICHMANN, F.: Notes on the development of treatment of schizophrenia by psychoanalytic psychotherapy. *Psychiatry*, 11:263-273, 1948.
8. ROSEN, J. N.: *Directed Analysis: Selected Papers*. New York: Grune & Stratton, 1953.
9. SULLIVAN, H. S.: *Conceptions of Modern Psychiatry*. New York: W. W. Norton, 1953.
10. HILL, L. B.: *Psychotherapeutic Intervention in Schizophrenia*. Chicago: University of Chicago Press, 1955.
11. LIDZ, T., FLECK, S. T., and CORNELISON, A. R.: *Schizophrenia and the Family*. New York: International Universities Press, 1965.
12. LAING, R.: Schizophrenia: Sickness or strategy? Lectures read at the W. A. White Institute, New York, N. Y., Jan. 1967.
13. ARIETI, S.: The structural and psychodynamic role of cognition in the human

psyche. In *The World Biennial of Psychiatry and Psychotherapy.* Edited by S. Arieti. New York: Basic Books, 1970, pp. 3-33.

14. LIDZ, T.: Family settings that produce schizophrenic offspring. In *Problématique de la Psychose.* Edited by P. Doucet and C. Laurin. Amsterdam: Excerpta Medica Foundation, 1969, pp. 196-210.

15. WYNNE, L. C. and SINGER, M. T.: Thought disorder and family relations of schizophrenics, I: A research strategy. *Arch. Gen. Psychiat.,* 9:191-198, 1963.

16. WYNNE, L. C. and SINGER, M. T.: Thought disorder and family relations of schizophrenics, II: A classification of forms of thinking. *Arch. Gen. Psychiat.,* 9:199-206, 1963.

17. JACKSON, D. D.: *The Etiology of Schizophrenia.* New York: Basic Books, 1960.

18. JACKSON, D. D.: Schizophrenia the nosological nexus. In *The Origins of Schizophrenia.* Edited by J. Romano. Amsterdam: Excerpta Medica Foundation, 1967, pp. 111-120.

19. BATESON, G., JACKSON, D. D., HALEY, J., et al.: Toward a theory of schizophrenia. *Behav. Sci.,* 1:251-264, 1956.

20. LIDZ, T.: The influence of family studies in the treatment of schizophrenia. *Psychiatry,* 32:237-251, 1969.

21. LIDZ, T.: *The Origin and Treatment of Schizophrenic Disorders.* New York: Basic Books, 1973.

22. ARIETI, S.: Conceptual and cognitive psychiatry. *Amer. J. Psychiat.,* 122:361-366, 1965.

23. ARIETI, S.: Special logic for schizophrenic and other types of autistic thought. *Psychiatry,* 11:325-338, 1948.

24. CHAPMAN, J.: The early diagnosis of schizophrenia. *Brit. J. Psychiat.,* 112:225-238, 1966.

25. NEALE, J. and CROMWELL, R. L.: Attention and schizophrenia. In *Annual Review of the Schizophrenic Syndrome,* Vol. 2. Edited by R. Cancro. New York: Brunner/Mazel, 1972, pp. 68-98.

26. PAYNE, R. W.: Cognitive abnormalities. In *Handbook of Abnormal Psychology.* Edited by H. J. Eysenck. New York: Basic Books, 1961, pp. 193-261.

27. PAYNE, R. W.: An object classification test as a measure of overinclusive thinking in schizophrenic patient. *Brit. J. Soc. Clin. Psychol.,* 1:213-221, 1962.

28. PAYNE, R. W., MATTUSSEK, P., and GEORGE, E. I.: An experimental study of schizophrenic thought disorder. *J. Ment. Sci.,* 105:627-652, 1959.

29. CAMERON, W.: Reasoning, regression and communication in schizophrenics. *Psychol. Monogr.,* 50 (1), 1938.

30. POLYAKOV, V. F.: The experimental investigation of cognitive functioning in schizophrenia. In *A Handbook of Contemporary Soviet Psychology.* Edited by M. Cole and I. Maltzman. New York: Basic Books, 1969, pp. 370-386.

31. VYGOTSKY, L. S.: Thought in schizophrenia. *Arch. Neurol. Psychiat.,* 31:1003-1077, 1934.

32. GOLDSTEIN, K.: The significance of psychological research in schizophrenia. *J. Nerv. Ment. Dis.,* 97:261-279, 1943.

33. VON DOMARUS, E.: The specific laws of logic in schizophrenia. In *Language and Thought in Schizophrenia: Collected Papers.* Edited by J. S. Kasanin. New York: Norton Library, 1964, pp. 104-114.

34. ARIETI, S.: *The Intrapsychic Self: Feeling, Cognition and Creativity in Health and Mental Illness.* New York: Basic Books, 1967.

35. SZASZ, T. S.: *The Manufacture of Madness.* New York: Harper & Row, 1970.

36. LAING, R. D.: *The Politics of Experience.* New York: Pantheon Books, 1967.

37. SHIRALA, M.: *Die Schizophrenie—des Einzeln und der Allgemeinheit.* Gottingen: Vandenhoeck & Ruprecht, 1961.

38. SIRALA, M.: Schizophrenia: A human situation. *Amer. J. Psycohanal.*, 23:39-58, 1963.
39. GOFFMAN, E.: *Asylums: Essays on the Social Situation of Mental Patients and other Inmates.* Garden City, N. Y.: Doubleday, Anchor Books, 1961.
40. ARIETI, S.: Psychodynamic search of common values with the schizophrenic. In *Proceedings of the IV International Symposium on the Psychotherapy of Schizophrenia, Turku, Finland, 1971.* Edited by D. Rubenstein and Y. O. Alanen. Amsterdam: Excerpta Medica Foundation, 1971, pp. 94-100.
41. SECHEHAYE, M. A.: *Symbolic Realization.* New York: International Universities Press, 1951.
42. BENEDETTI, G.: Ich-strukturierung und psychodynamik in der schizophrenie. In *Die Entstehung der Schizophrenie.* Edited by M. Bleuler and J. Angst. Bern: Huber, 1971.
43. ROSENFELD, H.: *Psychotic States: A Psychoanalytic Approach.* New York: International Universities Press, 1965.
44. BION, W. R.: *Second Thoughts.* London: Heinemann, 1954.
45. SEARLES, H. F.: *Collected Papers on Schizophrenia and Related Subjects.* New York: International Universities Press, 1965.
46. WILL, O. A.: The psychotherapeutic center and schizophrenia. In *The Schizophrenic Reactions.* Edited by R. Cancro. New York: Brunner/Mazel, 1970, pp. 153-167.
47. WILL, O. A.: Catatonic behavior in schizophrenia. *Contemporary Psychoanalysis,* 9:29-58, 1972.

2

Special Logic of Schizophrenic and Other Types of Autistic Thought

Published in 1948, this is my first paper devoted exclusively to schizophrenic cognition. Dissatisfied with the purely decriptive approach of Bleuler, I deal with the particular structures or forms of schizophrenic thought and introduce a special psychostructural approach to psychiatry, independently from the subsequent structural studies of Chomsky and others. This is the first paper which recognizes the merit of Von Domarus's studies, relates them to Piaget's contributions—then almost unknown in America—and correlates them to Freud's psychodynamic conceptions. Thus, at the same time that the paper differentiates and describes the particular forms which rule schizophrenic thought and language, it gives the first interpretation on how these particular forms are influenced by psychodynamic needs.

IN 1925 WILLIAM ALANSON WHITE (1) complained that there was almost nothing in the literature on the mechanisms of thought processes in schizophrenia—a subject which he considered of paramount importance. With due regard to a few exceptions—outstanding among which are the contributions of Vigotsky (2) and those published in the monograph edited by Kasanin (3), with Sullivan, Goldstein, Von Domarus and other authors collaborating—the same complaint could be repeated today. The same complaint would be even more justified in regard to researches concerning a particular aspect of thought processes in schizophrenia and other psychopathological states—namely, the study of logic.

From the time of Aristotle, it has been known that the healthy human mind follows the so-called laws of thought. It is also known that the deranged mind does not always respect these laws of thought: that is, it may think "illogically." With an important exception, Von Domarus, to be mentioned later, science has not gone much beyond this point. The lack of research in this field is partially due to a consuetudinary aversion which physicians in particular and biologists in general have for any method which is not strictly empirical. On the other hand, philosophers and logicians themselves have to be blamed and for the opposite reason— that is, on account of a nonpsychological attitude which to physicians seems almost untenable. Since they are interested in thought itself and not the thinker, they naturally have ignored the condition of health, illness, age, and the environmental situation in which the thinker happens to be.

It is my contention that the study of logic in mental illnesses may clarify several problems which have not yet been clarified by other methods of research. Furthermore, it is contended that it is not even necessary to be a logician in order to undertake such study. It will be shown in this paper that the application of a few elementary principles will open new avenues of research, the value of which cannot be properly estimated perhaps at the present time.

In the last half century, medical psychology has felt more and more the impact of psychoanalysis. The attention of an increasing number of workers has been concentrated upon the dynamics of emotional factors, conscious or unconscious, and has been more or less detracted from other aspects of psychological problems. Freudian psychoanalysis has made it possible to interpret the symptoms of the patient as a result of emotional forces or as attempts by the patient to fulfill psychologically what otherwise would be unfulfillable wishes. This interpretation and its derivatives have advanced tremendously knowledge and therapeutic means, especially in the field of psychoneuroses, but in the psychoses have led to a standstill. For instance, psychoanalysis may explain why a deluded patient wishes unconsciously that his delusion be reality, but has not explained how it is that he intellectually accepts his delusion as reality, in spite of contradictory evidence. An obsessive patient who has, let us say, the obsession that if he does not wear a special suit, his mother is going to die, recognizes fully the absurdity of such an idea. It is true that he will continue to wear that special suit, but he knows that the idea is illogical. He has retained sufficient logical power to recognize the unreal nature of such obsession. Psychoanalysis will help in explaining what unconscious emotional factors and dissociated ideas have determined this symptom. In the case of the deluded patient also, psychoanalysis may explain what unconscious emotional factors have determined the delusional idea but will not explain why such an idea is accepted as reality. It does not explain what change has occurred in the logic powers of the patient so that he is not able any longer to test reality. To say that the patient's ego is disintegrating is to satisfy oneself with obscure words.

In this paper, and in another one soon to follow (4), I would like to suggest that the schizophrenic does not think with ordinary logic. His thought is not illogical or senseless, but follows a different system of logic which leads to deductions different from those usually reached by the healthy person. The schizophrenic is seen in a position similar to that of a man who would solve mathematical problems not with our decimal system but with another hypothetical system and would consequently reach different solutions. In other words, the schizophrenic seems to have a faculty of conception which is constituted differently from that of the normal man. It can be further demonstrated that this different faculty of conception or different logic is similar to the one which is followed in dreams, in other forms of autistic thinking, and in primitive man. I, therefore, suggest that it be called paleologic, to distinguish it from our usual logic which is generally called Aristotelian, since Aristotle was the first to enunciate its laws. It is not meant in this article that Aristotelian logic is correct in an absolute sense. I am aware of the criticisms to which this logic has been subjected. Aristotelian logic is used only as a frame of reference, and only *relatively* to paleologic thinking.

In this paper the laws of paleologic, as they are deduced especially from the study of schizophrenic thought and dreams, will be examined in detail. I will then discuss in what situations and why a person may abandon a system of logic and adopt one which, as a rule, is repressed. This contribution should be considered preliminary in nature; further research is necessary to differentiate other laws of this archaic type of logic.

VON DOMARUS' PRINCIPLE

Paleologic is to a great extent based on a principle enunciated by Von Domarus (5). This author, as a result of his studies on schizophrenia, formulated a principle which, in slightly modified form, is as follows: *Whereas the normal person accepts identity only upon the basis of identical subjects, the paleogician accepts identity based upon identical predicates.* For instance, the normal person is able to conclude "John Doe is an American citizen," if he is given the following information: "Those who are born in the United States are American citizens; John Doe was born in the United States." This normal person is able to reach this conclusion because the subject of the minor precise, "John Doe," is contained in the subject of the major premise, "those who are born in the United States."

On the other hand, suppose that the following information is given to a schizophrenic: "The President of the United States is a person who was born in the United States. John Doe is a person who was born in the United States." In certain circumstances, the schizophrenic may conclude: "John Doe is the President of the United States." This conclusion, which to a normal person appears as delusional, is reached because the identity of the predicate of the two premises, "a person who is born in the United States," makes the schizophrenic accept the identity of the two subjects, "the President of the United States" and "John Doe."

The mechanisms or successive steps of this type of thinking are not necessarily known to the schizophrenic who thinks in this way automatically, as the normal person applies automatically the Aristotelian laws of logic even without knowing them. For instance, a schizophrenic patient thinks without knowing why that the doctor in charge of the ward is her father and that the other patients are her sisters. A common predicate—a man in authority—leads to the identity between the father and the physician. Another common predicate—females in the same position of dependency—leads the patient to consider herself and the other inmates as sisters.

At times the interpretation of this type of thinking requires more elaboration. For instance, a patient of Von Domarus' (5) thought that Jesus, cigar boxes, and sex were identical. Study of this delusion disclosed that the common predicate, which led to the identification, was the state of being encircled. According to the patient, the head of Jesus, as of a saint, is encircled by a halo, the package of cigars by the tax band, and the woman by the sex glance of the man.

At times paleologic thought is even more difficult to interpret because the principle of Von Domarus is applied only partially; that is, some partial identity among the subjects is based upon partial or total identity of the predicate. For instance, a person who is conceived by a schizophrenic as having a quality or characteristic of a horse may be thought of with a visual image consisting of part man and part horse. In this case one subject, the person, is partially identified with the other subject, the horse, because of a common characteristic—for instance, strength. It is well known how frequently similar distortions and condensation appear in hallucinations and drawings of schizophrenics. Similar conceptions appear in mythologies of ancient people and of primitives of today. As a matter of fact, anthropologic studies may disclose to the careful reader how often the principle of Von Domarus is applied in primitive thinking. Numerous studies, outstanding among which is the one by Storch (6), have emphasized the similarities between primitive and schizophrenic thought, but the common underlying principles of logic which rule this thought have received no mention. Werner (7) writes: "It is one of the most important tasks of the developmental psychology to show that the advanced form of thinking characteristic of Western civilization is only one form among many, and that more primitive forms are not so much lacking in logic as based on logic of a different kind. The premise of Aristotelian logic that, when a thing is *A* it cannot at the same time be *B*, will not hold true for the primitive. . . ." Werner, however, does not attempt to enunciate the principles of a different logic. He does not add that for the primitive *A* may be *B* if *A* and *B* have only a quality (predicate) in common, although in his outstanding book, *Comparative Psychology of Mental Development,* he gives numerous examples proving this fundamental fact.

A step forward toward the interpretation of this way of thinking has been made by Max Levin (8) who compares schizophrenic thought to that of young children. Levin concludes that the patient as well as the young child "cannot distinguish adequately between a symbol and the object it symbolizes." For example, a middle-aged schizophrenic, speaking of an actor whom she admired, said, "He was smiling at me." The patient had seen on the cover of a magazine a picture of the actor in the act of smiling. Thus she had confused a picture of the actor with the actor himself. Levin reports that a 27-month-old child, drinking milk while looking at the picture of a horse, said, "Give milk to the horse." At 25 months the same child, looking at the picture of a car, tried to lift the car from the picture and said to his father, "Daddy, get car out." For the child the pictured objects were real. Levin is correct in his observations. However, he has not been able to see them in the light of Von Domarus' principle. What appears to us as a symbol of the object is not a symbol for the schizophrenic or for the child but a duplication of the object. The two objects have been identified on account of the similar appearance. Levin makes other exceptionally interesting observations which, however, do not receive complete interpretation, and he is led to the conclusion that infantile and schizophrenic concepts "are the result of amusing mixtures of relevant and irrelevant." For instance, he reports that "a child of two knew the word 'wheel' as applied, for example to the wheel of a toy car. One day, at twenty-five months, as he sat on the toilet, the white rubber guard (supplied with little boys' toilet seats to deflect the urine) came loose and fell into the toilet bowl; pointing to it, he exclaimed, 'broke, wheel!' In explanation it is to be noted that he had many toy cars whose wheels, when of rubber, were always of white rubber. Thus he came to think that the word 'wheel' embraced not only wheels but also anything made of white rubber." Levin concludes that this example "shows how associations of the most ephemeral nature are permitted to enter into a concept when the child is too young to appreciate the non-essentiality." In view of what has been said before, it is obvious that an identification had occurred because of the same characteristic "white rubber."

The same principle of Von Domarus is applied in dreams. Freud (9) has demonstrated that a person or object A having a certain characteristic of B may appear in the dream as being B or a composite of A and B. In the first case there is identification; in the second, composition. The whole field of Freudian symbolism is based, from a formal point of view, on Von Domarus' principle. A symbol of X is something which stands for X, but also something which retains some similarity with X—common predicate or characteristic. For instance, penis may be identified with snake on account of the elongated shape of both, father with king on account of the position of authority they both enjoy, and so on. The reason why certain symbols are specific only for one person will be discussed later. It has to be pointed out again that what one, using psychiatric terminology, calls a symbol is not a symbol for the schizophrenic or for the dreamer, but is, consciously or unconsciously, a duplication of the object symbolized.

The study of Von Domarus' principle in schizophrenia, in primitive thought, and in dreams requires that more consideration be paid to the predicate which determines the identification. In fact it is obvious that the predicate is the most important part of this type of thinking. Since the same subject may have numerous predicates, it is the choice of the predicate in the paleologic premises which will determine the great subjectivity, bizarreness, and often unpredictability of autistic thinking. For instance, in the quoted example of Von Domarus, the characteristic of being encircled was the identifying quality. Each of the three subjects which were identified—Jesus, cigar boxes, and sex—had a potentially large number of predicates, but the patient selected one which was completely unpredictable and bizarre. The predicate which is selected in the process of identification is called the "identifying link." Why a certain predicate should be selected out of numerous possible ones as the identifying link will be discussed shortly. A predicate is, by definition, something which concerns the subject. One is used to recognizing as predicates abstract or concrete qualities of the subject or something which in a certain way resides or is contained in the subject—for instance, being white, red, fluid, friendly, honest, suspicious, having a tail, and infinite other possibilities. These are called predicates of quality. There are, however, other characteristics which are paleologically conceived as pertaining to the subject and, therefore, considered predicates, although they are not contained in the subject—for instance, the characteristic of occurring at a certain time or at a given place. For example, two completely different subjects may have as a common predicate the fact that they occur simultaneously or successively or in the same place. For instance, if a patient accidentally ate a certain exotic food on a day in which he had a pleasant experience, he may dream of eating again that special food because he wishes to relive the pleasant experience. Special food and pleasant experience are in the dream identified because they happen to be perceived at the same time. The identifying link in this case is a predicate of temporal contiguity. The predicate of contiguity may be not only temporal but also spatial. For instance, a patient may dream of being in her summer home in Connecticut. Nearby in Connecticut lives a man she loves. Home in Connecticut and loved man are identified because they both have the characteristic of residing in the same place. In this case the identifying link is a predicate of spatial contiguity. Two different subjects may be identified also because they originated from the same source or will give origin to the same event or to the same emotional reaction. For instance, a patient dreams of undressing a woman, with sexual intentions. In the dream he suddenly realizes that her vagina looks like an umbilicus. In his associations he remembers that when he was a child he thought that children were born from the umbilicus. In this dream vagina and umbilicus are identified because they both were thought of by the patient as organs which give birth to children. In this case the identifying link is a predicate of finality. In many cases the identifying link is a mixture of predicates of different types.

From the foregoing it appears that paleologic thinking is much less exact than Aristotelian. In the latter, only identical subjects may be identified. The subjects are immutable; therefore, only a few and the same deductions are possible. In paleologic thinking, on the other hand, the predicates lead to the identification. Since the predicates may be extremely numerous and one does not know which one may be chosen by the patient, this type of thought becomes unpredictable, individualistic, and often incomprehensible. If the identifying link is a predicate of quality, it will be relatively easy to understand the meaning of what the patient expresses. What are referred to in psychoanalytic literature as universal symbols are generally objects whose identifying link is a predicate of quality and, less frequently, of finality. If, however, the identifying link is an accidental predicate of contiguity, obviously the symbol is specific for the individual and many details concerning his life history are necessary in order to understand its meaning.

The unconscious choice of the predicate which is used as the identifying link, out of numerous possible ones, is often determined by emotional factors. In other words, emotional currents may determine which one of the predicates will be taken as the identifying characteristic. This extremely important point has been examined in detail in another of my publications (4) and will not be rediscussed here. It is obvious that if John Doe thinks that he is the President of the United States because he was born in the United States, he wishes to think so. His increased narcissistic requirements direct him toward the selection of that predicate—being born in the United States—out of many other possibilities. The same emotional factors described by Freud (10) in "Psychopathology of Everyday Life" and by Jung (11) in *Psychology of Dementia Praecox* are, of course, valid for paleologic thinking, also. However, these emotional factors do not explain the formal manifestations of this type of thinking. Conscious or unconscious emotions may be the directing motivation or the driving force of these thought processes, but the fact cannot be denied that these thoughts are molded according to a special pattern, which is conferred by the adoption of a different logic.

From the foregoing, the reader may have deduced the tremendous role played by Von Domarus' principle in non-Aristotelian thinking—a role whose importance escaped perhaps Von Domarus himself. For those interested in the problem mainly from a point of view of formal logic, I may add that of the four traditional laws of thought—law of identity, law of contradiction, law of excluded middle, law of sufficient reason—the first three are annulled by Von Domarus' principle. In one of the following paragraphs, it will be shown how the fourth law also is altered.

CONNOTATION, DENOTATION, VERBALIZATION

Before proceeding with this examination of paleologic thinking, I have to remind the reader of what is traditionally meant in logic by different aspects of terms, that is, by connotation and denotation. Let us take, for instance, the term *table*. The connotation of this term is the meaning of the term, that is, the concept *article of furniture with flat horizontal top, set on legs*. The denotation of the term is the object meant, that is, the table as a physical entity. In other words, the term *table* may mean table in general or it may mean any or all particular tables. Every term has both these aspects. It means certain definite qualities or attributes and it also refers to certain objects or, in the case of a singular term, to one object which has those qualities. The connotation is in a certain way the definition of the object and includes the whole class of the object, without any reference to a concrete embodiment of the object.

I feel that, in addition to the two aspects of the terms which are traditionally considered in logic, one has to consider a third aspect, if he wants to understand better the problem from a psychological point of view. This is the verbal aspect of the term, the term as a word or verbal symbol. I propose to call this aspect of the term *verbalization*. For instance, the term *table* may be considered from three aspects: its connotation, when one refers to its meaning; its denotation, when one refers to the object meant; its verbalization, when one considers the word as a word, that is, as a verbal representation or symbol of the object table or of the concept table.

Now it is possible to formulate a second important principle of paleologic. Whereas the healthy person in a weakened state is mainly concerned with the connotation and the denotation of a symbol but is capable of shifting his attention from one to another of the three aspects of a symbol, the autistic person is mainly concerned with the denotation and the verbalization, and experiences a total or partial impairment of his ability to connote. In view of this principle, two phenomena have to be studied in schizophrenia and other types of autistic thinking: first, the reduction of the connotation power; second, the emphasis on the verbalization.

Reduction of Connotation Power

For the person who thinks paleologically, the verbal symbols cease to be representative of a group or of a class, but only of the specific objects under discussion. For instance, the word "cat" cannot be used as relating to any member of the feline genus, but a specific cat, like "the cat sitting on that chair." Oftener there is a gradual shifting from the connotation to the denotation level.* This gradual regression is apparent if we ask a not too deteriorated schizophrenic to define words. For instance, following are some words which a schizophrenic was asked to define and her replies:

Q. Book.
A. It depends what book you are referring to.
Q. Table.
A. What kind of a table? A wooden table, a porcelain table, a surgical table, or a table you want to have a meal on?
Q. House.
A. There are all kinds of houses, nice houses, nice private houses.
Q. Life.
A. I have to know what life you happen to be referring to—*Life* magazine or to the sweetheart who can make another individual happy and gay.

From the examples it is obvious that the patient, a high school graduate, is unable to define usual words. She cannot cope with the task of defining the word as a symbol of a class or a symbol including all the members of the class, like all books, all tables, and so on. She tries first to decrease her task by limiting her definition to special subgroups or to particular members of the class. For instance, she is unable to define the word "table" and attempts to simplify her problem by asking whether she has to define various subgroups of tables—wooden tables, surgical tables, and so on. In the last example she wants to know whether I am referring to two particular instances, *Life* magazine or to the life of the sweetheart. This reply, which reveals impairment of connotation power, is complicated also by the emphasis on the verbalization, as will be demonstrated in the following paragraph.

This tightness to the denotation prevents the schizophrenic from using figurate or metaphorical languages, contrary to what it may seem at first impression. It has already been stated by Benjamin (12) that the schizophrenic is unable to interpret proverbs correctly. He will give always a

---

* This statement made by many logicians that there is an inverse ratio between connotation and denotation does not hold true if the problem is considered from a psychological point of view. In other words, a decrease in the connotation power is not accompanied by an increase in the denotation power and vice versa. Many logicians, too, have criticized this concept of inverse ratio, because objects (denotation) can be enumerated, but qualities and meanings cannot be measured mathematically. I might add that the study of primitive thought discloses that what would be called terms with great connotation (with meaning of specific objects) preceded terms with greater denotation, which originated at a higher level of development.

more or less literal interpretation of them. Figurate language increases the use of the term which acquires an unusual denotation and connotation. If one says, "When the cat's away, the mice will play," a normal listener will understand that by cat is meant a person in authority. A schizophrenic patient gave the following literal interpretation of that proverb: "There are all kinds of cats and all kinds of mice, but when the cat is away, the mice take advantage of the cat." In other words, for the schizophrenic the word "cat" could not acquire a special connotation.

The inability of the schizophrenic to use metaphorical language is revealed also by the following replies of a patient who was asked to explain what was meant when a person was called by the names of various animals, for instance:

Q. Wolf.
A. Wolf is a greedy animal.
Q. Fox.
A. A fox and a wolf are two different animals. One is more vicious than the other, more and more greedy than the other.
Q. Parrot.
A. It all depends what the parrot says.
Q. Peacock.
A. A woman with beautiful feathers. By the way, *Woman* is a magazine.

Many beginners in the field of psychiatry get the impression that schizophrenic language and thought are highly metaphorical and poetic. In reality it is not so. This impression is due to misinterpretation of the phenomena which were explained above in terms of Von Domarus' principle. For instance, a schizophrenic will be able to *identify* a man with a wolf on account of a common characteristic, greediness, but will not be able to accept the concept *wolf* as a symbol of greedy men. Two different mechanisms are employed. In the first instance, a very primitive paleologic mechanism is necessary; in the second instance a high process of abstraction is at play. If one understands fully this point, he understands also one of the fundamental differences between schizophrenic artistic productions and some manifestations of art of normal persons.

This restriction of the denotation power and decrease of the connotation power is very apparent in many instances reported by Goldstein (13). In the color sorting test, one of Goldstein's patients picked out various shades of green, but in doing so he named them—peacock green, emerald green, taupe green, bright green, bell green, baby green. He could not say that all might be called green. Another patient of Goldstein's said in the same situation: "This is the color of the grass in Virginia, this is the color of the grass in Kentucky, this is the color of the bark of the tree, this is the color of the leaves." The words used by the patients in naming colors belonged to a definite situation. "The words," Goldstein writes, "have become individual words, i.e., words which fit only a specific object or situation." In other words, the meaning or the connotation of the word includes not a class but only a specific instance. There is therefore a definite restriction of the connotation power.* Goldstein calls these phenomena expressions of "concrete attitude."

Emphasis on Verbalization

Whereas the word is normally considered just as a symbol to convey a meaning, in the autistic person it acquires a greater significance. In many cases the attention of the schizophrenic is focused not on the connotation or denotation of the term, but just on its verbal expression— that is, on the word as a word, not as a symbol. Other paleologic processes may take place after the attention has been focused on the verbalization. For instance, a schizophrenic examined during the past war said that the next time the Japanese would attack the Americans it would be at Diamond Harbor or Gold Harbor. When she was asked why, she replied: "The first time, they attacked at Pearl Harbor; now they will attack at Diamond Harbor or at Sapphire Harbor." "Do you think that the Japanese attacked Pearl Harbor because of its name?" I asked. "No no," she replied, "it was a *happy* coincidence." Note the inappropriateness of the adjective *happy*. It was a happy coincidence for her, because she could prove thereby the alleged validity of her paleophrenic thinking.

From this example, and from others which will follow, it is to be deduced that Von Domarus' principle is often applied when the emphasis is on the verbalization. Different objects are identified because they have names which have a common characteristic. The identification is very easily made if the terms are homonyms. Two otherwise different things are identified, or considered together, because they have the same verbalization, that is, the same phonetic or written symbol. In one of the examples mentioned above, the patient put together *Life* magazine and the life of the sweetheart. Another schizophrenic was noticed to have the habit of wetting her body with oil. Asked why she would do so she replied: "The human body is a machine and has to be lubricated." The

---

* Many logicians, on the other hand, would say that the connotation is increased. This point of view is psychologically wrong.

word *machine,* applied in a figurative sense to the human body, had led to the identification with man-made machines. It is obvious that for the schizophrenic and, to a minor degree, for persons who are in other autistic conditions, the term is considered not as a symbol but as a characteristic, a quality or a predicate of the object which is symbolized. The identification, due to the similar or common verbal expression, is based not only on Von Domarus' principle but also on the second principle of paleologic, that is, the emphasis on the verbalization and the decreased importance of the connotation.

Werner (7) thinks that a name is not merely a sign for the primitive; it is part of the object itself. The verbalization thus is conceived as part of the denotation. The word does not have the same connotation for the primitive as for the civilized man; the meaning is often restricted to the specific instance which is denoted.

Children, too, experience names as fused in the object they denote. Piaget (14) has illustrated this phenomenon very well. When he asked children not older than six, "Where is the name of the sun?" he elicited the following responses: "Inside! Inside the sun" or "High up in the sky!"

The emphasis on the verbalization together with the application of Von Domarus' principle may also be found in normal adults in the technique of jokes and witticisms. Some of the examples mentioned above, such as the schizophrenic who was wetting her body with oil, have definite comical characteristics. The important point, however, is that what is comical for the healthy person is taken seriously by the schizophrenic. In a future publication the relation between wit and paleologic rules will be discussed. Freud (15) also, in his important monograph on wit, has described many mechanisms involved in the technique of witticisms but could not reduce them to the few principles of paleologic thinking.

The emphasis on verbalization appears also in many dreams, as revealed first by Freud (9) in his monograph on dream interpretation. I report here one of the numerous examples he gives. C. dreams that on the road to X he sees a girl, bathed in a white light and wearing a white blouse. The dreamer began an affair with a Miss White on that road.

CAUSALITY

I mentioned before that the first three laws of thought of traditional logic were eliminated by Von Domarus' principle. On the other hand, there is retained in paleologic thinking the fourth law, the law of sufficient reason: "We must assume a reason for every event." The methods, however, by which a reason for, or a cause of, an event is searched are different from those used by the normal mind. The works of Piaget (16) on the mentality of the child help in understanding this problem. The autistic person, as well as the child, confuses the physical world with the psychological. Instead of finding a physical explanation of an event, the child, as well as the primitive and the autistic, looks for a motivation or an intention as the cause of an event. Every event is interpreted as caused by the will of an animated being. Of course, similar explanations of incidents are justified many times. For instance, if one says "I read this book of geometry because I want to learn this subject," this psychological causality is justified. The child, however, invokes to a much larger extent motives and intentions as causes of phenomena. He is always in search for a motivation which leads to an action. Children, examined by Piaget in Switzerland, thought that God made the thunder in the sky, that the Negroes were made in that way because they were naughty when they were little and God punished them; that there were a great and a little Salève lakes, because some people wanted to go into the little one and some into the great one. Werner (7) reports other examples. A boy, five years of age, thought that in the evening it got dark because people were tired and wanted to sleep. The same child thought that the rain was due to the fact that the angels swept the heavens with their brooms and lots of water.

The intentions are ascribed first to other people, then to things. The moon follows the child, the sun goes up in the sky, the rivers run. The world becomes peopled in various degrees.

An animistic and anthropomorphic conception of the world thus originates. Many works of anthropology and comparative psychology fully illustrate how the same conception of psychological causality is present in the primitive of today and in the mythology of ancient peoples.

In dreams, too, events are engendered by wishes, intentions, or psychological motivations. Paranoiacs and paranoids interpret almost everything as manifesting a psychological intention or meaning related to their delusional complexes.

One may conclude therefore that whereas the normal person is inclined to explain phenomena by logical deductions, often implying concepts involving the physical world, the autistic person, as well as the primitive and the child, is inclined to give a psychological explanation to all phenomena.

Between causality by psychological explanation and causality by logical deduction there are many other intermediate types of explanation which are described by Piaget. For instance, moral causality, magical causality, and so on. In a future contribution I will deal with this difficult problem.

This subject will be dealt with very briefly here, because it was elaborated in one of my previous publications (17). Whereas the normal adult is able to think of the present, to revive the past, and to anticipate the future, or, in other words, is able to transport chronologically remote phenomena to the only possible subjective or psychologic tense—present —the autistic person thinks mostly about the present.

Animals are unable to prospect a distant future. Experiments with delayed reactions have disclosed that they cannot keep in mind future events for more than a few minutes (18, 18a). They can foresee only the very immediate future—that is, only the reaction to a stimulus as long as the stimulus is present or was present not longer than a few minutes before. Pre-human species may be called biologic entities without psychic tomorrow. Cattle go to the slaughterhouse without feelings of anxiety, being unable to foresee what is going to happen to them. In humans, ability to anticipate the future begins during the anal period. At that stage of development the child becomes able to postpone immediate pleasure for some future gratification. In other words, it is when the ability to anticipate is developed that "the reality principle" originates.

Phylogenetically, anticipation appeared at the primordial eras of humanity when man became interested not only in cannibalism and hunting, which are related to immediate present necessities, but also in agriculture and in hoarding in order to provide for future needs. It is in this period that culture—that is, knowledge to be used in future times or to be transmitted to future generations—originated. A person who would be able to conceive mentally only the present time would aim only toward what Sullivan (19) calls "satisfaction." A person who is able to prospect the future as well would aim also toward what Sullivan calls "security."

Autistic phenomena always occur as present phenomena without any reference to the future, although they may be motivated by wishes for the future. As Freud has emphasized, in dreams the situation is always lived in the present. In schizophrenia too, there is what I have called a "restriction of the psychotemporal field." The patient withdraws more or less to a narcissistic level, and his temporal orientation becomes also more and more similar to that of the narcissistic period, that is, related to the present time. Balken (20), in her study with the Thematic Apperception Test, found that the schizophrenic does not distinguish between past, present, and future. According to her, the schizophrenic, in the attempt "to relieve the tension between the possible and the real" clings "desperately and without awareness to the present." In early schizophrenia, however, and especially in the paranoid type, the patient is still able to concern himself with past and future. Some delusions, especially with persecutory content, may involve the future rather than the present. The more the illness progresses, however, the more grandiose and related to the present time the delusions become. "I *am* the emperor of China; I *am* a millionaire."

To use Sullivan terminology, the schizophrenic, in a desperate attempt to regain security, uses more and more autistic mechanisms.

PERCEPTUALIZATION OF THE CONCEPT

From the foregoing the reader has certainly inferred that the autistic person has the tendency to live in a world of perception rather than in a world of conception. The more autistically a person thinks, the more deprived he becomes of concepts or of Plato's universals. His ideas become more and more related to specific instances, and not concerned with classes, groups, or categories. Naturally, all gradations are possible and could be retraced in primitives.

When the pathologic process progresses further, the ideational formations will contain more and more concrete elements, representing reality as it appears to the senses rather than to the intellect. Perceptual elements finally eliminate completely higher thought processes. Storch (6) has demonstrated that the same process of perceptualization is found in the primitive as in the schizophrenic. Ideas are represented by sensory images. The wealth of vivid sensory images which are found in old myths was not the work of art but of necessity. The normal artist, too, uses perceptualization of concepts in his artistic productions but retains that ability to abstract which has not yet been acquired by the primitive and which has been lost by the schizophrenic. Perceptualization of the concept has its fullest expression in dreams and in hallucinations. As Freud and others have pointed out, the dream is just a translation of thoughts into visual images. Thoughts become visual perceptions. If the dreamer thinks about himself he sees himself in the dream. He sees himself as a physical entity or as a visual image, not as an abstract concept symbolized by the pronoun "I." These visual images use sensorial material. Since, for anatomical reasons, nobody can see his own face, the dreamer cannot recall the visual image of his face. This explains why the dreamer usually sees himself in the dream, but not his face. The sensorial material is revisualized and elaborated in accordance with paleologic and other archaic mechanisms. The same thing could be repeated about hallucinations, except that in them auditory images are by far more common than visual.

This paragraph can therefore be summarized by stating that in autistic thought concepts have the tendency to disappear as concepts, inasmuch as their content tends to assume a perceptual expression. This process of perceptualization is completed in dreams and in hallucinations.

FURTHER APPLICATION AND LIMITATION OF PALEOLOGIC RULES—
REFERENCE TO MORE PRIMITIVE MECHANISMS

The few principles of paleologic thought which were expounded above have a much vaster application than it may seem from the few examples given. The whole way of thinking may be so entirely transformed as to become completely inaccessible.

Von Domarus' principle may lead to what may be called self-identification. Self-identification, or identification of the self with another person, may occur unconsciously in normal and in neurotic persons, or consciously as in the delusional psychotics. The formal mechanism is the following: "If X will be identified with Y, because they have a common quality, it will be sufficient for me to acquire a quality of the person I want to be identified with, in order to become that person."

The very common hysterical identifications follow this mechanism. Freud's patient, Dora, developed a cough like that of Mrs. K. with whom she wanted to identify (21). A patient, mentioned by Fenichel (22), felt an intense pain in one finger. She felt as if she had her finger cut with a knife. She identified herself with her loved cousin, a medical student, who, she imagined, might have cut himself while dissecting.

The deluded patient discovers in himself a quality possessed also by a hero, a saint, a general, and identifies himself with the person who has that given quality. Other deluded patients try to acquire or to confer on others identifying qualities. A paranoid schizophrenic wanted her child to become an angel. Since angels are nourished only "by spiritual food," she did not feed her child for a few days—that is, until her relatives became aware of her acutely developed condition.

Von Domarus' principle in reverse is also applied in paleologic thinking as well as in primitive and infantile thinking. If A has not a given quality of A′, A cannot be A′. I shall resort again to one of the very interesting examples given by Levin (23), although he has not fully interpreted it.

A bright six-year-old boy asked Levin whether twins are always boys. He replied that they may be either boys or girls, or a boy and a girl. When the child heard that twins may be a girl and a boy, he asked with surprise: "Then how could they wear the same clothes?" Levin concludes that the child had seen identical twins dressed alike, and his concepts of twins included an irrelevant detail, identity of raiment. If we apply Von Domarus' principle in reverse, the mental mechanism seems to be the following: "Twins have a common quality—identical raiment. If two people have not or cannot have identical raiment, they cannot be twins."

The five principles mentioned above—namely, 1) Von Domarus' principle, 2) the changed emphasis on the connotation, denotation, and verbalization of symbols, 3) psychological causality, 4) the narrower conception of time, and 5) the tendency to perceptualize concepts—obviously have a tremendous importance. These specific principles are representative of a power of perception and conception completely different from those usually possessed by the normal modern adult in waking status. These mechanisms offer to the thinker a completely different vision of the external universe as well as of his own inner experiences.

Throughout this paper the reader has probably been impressed by the continuous references to primitive and infantile thought. This has been done to convey the notion that the type of thought which uses a non-Aristotelian logic is representative of a certain stage of phylogenetic and ontogenetic development. Unfortunately, many modern studies of anthropology and of child psychology, influenced by orthodox Freudian psychoanalysis, have not gone at all into this type of research. The character structure of a primitive society is interpreted by some orthodox analysts as due to a reproduction at a phylogenetic level of an ontogenetic Freudian complex such as in Freud's "Totem and Taboo" (25). Fromm rightly calls this method the naive Freudian approach to anthropology. Other orthodox psychoanalysts, like Róheim (26) and Kardiner (27), interpret the character structure and the whole primitive culture as the result of the special upbringing of children in that given culture. The fact that the primitive interprets the world paleologically and therefore has a completely different vision of the universe, and that this completely different vision of the universe, in its turn, has its influence upon the upbringing of children, is completely ignored by these orthodox authors. For instance, the projective mechanisms described by Kardiner have not been interpreted as at least partially due to a different type of causality—namely, to that psychological causality mentioned in a previous paragraph of this paper.

Since I have mentioned that this type of paleologic thinking is typical in autistic states and especially of schizophrenics, does it follow that the characteristics of schizophrenic thought can all be interpreted in view of the paleologic principles expounded above?

These principles explain a great deal but certainly cannot explain every characteristic of schizophrenia or even of schizophrenic thought. This limitation is due to two different reasons. The first one is that not all paleologic rules have yet been discovered. For instance, some of the paleologic laws, discussed above, may explain the formal mechanisms of delusions of misidentification or of grandeur, but cannot explain why the homosexually loved person is transformed into the persecutor. The emotional mechanism, which is at play in this transformation, is understood very well because of the contributions of Freud, and especially his work on the Schreiber case (28). The concomitant paleologic mechanism is not yet clear, although some hypotheses are now under study.

The other reason is that schizophrenia involves the resurgence of archaic mechanisms, some of which are even more primitive than the paleologic. Paleologic thought is, by definition, thought that follows an archaic type of logic, which phylogenetically preceded the Artistotelian. However, not all thought is logical; primitive forms of thought follow no logic whatsoever, either Aristotelian or paleologic, but only associations. Associational thought, in contrast to logic thought, shows no signs of direction toward an end or conclusion. It consists generally of recollections which are at the mercy of the laws of association* and of primitive emotions.

---

* Many readers may be surprised that I dare to mention the laws of association of ideas. Some psychological schools have tried to get rid of two fundamental characteristics of psychological phenomena: consciousness, denied by the behaviorists; and association of ideas, denied by those who are obsessively afraid of mental atomism. Nobody today would deny any longer that consciousness is a quality of some psychological processes. A two-minute observation can convince anyone of the fact that ideas do associate. I see my old high school and think of my adolescence; I hear somebody mention the name of Chopin, and I think immediately of an acquaintance of mine who is a pianist. The psychoanalytic treatment is based on free *associations* of ideas. In reality, associations in the analytic situation are free only from (Aristotelian) logic;

Mrs. Nickleby, Dickens' character, is certainly remembered by the reader for her sparing use of logical processes in her conversational ac- activities and for her conspicuous use of associational thought. In this type of thought ideas are expressed as they are recalled; they follow no logic rules but only the laws of associations—laws of contiguity and similarity —and underlying emotional currents. In advanced schizophrenia, im- pairment is to be noted, not only in logic thought, but also in associa- tional thought. Even the simplest ideas cannot associate properly, as pointed out by Bleuler (29).

PALEOLOGIC AND PSYCHOPATHOLOGICAL STATES

Now that the principal known laws of paleologic have been examined, it is appropriate to consider in what circumstances and why the normal adult abandons the Aristotelian way of thinking and adopts a more primitive type.

As mentioned before, logic (Aristotelian) thought is rigid and exact. In this type of thought only identical subjects can be identified. *A* is only *A* and cannot be *B*. The immutability of the subjects and the other char- acteristics described above make only few deductions possible. The person who thinks logically may find reality very unpleasant as long as he continues to think so. John Doe cannot think that he is the President of the United States just because he was born in the United States, but he may think so if he abandons this method of logic and embraces a new one. Once he sees things in a different way, with a new logic, no Aristotelian persuasion will convince him that he is wrong. He is right, according to his own logic.

The maiden may not dare to think that she wishes sexual relations, but if in the dream the penis assumes the form of a terrifying snake, her objections will be temporarily removed. These examples disclose that one has the tendency to resort to paleologic thinking when one's wishes cannot be sustained by normal logic. If reality cannot grant gratification of

---

they are not free from emotional currents, from paleologic mechanisms, and from the laws of association.

In a future contribution the transition will be studied from associational to paleo- logic thought. It will be demonstrated that the "associational link" becomes "the identifying link" in paleologic thought. In associational thought, if the associational link is a predicate of contiguity, the two ideas associate because of the law of con- tiguity. If the associational link is a predicate of quality, the ideas associate because of the law of similarity.

wishes, a new system of logic, which will transform reality into a more complacent form may be adopted.

This tendency, which each person has, to think paleologically, is, of course, usually corrected by Aristotelian thought. The laws of paleologic are unconsciously applied in neurotic manifestations and in dreams, but are rejected by the patient and by the waking person. This is possible because the neurotic and the waking person retain their normal Aristotelian logic. Only dissociated tendencies in the neurotic retain autistic mechanisms.

In schizophrenia, instead, the paleologic way of thinking has the upper hand and seems to the patient a sound interpreter of reality. Because of the above-described, individual, and often unpredictable characteristics of this type of thinking, the schizophrenic will not be able to obtain consensual validation, but will reach that inner security derived by the newly established agreement between his logic and his emotions. He will have to withdraw more and more from this Aristotelian world, but will be finally at peace with himself.

The situation is not so clear-cut in the beginning of schizophrenia. The important contributions of Sullivan about the onset of schizophrenia will help one understand what is taking place at this stage of the illness.

After the state of panic which the new schizophrenic has undergone, the patient becomes aware of dissociated tendencies. He becomes aware not only of what was accepted and incorporated in his self-system but also of another and great part of his personality which was obscure to him.

It appears natural to Sullivan that the patient does not accept immediately this state of affairs, this new personality, and suffers terrifying experiences: "The structure of his world was torn apart and dreadful, previously scarcely conceivable, events injected themselves" (19). This description of Sullivan's is even better understood if one accepts the fact that the new schizophrenic realizes that his mind has started to think in a different way, obscure to him. He realizes that he is inclined to interpret the world in a different way, at variance from his previous way of thinking and from that of other people, and he is afraid that he will become insane. The schizophrenic fear of becoming insane is not just the obsessive idea of insanity found in neurotics, but is a realization that some change in his way of thinking is actually taking place. At this stage the patient is able to think at the same time logically and paleologically, but his logic is not able any more to control the paleologic thoughts. Paleologic thinking will be first limited only to ideas connected with the patient's complexes, especially if the illness takes a paranoid course. The more progressed is the illness, however, the greater will be the percentage of paleologic thinking in the schizophrenic mixture of these two types of thoughts. Finally, when hebephrenic dilapidation approaches, there is a resurgence of thought mechanisms even more primitive than the paleologic.

REFERENCES

1. WHITE, W. A.: The language of schizophrenia. In *Schizophrenia (Dementia Praecox)*. New York: Paul Hoeber, 1928, pp. 323-343.
2. VIGOTSKY, L. S.: Thought in schizophrenia. *Arch. Neurol. & Psychiat.*, 31:1036, 1934.
3. KASANIN, J. S. (Ed.): *Language and Thought in Schizophrenia: Collected Papers*. University of California Press, 1944.
4. ARIETI, S.: Autistic thought: Its formal mechanisms and its relations to schizophrenia. *J. N, and M. Disease*, 111:288-303, 1950.
5. VON DOMARUS, E.: Über die beziehung des normalen zum schizophrenen denken. *Arch. Psychiat.*, Berlin, 74:641, 1925; and The specific laws of logic in schizophrenia, reference footnote 3 (in Kasanin).
6. STORCH, A.: *The Primitive Archaic Forms of Inner Experiences and Thought in Schizophrenia*. New York and Washington: Nervous and Mental Disease Publishing Company, 1924.
7. WERNER, H.: *Comparative Psychology of Mental Development*. New York: Harper & Bros., 1940.
8. LEVIN, M.: Misunderstanding of the pathogenesis of schizophrenia, arising from the concept of "splitting." *Amer. J. Psychiat.*, 94:877-889, 1938.
9. FREUD, S.: The interpretation of dreams. In *The Basic Writings of Sigmund Freud*. New York: Modern Library, 1938.
10. FREUD, S.: Psychopathology of everyday life. In *The Basic Writings of Sigmund Freud*. New York: Modern Library, 1938.
11. JUNG, C. G.: *The Psychology of Dementia Praecox*. New York: Nervous and Mental Disease Monograph Series No. 3, 1936.
12. BENJAMIN, J. D.: A method for distinguishing and evaluating formal thinking disorders in schizophrenia, reference footnote 3 (In Kasanin [3] above)
13. GOLDSTEIN, K.: The significance of psychological research in schizophrenia. *J. N. and M. Disease*, 97:261-279, 1943.
14. PIAGET, J.: *The Child's Conception of the World*. London: Routledge and Kegan Paul Ltd., 1929.
15. FREUD, S.: Wit and its relation to the unconscious. In *The Basic Writings of Sigmund Freud*. New York: Modern Library, 1938.
16. PIAGET, J.: *The Language and Thought of the Child*. London: Routledge and Kegan Paul, 1948. Also, *The Child's Conception of Physical Causality*. London: Kegan, Trench, Trubner, 1930. (Also see [14] above)
17. ARIETI, S.: The processes of expectation and anticipation. *J. N. and M. Disease*, 100:471-481, 1947.
18. HUNTER, W. S.: The delayed reaction in animals and children. *Behav. Monogr.*, 2:86, 1913.
18a. HARLOW, H. F., WEHLING, H., and MASLOW, A. H.: Comparative behavior of primates: Delayed reaction tests on primates. *J. Comp. Psychol.*, 13:13, 1932.

19. SULLIVAN, H. S.: *Conceptions of Modern Psychiatry.* Washington, D. C.: The William Alanson White Psychiatric Foundation, 1946.
20. BALKEN, E. R.: A delineation of schizophrenic language and thought in a test of imagination. *J. Psychol.,* 16:239, 1943.
21. FREUD, S.: Fragment of an analysis of a case of hysteria (1905). In *Collected Papers,* Vol. 3., 13-146. London: Hogarth Press, 1946.
22. FENICHEL, O.: *The Psychoanalytic Theory of Neurosis.* New York: W. W. Norton & Co., 1945.
23. LEVIN, M.: On the causation of mental symptoms. *J. Mental Sci.,* 82:1-27, 1938.
24. FREUD, S.: Totem and taboo. In *The Basic Writings of Sigmund Freud.* New York: Modern Library, 1938.
25. FROMM, E.: Unpublished lectures given at Seminar on Social Psychology, 1948. William Alanson White Institute of Psychiatry, New York.
26. RÓHEIM, G.: *The Riddle of the Sphinx.* London: International Psycho-analytical Library, No. 25, 1934.
27. KARDINER, A.: *The Individual and His Society.* New York: Columbia Press, 1939.
28. FREUD, S. Psycho-analytic notes upon an autobiographical account of a case of paranoia (dementia paranoides) (1911). In *Collected Papers,* Vol. 3:387-470. London: Hogarth Press, 1946.
29. BLEULER, E.: *Dementia Praecox, oder Gruppe der Schizophrennen.* Leipzig und Wien: Franz-Deutsche, 1911.

3

Hallucinations, Delusions, and Ideas of Reference Treated with Psychotherapy

Written in 1961, this is the first paper applying to psychotherapy my findings on the special structures and forms of schizophrenic cognition. It describes the treatment of hallucinations which I had devised in treating Geraldine, a patient whose complete case report I later included in the second edition of Interpretation of Schizophrenia. *Here also is the first presentation of the method of acquiring awareness of the punctiform insight, as I first developed it in treating the patient Violet.*

SINCE JUNG'S (1) FORMULATIONS, schizophrenic symptoms have often been compared to dreams of normal or neurotic persons and have been interpreted similarly. However, whereas dreams are interpreted while the patient is awake and has reacquired his normal cognitive functions, the schizophrenic has to be treated while he is still in the "dream" of the psychosis.

Bringing light into the obscure complexity of the lived dream of the psychosis is a difficult task, attempted by different authors in different ways. Some of them have tried to enter "the dream," that is, to enter directly into "the psychotic reality." Rosen (2, 3) has made this attempt with his own method of direct analysis and Sechehaye (4, 5, 6) with her method of symbolic realization. Although these methods have been successful with some patients, they seem to be difficult to use or ineffective with other patients. "The psychotic world" is often irreducible and unique; moreover, a part of the patient is still in contact with the realistic world and will distrust any attempt "to share" the psychosis. In Sullivan's (7, 8) and Fromm-Reichmann's (9, 10) methods, on the other hand, the therapist assumes the role of "ambassador of reality," as

46

Racamier (11) aptly wrote, by interpreting the symptom to the patient as a way of remodeling his life in accordance with past or present thwarted interpersonal relations.

The techniques to be described in this paper apply only to an early stage of the treatment—as soon as relationship has been established (12) —and consist chiefly of making the patient aware of certain processes that he himself brings about or over which he retains some control. In other words, an attempt is made to make the patient realize that he no longer needs to transform or translate his psychodynamic conflicts into psychotic symptoms, in spite of a strong tendency to do so: that is, both the "world" of reality and the "world" of psychosis are, in certain circumstances, still accessible to him.

Although this method must be considered only a part of the total treatment of schizophrenia, it should not be considered symptomatic in the usual sense of this word. Psychotic symptoms tend not only to be self-perpetuating, but also to facilitate progressive regression and to bring about an increasing lack of consensual validation. Needless to say, this method does not exclude the traditional interpretations of the psychodynamic content of the symptoms. On the contrary, at a later stage of the treatment traditional interpretations are given in addition to those outlined in this paper.

For the purpose of this paper the author has reviewed the records of the last ten cases treated by him. The cases involved actively psychotic patients with hallucinations, delusions, and ideas of reference; however, they were not so acutely disturbed as to make hospitalization mandatory. In one case of chronic, well-systematized paranoid condition, no improvement was obtained. In another case, complicated by overt homosexuality, relapse of all symptoms occurred after a period of remission. In eight cases, either complete removal of psychotic symptoms or great improvement was obtained.

HALLUCINATIONS

Only auditory hallucinations will be taken into consideration, but the same procedures could be applied to other types of hallucinations, after the proper modifications have been made.

With the exception of patients who are at a very advanced state of the illness or with whom no relatedness whatsoever can be reached, it is possible to recognize that the hallucinatory voices occur only in particular situations, that is, *when the patient expects to hear them.*

For instance, a patient goes home, after a day of work, and expects the neighbors to talk about him. As soon as he expects to hear them, he hears them. In other words, he puts himself in what I have called *the listening attitude* (12, 13). If we have been able to establish not only contact but relatedness with the patient, he will be able under our direction to distinguish two stages: that of the listening attitude and that of the hallucinatory experience. At first he may protest vigorously and deny the existence of the two stages, but later he may make a little concession. He will say, "I happened to think that they would talk and I proved to be right. They were really talking."

A few sessions later, however, another step forward will be made. The patient will be able to recognize and to admit that there was a brief interval between the expectation of the voices and the voices. He will still insist that this sequence is purely coincidental but eventually he will see a connection between his putting himself into the listening attitude and his actually listening. Then he will recognize that he puts himself into this attitude when he is in a particular situation or in a particular mood, for instance in a mood where he perceives hostility, almost in the air. He has the feeling that everybody has a disparaging attitude toward him, then he finds corroboration for this attitude of the others: he hears them making unpleasant remarks about him. At times he feels inadequate and worthless, but he does not sustain this feeling for more than a fraction of a second. The self-condemnation almost automatically induces him to put himself into the listening attitude and then he hears other people condemning him.

When the patient is able to recognize the relation between the mood and putting himself in the listening attitude, a great step has been accomplished. He will no longer see himself as a passive agent, as the victim of a strange phenomenon or of persecutors, but as someone who still has a great deal to do with what he experiences. Moreover, if he catches himself in the listening attitude, he has not yet descended to or is not yet using abnormal or paleologic ways of thinking from which it will be difficult to escape. Although he is in the process of falling into a seductive trap, he may still resist the seduction.

I have found that if an atmosphere of relatedness and understanding has been established, patients learn with not too much difficulty to catch themselves, several times during the day, in the act of putting themselves into a listening attitude at the least disturbances. At times, although they recognize the phenomenon, they feel that it is almost an automatic mechanism which they cannot prevent. Eventually, however, they will be able to establish more and more control over it. Even then, however, there will be a tendency to resort again to the listening attitude and to the hallucinatory experiences in situations of stress. The therapist should never be tired of explaining the mechanism to the patient again and again, even when such explanation seems redundant. It is seldom redundant, as the symptoms may reacquire an almost irresistible attraction.

RE-ENLARGEMENT OF THE PSYCHOTEMPORAL FIELD

Another therapeutic difficulty may be encountered later, when we attempt more classic psychodynamic interpretations of the symptoms—for instance, when we try to explain to the patient that what he hears the voices saying is an attributing to others of the feelings he nourished about himself. Thus an infuriated patient could say, "How could you think that I consider myself a bad woman, a prostitute, as the voices say? This is a lie. I am a good woman." The patient is justified in having such a belief and in thinking that the psychiatrist who makes such an interpretation talks nonsense. For when the patient hears a disparaging voice, she no longer has a disparaging opinion of herself. The projection mechanism saves her from self-disparagement. We must instead point out to the patient that there was one time when she had a bad opinion of herself. Even then she did not think she was a prostitute but had a low self-esteem, such as she probably thought a prostitute would have about herself. In other words, we must try to re-enlarge the patient's psychotemporal field (14, 15). As long as he attributes everything to the present, he cannot escape from the trap of the symptoms. Although at this point of the illness, he already tends to live exclusively in the present, he retains a conception of the past, and such conception must be exploited (14, 15).

IDEAS OF REFERENCE AND DELUSIONS

Four methods of interpreting the formal mechanisms of ideas of reference, or delusions, or both, will be mentioned.

The first extends what I have said about the listening attitude to ideas of reference and delusions. Before the delusions are in full swing, or ideas of reference are well formulated, the patient must learn to recognize that he is in what I call *the referential attitude*. He is searching, looking for references which will corroborate the pre-existing mood. For instance, if the patient tells us that while he was in the subway he observed peculiar faces, some gestures that some people made, an un-

usual crowd at a certain station, and that all this is part of a plot to
kidnap and kill him, it is useless to reply to him that these are imaginary or false interpretations of certain occurrences. At this point he is
forced to believe that these events refer to him. We must instead help
the patient to recapture the mood and attitude which he had prior to
those experiences, that is, to become aware of his referential attitude.
He will be able to remember that before he went into the subway, he
looked for the evidence, he almost hoped to find it, because if he could
have found that evidence, he would be able to explain that indefinite
mood of being threatened he was experiencing. He had the impelling
need to transform a vague, huge menace into a concrete threat. The
vague menace is the anxiety of the interpersonal world, which in one
way or another constantly reaffirms the failure of his life.

The patient is then made aware of his tendency to concretize the
vague threat. The feelings of hostility and inadequacy which he experienced before the onset of the psychosis have become concretized not to
the point of hallucinations, but to the point of delusions or ideas of
reference. No longer does the patient feel surrounded by an abstract
world-wide hostility. It is no longer the whole world which considers
him a failure—now "they" are against him, "they" call him a failure, a
homosexual, a spy. . . . This concretization is gradual. The "they" obviously refers to some human beings who are not clearly defined. The
"they" have become concretized even more, may become definite persecutors.

The second method of therapy of delusions and ideas of reference
consists in fact of making the patient aware of his *concretizing attitude,*
in accordance with the processes I have described in other writings (13,
15, 16). In other words, although the delusions are symbolic, we generally avoid complicated explanations of symbols, along classic psychoanalytic lines. Instead, we help the patient to become aware of his own
concretizing, of substituting some ideas and feelings for others which
are easier to grasp or to contend with in his distress. He may often
learn to check himself, as he may learn to check his listening attitude.
For instance, we may explain to him that the feeling he has that some
people control his thoughts is a concrete representation and reactivation
of the feeling he once had that the surrounding adults were controlling
his life and even obligating him to orient his thinking in a certain
direction.

The third method consists in showing to the patient that in order to
sustain his delusional or referential beliefs he must resort to a special

form of abnormal cognition or paleologic. Again since I have treated this matter in detail elsewhere, I shall omit it here entirely (13, 15, 16, 17). In order to avoid misunderstandings, however, I must add that this method works mainly in two situations: 1) when the patient is at an advanced stage of treatment, 2) when he has recognized his listening, referential, or concretizing attitude. For instance if the patient has learned to catch himself while he is searching for the referential attitude, he will recognize that the evidence he searches for is based on paleologic.

I want to move instead to a fourth method which I have not yet described, and which in a certain way may be considered a special subtype of the second method—that is, of interpretation, based on the concretization of the concept. This is the method of *acquiring awareness of the punctiform insight.* An example will illustrate what I mean.

A patient, a 35-year-old single woman, whom we shall call Violet, was suffering from a relatively mild form of paranoid schizophrenia, which permitted her to maintain a not-too-inadequate social life and to keep her job, in spite of her many symptoms. She had occasional hallucinations, some delusions, and numerous ideas of reference.

On her birthday she received a bouquet of roses from the company for which she works. When she opened the package and saw beautiful yellow roses, instead of being happy she started to concentrate on the color yellow. The color means jealousy, and she felt that by giving her yellow roses the people in the office wanted to communicate to her that they knew she was jealous of the wife of the boss. The following day she heard one of the workers humming the tune of the song, "The Yellow Rose of Texas," and she felt this was done purposefully to expose her.

Eventually everything which was yellow in color acquired the same meaning for her and had to be avoided. Finally she even got rid of two of her dresses, which were yellow.

In her office there was a water cooler which was out of order and which had to be hit in order to permit the water to flow. When people, especially the boss of a certain department, were hitting the cooler, she thought they meant to hit her. When I asked her why she thought so she said, "I never walk, I run, like water, and I deserve to be hit." I explained to her that when she was in a state of anxiety she resorted to a special type of thinking to demonstrate her unworthiness, and that she attributed to others the feelings she had about herself. This explanation helped, and for some time there was considerable improvement, but then similar symptoms came back, although much more infrequently. For instance, when people in the office and especially the boss in the department were using the word "machine," she was sure they were referring to her. She said, "I work like a machine. I am sure they refer to me."

One day Violet came to my office in an angry mood, and told me that she was very angry because the previous day her friend Lucy had gone to visit her and had taken along her dog, a little cocker spaniel. She added, "You see! She thinks my home is a dog house. She thinks I am a dog."

Now, occasionally, I use some examples taken from one patient in my explanations to other patients, with whom I have established relatedness, in order to make them aware of the mechanisms they are liable to use when they are in distress. It happened that I reported this episode of the dog to another very articulate and sensitive schizophrenic patient who told me, "Your patient is probably right. Her friend probably treats her as a dog. Do you know that dog owners own dogs because they want to treat people like dogs? A human being does not obey them easily, but a dog does. I keep away from people who own dogs."

Of course, I did not accept my patient's point of view that dog owners necessarily have those characteristics, but I remember that a small percentage of dog owners, whom I have treated, do own dogs for the reasons mentioned by my patient. It occurred to me also that Lucy, Violet's friend, fitted that description very well. She was a domineering, aggressive person who was treating people like dogs, especially masochistic and compliant persons like my patient, who were willing to accept her behavior unconditionally. I realized then that Violet had had insight in thinking that Lucy was treating her like a dog, but this insight was sustained by a concrete representation, by the evidence brought forth by a small, otherwise insignificant episode. I re-examined all the bizarre symptoms Violet had experienced and discussed them with her. The chief of the department who was hitting the water cooler in a forceful manner was then recognized as a hostile and demanding person who gave Violet a tremendous amount of work and showed hostility at the least provocation, taking advantage of her submissive and masochistic characteristics. It is probable that by hitting the cooler after talking to her, he was letting off hostility. Perhaps he was doing something emotionally equivalent to a desire to hit Violet, when she dared not to comply in an absolute manner. Most probably my patient had intuitively recognized in this apparently harmless act of the boss a gesture of displaced hostility. My patient thus had insight, but the insight was sustained by paleologic thinking and concretization. She was more intuitive than the average person in recognizing this gesture of the boss as an act of hostility directed toward her, but for her the act had become equivalent to an overt act of hostility, just as it was for the boss. For us, the act is not equivalent to an act of hostility, but only symbolic, because at a reality level hitting the cooler is different from hitting Violet. Continuing in her paleologic thinking, the patient was then extending to all members of the firm the intention intuitively perceived in the boss.

The patient also had the conviction that when they were using the word "machine," they were referring to her. In fact, they actually were treating her as a machine, not as a person, by taking advantage of her efficiency and willingness to do a large amount of work, without protest, like a machine.

A reconsideration of her symptoms disclosed that in her ideas of reference there was always some truth—I would say at least a grain of truth. This grain of insight, however, remained a grain, a punctiform insight, and did not expand into a complete insight, for the following reasons.

1. It could not transcend the level of immediate reality which made the insight possible. Although the insight was obviously derived from a more general or abstract evaluation of the total situation, this total evaluation had become unconscious and the patient was aware only of the significance of the concrete event, which was accepted as expression of reality, not as a symbol. Thus Violet felt hit as the cooler was, literally treated as a dog, etc.

2. The patient tried to attune or to accord with the symptom the rest of her life, but this cannot be done, the symptom remaining incongruous with reality. In other words, instead of enlarging the insight to an abstract level, the patient generalizes it to a concrete level, actually distorting the rest of reality to fit the concreteness of the manifestation.

This partial insight can be exploited psychotherapeutically. The patient must be told that he has insight, that he saw some truth. When we re-examined the symptoms, I told Violet that she had unusual understanding in perceiving that the boss wanted to hit her and in realizing that Lucy was treating her like a dog, and praised her for such understanding.

This is, of course, interpretation, but from a new slant. The interpretations we generally give the patient concern their inner reality; here it is suggested instead that we tell him how the inner reality coincides with his appreciation of the external world, and how accurate this appreciation is at times. The insight is not given as something which the patient will passively accept, but as something he has actively created. As in the case of the recognition of the listening attitude, the patient changes from a passive to an active role. In other words, we exploit the little gaps of reality in the realm of the psychosis, or, to put it in a way which I prefer, we exploit the points of agreement between psychosis and reality. By doing so we make the best contact with the patient. Violet, for instance, felt much better and no longer alone in the peculiarness of her symptoms. She felt that I shared her feelings. I did not pretend to do so.

The benefit the patient receives from this method is not just the result of some kind of intellectual agreement between two debating persons. The anguish of the psychotic patient is increased by the fact that nobody can reach him, that "no consensual validation" is possible. If such consensual validation is obtained in at least a few instances, the patient will feel almost as if the first blow had been struck against the inaccessible barrier, and a path toward togetherness had again been opened.

This method, of course, should not be confused with the situation in which the regressed patient is aware of his normally unconscious symbolism, which is completely disconnected from reality. In these situations "the insight" is more harmful than beneficial, and at times has to be repressed (18).

We must not overlook, however, that the way of interpreting which I have just described may also present risks, if not applied appropriately. For instance, if the patient accepts the insight only at the level of concretization he may act out in accordance with his psychosis. We must work intensively to help him move away from the point where psychosis and reality converge. This is possible in an atmosphere of relatedness and under the impulse received from the conviction that some points of view are shared with the therapist.

For instance, Violet was told that it was true she was treated as a machine and what a sensitivity she had in realizing that they talked of her and treated her as if she were a machine! But what could she do now to change the situation? How could she change her behavior, her attitude, so that she would no longer be treated as a machine?

CONCLUSIONS

Some methods have been described by which some schizophrenic patients who are actively psychotic but not too acutely disturbed are helped to become aware of and to control some of their psychopathologic mechanisms. The interpretations are effective, not as abreacting insights passively received from the therapist, but as tools with which the patient has to work actively.

With the use of this technique the patient often loses his overt symptomatology and becomes capable of acquiring that deeper knowledge of himself which is a prerequisite for recovery.

REFERENCES

1. JUNG, C. G.: *The Psychology of Dementia Praecox.* New York: Nerv. & Ment. Disease Monograph Series, 1936.
2. ROSEN, J. N.: The treatment of schizophrenic psychosis by direct analytic therapy. *Psychiat. Quart.,* 2:3, 1947.
3. ROSEN, J. N.: *Direct Analysis. Selected Papers.* New York: Grune & Stratton, 1953.
4. SECHEHAYE, M. A.: *Symbolic Realization.* New York: International Universities Press, 1951.
5. SECHEHAYE, M. A.: *Autobiography of a Schizophrenic Girl.* New York: Grune & Stratton, 1951.
6. SECHEHAYE, M. A.: *A New Psychotherapy in Schizophrenia.* New York: Grune & Stratton, 1956.
7. SULLIVAN, H. S.: *Conceptions of Modern Psychiatry.* Washington: W. A. White Foundation, 1947.
8. SULLIVAN, H. S.: *Clinical Studies in Psychiatry.* New York: W. W. Norton, 1956.
9. FROMM-REICHMANN, F.: Some aspects of psychoanalytic psychotherapy with schizophrenics. In *Psychotherapy with Schizophrenics.* Edited by E. B. Brody and F. C. Redlich. New York: International Universities Press, 1952.
10. FROMM-REICHMANN, F.: The psychotherapy of schizophrenia. *Amer. J. Psychiat.,* 111:410, D, 1954.
11. RACAMIER, P. C.: Psychoanalytic therapy of the psychoses. In *Psychoanalysis Today.* Edited by S. Nacht. New York: Grune & Stratton, 1959.
12. ARIETI, S.: Introductory notes on psychoanalytic treatment of schizophrenics. In *Psychotherapy of Psychoses.* Edited by A. Burton. New York: Basic Books, 1961.
13. ARIETI, S.: *Schizophrenia. In American Handbook of Psychiatry.* Edited by S. Arieti. New York: Basic Books, 1959.
14. ARIETI, S.: The processes of expectation and anticipation; their genetic development, neural basis and role in psychopathology. *J. Nerv. & Ment. Dis.,* 106: 471, 1947.
15. ARIETI, S.: *Interpretation of Schizophrenia.* New York: Brunner, 1955.
16. ARIETI, S.: Schizophrenic thought. *Amer. J. Psychother.,* 13:537, 1959.
17. ARIETI, S.: Special logic of schizophrenic and other types of autistic thought. *Psychiatry,* 11:325, 1948.
18. FEDERN, P.: *Ego Psychology and the Psychoses.* New York: Basic Books, 1952.

4

The Schizophrenic Patient in Office Treatment

Expanding on the techniques described in the previous paper and adding others, this paper, published in 1965, discusses the relevance of attacking the single psychological symptoms in schizophrenia. It also points out how important in the treatment of the psychotic are not only psychodynamic interpretations, as they are given traditionally in classic psychoanalysis, but also interpretations concerning mechanisms and forms.

AS YOU ALL KNOW, long, laborious, tortuous, unpredictable and multifaceted is the psychotherapeutic treatment of schizophrenia. What I shall be able to report to you here will be only fragments of a therapeutic technique, whose presentation will be distorted not only by the limitation of time, but also by my personal bias in selecting the material and by the fact that here and there I shall feel obligated to make short excursions into theoretical ground. I hope that in spite of these fragmentations and detours a certain continuity will be maintained and a certain organization recognized.

First of all I must dispel some doubts which you may have about the office treatment of schizophrenics. What type of patients do I refer to in particular? In which way do they differ from hospitalized patients? Although many of us in private practice treat borderline, prepsychotic and so-called pseudoneurotic patients, these categories will not be the object of this report. I want to make clear that the patients to whom the content of the present paper applies, are full-fledged psychotics, with the classic symptoms of schizophrenia, such as hallucinations, delusions and ideas of reference. However, they have never been antisocial nor have they been of public scandal, and their symptomatology is not so

56

acute or unmanageable as to make hospitalization an absolute necessity. One of my aims in fact is to avoid hospitalization. Although my paper refers in particular to office patients what I am going to say can be applied also to hospitalized patients.

The therapeutic procedure which will be outlined can be seen in two separate aspects. The first aspect is the establishment of relatedness; the second is an actual attack on the psychotic symptoms, followed by a psychodynamic understanding.

This division is undoubtedly artificial and made for didactical purposes. Actually it reflects a double aspect of the schizophrenic process, a dual character, the interpersonal and the intrapsychic, which at the present stage of our knowledge is difficult to synthesize or to transform into what would appeal more to our own esthetic or philosophic conceptions; namely a unitarian aspect of the disorder or even of normal man. We know that these two psychologies and psychopathologies, the interpersonal and the intrapsychic, are interconnected, but as much as we would like to unite them in a superior synthesis, we are not yet able to do so in a manner which would satisfy our scientific standards.

ESTABLISHMENT OF RELATEDNESS

The establishment of relatedness, or, if we adopt a more classical terminology, the re-establishment of object-relations with a patient who not only shows a disorder in such relations but seems to be motivated toward a greater disorganization of them, is an important part of the treatment of schizophrenia. As a matter of fact, it is perhaps the most difficult part to teach, as it is not fully understood and to some extent still relies on intuitional procedures.

In his recent writings Tarachow (11, 12) describes two types of therapy: the first type is the classic psychoanalysis in which the analyst rejects the patient as object and teaches the patient to reject the analyst as object. The second type is what he calls psychotherapy, in which therapist and patient retain each other as object; often as infantile objects. Now, if we follow Tarachow's classification, it is obvious that the therapy of the schizophrenic belongs to the second type. Patient and therapist must work against the tendency of the disorder and try to resume toward each other the role of objects.

How can we re-establish object-relations in schizophrenic patients? The procedure is different according to the type of patients. In patients who are acutely decompensating, like, for instance, in some cases of post-partum psychosis, the therapist must assume an attitude of active and intense intervention. A strong and healthy person must enter the life of the patient and convey a feeling of basic trust. The patient must be approached with very simple, at times even preverbal ways, that I have described elsewhere (4, 5). This approach is not an appeal to the unconscious of the patient, à la Rosen (8). I don't think we can directly touch the unconscious. It is a communication with the basic, unsophisticated and genuine part of the patient. If I could paraphrase the words of the poet Wordsworth, used in a completely different context, I could say that it is a communication with "the naked and native dignity of man." The patient must acquire a feeling of reliance and trust. In normal development the mother-child relation engenders what has been called basic trust: a complex, interpersonal feeling which consists of the expectation, on the part of the child, that the mother will be there to give and love; and of the taken for granted idea, on the part of the mother, that the child will grow up to be a normal and worthy and loving person.

In the therapeutic situation the patient must experience something reminiscent of this basic trust, as perhaps he never experienced. This trust must be conferred by the simplicity, strength and forwardness of the therapist, not by his solicitous benevolence. In some cases the patient needs to lean and cling, to be talked to for hours and hours. The therapist has the feeling he has to perform almost a psychological blood transfusion. The needs of the patient may be so great, as to be indeed impossible to satisfy if we adhere to our schedule or to the conventional ways of private practice.

This attitude of active and intensive intervention that I have just referred to, is not only not indicated in some cases, but can be harmful. This type of intervention may be experienced as an intrusion, and even more than that, as an attack. The patient may be scared, and may withdraw or disintegrate even more. The typical schizophrenic defense, in fact, is withdrawal or psychological isolation, which, like the recently devised experimental sensory deprivations, makes the symptoms flourish. Let us remember that in these cases too the patient does not really want to be isolated. His need for communion with people is great, but his fear is even greater. In these cases the therapist must give himself small doses; the session must be of shorter duration than usual, and the main aim must be that of imparting to the patient the feeling that at least one interpersonal contact, the one with the therapist, needs not to provoke overwhelming fear. The therapist must be, at the same time, close and distant, close enough to give, distant enough not to scare. Neutral material may be the object of the verbal relationship. Although it may not be pertinent to the basic problems of the patient it may decrease the isolation and object-deprivation, and may help the patient to accept the therapist, so that the closeness will increase and the distance diminish.

I must add, however, that even in the treatment of these not too acute cases, we may have occasionally re-exacerbations with rapid disintegration, at times provoked by a sudden anxiety engendered by the treatment, without the therapist realizing what was happening. In these cases the therapist must either shift to that intense intervention which I have outlined above, or, to the opposite, and become more distant. I must admit that I have not yet succeeded in objectivizing in which cases I must adopt one procedure rather than the other, and that, much to my regret, I must resort to my intuition—an unscientific procedure.

We must frankly acknowledge that this part of the treatment, the establishment of relatedness, is still in several aspects at a prescientific level of development. On the other hand we should not be discouraged or exaggerate its difficulties. One thing has to be remembered which is ignored by many people because of their theoretical approach to schizophrenia. Before the patient became psychotic he had some type of object-relations or of relatedness. Undoubtedly this object-relation was not the healthiest, and it proved to be vulnerable; but nevertheless it existed. Only people suffering from severe child-schizophrenia or from those conditions described by Leo Kanner (7) as early infantile autism, had practically no object-relationships. All the other patients did, but it was a kind of vulnerable object-relation, because not founded on security, optimism, and basic trust. The psychosis makes this type of object-relatedness collapse. With our intervention we can rebuild it, but it will be again like a paper castle, unless it will be rebuilt on better foundations: basic trust for oneself and the therapist, insight into one's psychological mechanisms, in both their formal aspects and psychodynamic content.

There are many worthwhile techniques to be taken into consideration in detail in the establishment of relatedness with the schizophrenic, but I still have many things to cover in this paper and I must refer the reader to my writings for my point of view on this subject (4, 5). I shall add, however, the following general remarks:

1. The patient-therapist relationship is a special object-relationship. Although the therapist must avoid the mistakes the parent made, the

relationship must at first bear some resemblance to the parent-child relationship.

2. Eventually this relationship will be less and less modeled after the parent-child relationship and more and more after one of peer-relationship. When this transformation occurs the relationship may no longer be well represented by the word "object" but by Martin Buber's I-Thou formula, which implies no longer subjects and objects, but two subjects which interrelate.

3. The establishment of relatedness is often enhanced by the use of a therapeutic assistant, generally a psychiatrically trained nurse or a former patient. I shall come back to this third point later.

ATTACK AGAINST PSYCHOPATHOLOGIC MECHANISMS AND CONTENT

I wish now to discuss the direct attack on the mechanisms and content of the psychosis. I must add that many people rely only on the establishment of relatedness in the treatment of schizophrenia, especially in very acute cases. The symptoms seem to drop at times as soon as this relatedness is established. In my experience, although this is true in some cases, in the majority of cases the symptoms persist or return if the patient has not acquired insight into his psychological mechanism, and has not changed his vision of himself, the others, life, and the world. Although psychodynamic interpretations are much better known, I believe that interpretations concerning mechanisms and forms are also important, especially at an early phase of the treatment and I shall devote most of the rest of this paper to this topic.

With some special technical procedures which I have devised, the patient is helped to become aware of the ways with which he transforms his psychodynamic conflicts into psychotic symptoms. Although form and content are interrelated, a fundamental distinction remains between content interpretations given in accordance with more traditional psychodynamic methods and interpretations of forms and mechanisms. Whereas the benefit from traditional interpretations is due or believed to be due to acquisition of insight into repressed experiences and to the accompanying abreaction, and therefore is supposed to be immediate, the effectiveness of the second type of interpretation consists of the acquisition of methods with which the patient can work at his problems. They do not consist exclusively of insights passively received, but predominantly of tools with which the patient has to actively operate.

In what follows I am going to discuss this type of treatment in such symptoms as hallucinations, delusions, ideas of reference and related manifestations. Before doing so, however, I would like to make another short theoretical detour.

My insistence on attacking the schizophrenic symptom may appear a restricted if not an antiquated procedure. In fact not only in our psychiatric training but even in medical school we have learned that it is not the symptom but the cause of the disease which we should be mostly concerned with. Symptomatic treatment is secondary to causal treatment. I agree with this general principle which I think should be followed most of the time. In the most serious psychiatric conditions, however, we find ourselves in unusual circumstances. The symptom is more than a symptom. Often it is a maneuver which tends to make consensual validation impossible and to maintain interpersonal distance. What may have originated as a defense actually makes the whole situation of the patient more precarious and may enhance regression.

Secondly, the symptom stands for a great deal more, actually for what it wants but cannot eliminate. I shall explain what I mean by taking as example a typical and common symptom. A patient has an olfactory hallucination; he smells a bad odor emanating from his body. In this symptom actually a great deal of pathology is encapsulated. The patient feels he has a rotten personality, he stinks as a person. A schizophrenic process of concretization takes place and an olfactory hallucination results. This olfactory hallucination stands for or summarizes the whole life history, the whole evaluation of the self, the whole tragedy of the patient. Sophisticated as we are, we usually say that the hallucination is symbolic of what the patient feels about himself. This is correct, provided we understand that the symbol is a symbol for us, not for the patient. The patient, by virtue of the symptom, stops worrying about his personality and worries only about his stinking body. What we call a symbol, actually has a realistic, not a symbolic value for the patient. It tends to replace the reality which it wants to substitute. The symptom is not, for instance, like a flag which represents a country. The flag is not the exact equivalent or a duplication of the country it represents. This process of concretization, as exemplified in the hallucination of the above-mentioned patient, is perhaps the most common mechanism in schizophrenia, and, as we shall see later in detail, related to altered cognition. Whatever cannot be sustained at an abstract level, because too anxiety-provoking, is reduced to or translated into concrete representations.

Now at this point, I am sure, most of you, if not all of you, think that I have contradicted myself. In fact if the symptom is a substitution for such a great part not only of the illness but also of the life of the patient is it not true that the patient needs this substitution? He needs to eliminate so much mental pain, and I, in a cruel and antitherapeutic way, want to deprive him of his precious defense.

The point is that if an atmosphere of basic trust is developed in which the patient feels he obtains a great deal from the therapist in human relatedness, he is willing to relinquish his symptoms, or to convert them into less psychotic or neurotic ones. The new symptoms, like the recognition of being concerned with one's own personality and not body, may be more difficult to bear, but can be more easily shared by the therapist. In other words, the therapist will be able to help the patient to bear his cross, if this cross is a less autistic, or less psychotic one. Later in this paper I shall give examples. At this point I want to show how the therapist can help the patient to unravel some psychotic symptoms. Some of you may have already heard or read these procedures, as I must borrow from my previous writings (1, 2, 3, 4, 5, 6). I shall start with the treatment of hallucinations.

Only auditory hallucinations will be taken into consideration, but the same procedures could be applied to other types of hallucinations, after the proper modifications have been made.

With the exception of patients who are at a very advanced stage of the illness or with whom no relatedness whatsoever can be reached, it is possible to recognize that the hallucinatory voices occur only in particular situations, that is *when the patient expects to hear them.*

For instance, a patient goes home, after a day of work, and expects the neighbors to talk about him. As soon as he expects to hear them, he hears them. In other words, he puts himself in what I have called *the listening attitude.*

If we have been able to establish not only contact but relatedness with the patient, he will be able under our direction to distinguish two stages: that of the listening attitude and that of the hallucinatory experience. At first he may protest vigorously and deny the existence of the two stages, but later he may make a little concession. He will say, "I happened to think that they would talk and I proved to be right. They were really talking."

A few sessions later, however, another step forward will be made. The patient will be able to recognize and to admit that there was a brief interval between the expectation of the voices and the voices. He will still insist that this sequence is purely coincidental but eventually he will see a connection between his putting himself into the listening attitude and his actually hearing. Then he will recognize that he puts himself into this attitude when he is in a particular situation or in a particular mood, for instance in a mood on account of which he perceives hostility, almost in the air. He has the feeling that everybody has a disparaging attitude toward him, then he finds corroboration for this attitude of the others; he hears them making unpleasant remarks about him. At times he feels inadequate and worthless, but he does not sustain his feeling for more than a fraction of a second. The self-condemnation almost automatically induces him to put himself into the listening attitude and then he hears other people condemning him.

When the patient is able to recognize the relation between the mood and putting himself in the listening attitude, a great step has been accomplished. He will not see himself any longer as a passive agent, as the victim of a strange phenomenon or of persecutors, but as somebody who still has a great deal to do with what he experiences. Moreover if he catches himself in the listening attitude, he has not yet descended to or is not yet using abnormal or paleologic ways of thinking from which it will be difficult to escape. He is in the process of falling into the seductive trap of the world of psychosis but may still resist the seduction and remain in the world of reality.

I have found that if an atmosphere of relatedness and understanding has been established, patients learn with not too much difficulty to catch themselves in the act of putting themselves into the listening attitude at the least disturbances, several times during the day. At times, although they recognize the phenomenon, they feel that it is almost an automatic mechanism, which they cannot prevent. Eventually, however, they will be able to control it more and more. Even then, however, there will be a tendency to resort again to the listening attitude and to the hallucinatory experiences in situations of stress. The therapist should never be tired of explaining the mechanism to the patient again and again, even when such explanations seem redundant. It is seldom redundant, as the symptims may reacquire an almost irresistible attraction.

But now that we have deprived the patient of his hallucinations, again you can ask, how can he manage with his anxiety? How can we help him to bear his burden or a heavier but less unrealistic cross? An example will perhaps clarify this matter. A woman used to hear a hallucinatory voice calling her a prostitute. Now, with the method I have described we have deprived her of this hallucination. Nevertheless she experiences a feeling, almost an abstract feeling coming from the external environment, of being discriminated, considered inferior, looked upon as a bad woman, etc. She has almost the wish to crystallize or concretize again this feeling into a hallucination. If we leave her alone she will hallucinate again. If we tell her that she projects into the environment her own feelings about herself, she may become infuriated. She says, "The voices I used to hear were telling me I am a bad woman, a prostitute, but I never had such a feeling about myself. I am a good woman." The patient, of course, is right, because when she hears a disparaging voice, no longer has she a disparaging opinion of herself. The projective mechanism saves her from self-disparagement. We must instead point out to the patient that there was one time when she had a bad opinion of herself. Even then she did not think she was a prostitute but had a low self-esteem, such as she probably thought a prostitute would have about herself. Now what we have to carry and bear and share is the cross of a deep feeling of inadequacy. The therapist with his general attitude and firm reassurance and sincere interest in the patient will be able to share or to decrease the burden of this cross. At this point the therapeutic assistant is also very useful, as I shall discuss later.

The realization of the low self-esteem is not yet a complete psychodynamic explanation of the symptom, but at this stage of the treatment we stop at this explanation. The matter will be pursued later, when we shall examine the factors in the early family environment which led to this negative self-appraisal.

What I have said about hallucinations could with the proper modifications be repeated for ideas of reference and delusions. Before the delusions or ideas of reference are well formulated, the patient must learn to recognize that he is in what I call the referential attitude. For instance, he is taking a stroll in Central Park on a beautiful Sunday afternoon, when all of a sudden peculiar events begin to take place. People sitting on the benches start to talk with animation and to look at him with strange eyes. They make some gestures which have obvious reference to him. Children who were running all over or playing in the contiguous playground now all run toward the opposite direction avoiding being near him. An American flag which could be seen from the distance, open to the wind and waving on top of a pole, is now drooping. All this is an indication that people think that a horrible man, perhaps a pervert who attacks children and women, is in the park. The patient is supposed to be that man. The news is spreading. He rushes back home in a state of intense, agonizing turmoil.

And yet, we must ask him when he comes for the session, what happened before he went into the park? In what mood was he? Was he not looking for a certain evidence? Did he not almost hope to find it, so that he would be able to explain that indefinite mood of being thought of as a horrible creature? He had the impelling need to transform a vague, huge menace into a concrete threat, to restrict to a specific event a spreading feeling of being humiliated, disparaged, discriminated.

The direct attack on the symptom consists again in making the patient aware of his concretizing the vague threat. He must recognize how he substitutes ideas and feelings for others which are easier to grasp or to contend with in his distress. He will learn to check himself, as he may learn to check his listening attitude.

But again we made him retranslate the concrete into the abstract, and reintroject what he had projected. Will he be able to do so? He will, if we share the burden of the cross with the ultimate aim of removing the cross altogether.

I want to talk now briefly about another group of symptoms: the thought disorder of the schizophrenic. The thought disorders constitute indeed the most important part of the regression, what Bleuler called autism; what in Freudian terminology is referred to as the reemergence of the primary process. And yet many people discuss schizophrenia as if such thought disorders would not exist. Others make some concessions and believe that the schizophrenic thinks irrationally because the irrationality of the mother or of the family is transmitted to him. There is some truth in these allegations, but unless this partial truth is clarified, knowledge of it may become more confusing than revealing. For instance, the mother of a paranoid schizophrenic may be a hostile, suspicious person, whose vision of the world is one permeated by pessimism, distrust and hate: the world is a jungle; people are ready to cheat you. If you want to survive you must be careful and be prepared to defend yourself. This point of view is not necessarily psychotic. It may even be called a philosophy of life, which may very well be transmitted to the child. However, when the son of this woman not only sees the world as hostile but starts to think that people are plotting to kidnap him or to poison him, he goes further than the mother. To the irrationality of the mother he has added his psychotic, autistic, primary process twist. In Sullivanian terminology the attitude of the mother would be called a parataxic distortion (9, 10) but the way of thinking of the child was more than parataxic; it was prototaxic, a Sullivanian word for autistic. To study only the influence of the environment in reference to the alteration in cognition is not to go to the core of the problem. The same criticism could be repeated for those theories according to which thought disorders are due only to poor communication or to the so-called double-bind communication between mother and child.

When I was discussing hallucinations, delusions and ideas of reference, I was implicitly referring to some aspects of schizophrenic cognition. I would be tempted now to enter into a long disquisition about the logic of the schizophrenic. But I must be extremely brief and simplify as much as I can. At a certain stage of schizophrenic regression, the patient identifies not in virtue of identical subjects, as Aristotelian logic requires, but in virtue of identical predicates, that is in accordance with the principle of von Domarus. As we shall see from the examples which follow, this need to identify subjects which should not be identified is extremely strong in the schizophrenic and has at least two motivations or purposes. The first is of a general character: that of recapturing some order or cognitive organization in the confused or fragmented schizophrenic world; the second, specific in each patient, to believe as true and rational what he wishes to be true. An example that I often quote is that of a patient who thought she was the Virgin Mary. Asked why, she replied, "I am a virgin; I am the Virgin Mary." The common predicate "being virgin" led to the identification of the two subjects, the Virgin Mary and the patient. Obviously, the patient had the need to identify with the Virgin Mary, who was her ideal of perfection and to whom she felt close. At the same time she had the need to deny her feeling of unworthiness and inadequacy.

Following are a few more examples. A red-haired 24-year-old woman in a post-partum schizophrenic psychosis developed an infection in one of her fingers. The terminal phalanx was swollen and red. She told the therapist a few times, "This finger is me." Pointing to the terminal phalanx she said, "This is my red and rotten head." She did not mean that her finger was a representation of herself, but, in a way incomprehensible to us, really herself or an actual duplicate of herself. Another patient believed that the two men she loved in her life were actually the same person, although one lived in Mexico City and the other in New York. In fact both of them played the guitar and both of them loved her. By resorting to a primitive cognition which followed the principle of Von Domarus, she could reaffirm the unicity or univocality of the image of the man she wanted to love. Many patients at this stage indulge in what I call an orgy of identifications. As a last example, I shall mention a new patient who while waiting for the first time in the waiting room of my office, saw in one of the magazines which were there an advertisement with the picture of a baby in the nude. He remembered that he too, when he was a small child, had a picture of himself taken in that way, and the bastard of his father had not too long ago threatened to show that picture to the patient's girl friend. Seeing that picture in my waiting room, he thought, was not a fortuitous coincidence. The patient presented the phenomenon commonly found in schizophrenics of seeing non-fortuitous coincidences all over. The terrible coincidences for which there was no explanation were pursuing him relentlessly. The phenomenon of the coincidences is related also to the principle of von Domarus. A coincidence is a similar element occurring in two or more instances at the same time or after a short period of time. The patient tries to find glimpses of regularities in the midst of the confusion in which he now lives. He tends to register identical segments of experience and to build up systems of regularity upon such identical segments. At times the alleged regularity that the identical segments suggest gives sustenance to a complex which, although by now disorganized, retains a strong emotional investment. Contrary to what we do in the presence of less serious cognitive disorders, often we cannot explain to the patient the structure of the formal mechanisms he is using. We must help him in other ways. The patient must find some clarity not in the recurrence of similar fragments of experience, but from the feeling of relatedness with the therapist, as I have mentioned at the beginning of this paper. Interpersonal security must substitute the precarious intrapsychic security of the psychopathologic process.

There are, however, some ways of thinking which the schizophrenic shares with the normal person and which can be better explained to the patient. One of them is the rationalization. I shall compare the rationalization of a normal person to that of a schizophrenic, to show in which way they are similar and in which way they differ. As a rationalization of a normal man I shall take that of a colleague of ours who intended to attend a lecture without fully realizing that that evening he would have preferred to remain home with his family and relax. He looked out of the window, saw that it was raining and said, "The weather is bad. It is wiser to stay home." Now, not he but the weather is responsible for his not attending the lecture. I shall mention now a rationalization of a patient. A woman who was born and raised in a South American country in a well-to-do family, came to the United States in her early twenties, after having completed her college education. While in the United States, she married an American citizen, from whom she had a child. When I first saw her she was in her middle thirties, had been sick for several years and showed signs of moderate regression. She appeared apathetic, except when she was talking about her husband, for whom she nourished bitter resentment. She would repeatedly say that her husband was a bad man and she always knew it. When she was asked why she had married her husband if she knew he was such a bad man, she replied, "The wedding ceremony took place in this country. When the priest asked me if I wanted to marry my husband, he spoke English and I did not understand him. I said 'I do.' If he had spoken in Spanish, my own language, I would have never agreed to marry such a man." This rationalization would be facetious if it were not pathetic. It would be logical if it would not be based on illogical premises. The patient obviously understood the question at the wedding ceremony and replied "I do" in English. Moreover she spoke English fairly well, even at the time of her wedding. Her rationalization, however, cannot be interpreted just at face value as an attempt to justify herself, or disavow her responsibility or to make her marriage almost illegal. There was much more than that in this apparently absurd rationalization. The years spent in the United States had a flavor of unreality for her, or at least they seemed lived in an atmosphere of fogginess and confusion. They were characterized by a series of unfortunate events, which culminated in her unhappy marriage. Only life prior to her coming to the United States, that is that period of her life when she was speaking Spanish, made sense to her. In her mind, thus, what was confused or unclearly motivated became associated with the English language. Again, following our theoretical framework, we could say that the patient made a gigantic concretization. She reduced the uncertainty and fogginess of her North American life to a linguistic difficulty. Again this symptom, a rationalization, is not just a technical device to avoid responsibility; it is also and predominantly an expression of her whole life history, of her whole tragedy, of the difference between the peace or apparent peace of her early life and the turbulence or apparent turbulence of her married life.

In a way comparable to the work of the fine artist and of the poet, a little episode, or a little symptom becomes representative of a much larger segment of reality.

But let us examine again the rationalization of our colleague, who did not attend the lecture. We cannot take even his rationalization literally. The bad weather, the storm, his going out at night may be for him symbolic of the hard professional competitive world where you always have to keep abreast, where you have challenges to meet. Staying home is being protected, being with your wife, or with mother or in mother's womb, whatever level of interpretation you prefer. His rationalization again represents a dilemma between the two types of life he has to cope with.

However, there are important differences between his rationalization and the patient's. Our colleague's rationalization could stand on its own merit. People at times do stay home because of the bad weather. There is thus concordance between the obvious reality, although a superficial reality, and the psychodynamic reality which is suppressed. That is, the colleague can stay home for both reasons, because of the weather and because he does not want to meet the challenge of the professional life.

In the rationalization of the patient there was no congruence or concordance between the external or superficial reality and the psychodynamic. The rationalization becomes plausible only if we understand what is suppressed, substituted or concretized, if we know the complicated experiences the patient went through. It is only when the patient is told what he is doing and when we share with him the anxiety of the knowledge of what was once repressed, that he will not resort to implausible rationalizations any longer.

GENERAL PARTICIPATION IN PATIENT'S LIFE

I must add now a few remarks on the general participation in the patient's life. The treatment of the very sick schizophrenic cannot consist only of the sessions, but an active participation in his life is necessary, as many authors have reported. In the beginning of the treatment the patient must feel that many events are shared by the therapist. In many instances the patient's requirements are immense and the help of a therapeutic assistant may be necessary. A psychiatrically trained nurse or former patients are the best qualified to act as therapeutic assistants, as Federn and Rosen have previously reported.

The assistant is there to help, to support, to share. It is particularly at a certain stage of the treatment that the therapeutic assistant is valuable. When he patient has lost concrete delusions and hallucinations, by virtue of the methods which I have outlined, and has decreased the tendency to concretize, he may nevertheless retain a vague feeling of being threatened, which is abstract, diffuse, and from which he tries to defend himself by withdrawing. The assistant is there to dispel that feeling. That common exploration of the inner life in which the patient and therapist are engaged is now complemented by an exploration of the external life, effectuated with the therapeutic assistant.

Although the therapist and his assistant participate in many aspects of the patient's life, they do not stultify the growth of the patient, who is allowed to take his own initiative whenever possible. At a late stage of the treatment the patient wants tasks to be given to him, contrary to the way he felt at the beginning of the treatment. By fulfilling these tasks, at first easy ones, later more difficult, the patient will gain in self-evaluation. At the same time that he wants the therapist to share his life, he wants to a certain extent to share the therapist's life. Thus questions concerning the therapist's life should not be dismissed but answered with sincerity whenever possible.

PSYCHODYNAMIC FORMULATIONS

I do not want to convey the impression that the treatment is over when we have established relatedness, interpreted the formal mechanisms or translated them into non-psychotic ones. Although given even at the beginning of the treatment, at a more advanced stage more and more interpretations refer to psychodynamic mechanisms. They refer to the life struggle of the patient, are based on the genetic history, on the pathologic ways with which the patient has tried to solve his conflicts, and therefore do not vary very much from the interpretations given to neurotics. The psychodynamic history and life-pattern of the schizophrenic, if we ignore the personal variables which are many and important, can be reconstructed, and interpreted as consisting of three stages:

Stage one: In early childhood, at times even later, the future patient is at war with his family. Early interpersonal relations are characterized by intense anxiety, devastating hostility, or false detachment.

Stage two: The future patient introjects and acquires toward himself the same attitude that he felt the family had toward him. He grows with low self-esteem and a shaky self-identity. But somehow he cannot accept this self-appraisal. He is now at war with himself.

Stage three, or psychotic stage: The patient now rejects the vision of himself that he had introjected and, through cognitive alteration, projects it to others. Now the others accuse him, no longer does he accuse himself. At this point he is at war with the world. He may go to the point of destroying the world by altering deeply his cognitive and symbolic understanding of it. In the catatonic type of schizophrenia this third stage is somewhat different.

What do we try to do in the treatment that I have outlined? We attack the sequence of events in reverse. In the first stage of treatment we are concerned predominantly with the third or psychotic stage of the life history of the patient. We help the patient retranslate the psychotic symptoms into non-psychotic; that is, he must reintroject. But, as we have already seen, if the patient reintrojects, his anxiety may increase again with tendency to project again. The second stage of the treatment, which actually starts at the same time that the first starts, although it continues much longer, consists of making the patient increasingly aware of the fact that we share the burden of this anxiety and want to help him rebuild his self-esteem. This task will be less difficult if the patient will introject and incorporate healthy influences from the therapist. At the third stage of the treatment we attack the first stage of the life-history of the patient. We complete the psychodynamic understanding of the early intrafamily war, that is, of the early interpersonal factors which led to the unfortunate outcome. But at this point, the therapy is not fundamentally different from that used with psychiatric patients belonging to other categories.

REFERENCES

1. ARIETI, S.: Special logic of schizophrenic and other types of autistic thought. *Psychiatry*, 11:325, 1948.
2. ARIETI, S.: *Interpretation of Schizophrenia*. New York: Robert Brunner, 1955.
3. ARIETI, S.: Schizophrenia: The manifest symptomatology, the psychodynamic and formal mechanisms. In *American Handbook of Psychiatry*. Edited by S. Arieti. New York: Basic Books, 1959.
4. ARIETI, S.: Introductory notes on psychoanalytic treatment of schizophrenia. In *Psychotherapy of Psychoses. Edited by A. Burton*. New York: Basic Books, 1961.
5. ARIETI, S.: Psychotherapy of schizophrenia. *Arch. Gen. Psychiat.*, 6:112, 1962.
6. ARIETI, S.: Hallucinations, delusions and ideas of reference treated with psychotherapy. *Amer. J. Psychother.*, 16:52, 1946.
7. KANNER, L.: Irrelevant and metaphorical language in early infantile autism. *Amer. J. Psychiat.*, 103:242, 1946.
8. ROSEN, J. N.: *Direct Analysis*. New York: Grune & Stratton, 1953.
9. SULLIVAN, H. S.: *Conceptions of Modern Psychiatry*. New York: Norton, 1953.
10. SULLIVAN, H. S.: *The Interpersonal Theory of Psychiatry*. New York: Norton, 1953.
11. TARACHOW, S.: Interpretation and reality in psychotherapy. *Int. J. Psychoanal.*, 43:377, 1962.
12. TARACHOW, S.: *An Introduction to Psychotherapy*. New York: International University Press, 1963.

5

Anxiety and Beyond in Schizophrenia and Psychotic Depression

This paper aims at clarifying the role of anxiety in those severe conditions, like schizophrenia and depression, that proceed to a stage beyond anxiety.

FOR YOUNG PSYCHIATRISTS it is hard to believe that before the advent of psychodynamic psychiatry, and even later in some extremely conservative schools, the presence of anxiety in schizophrenia was not acknowledged. Blunting of affect, apathy, indifference, alienation from one's own feelings, affective incongruity were the main expressions used to characterize the schizophrenic.

Still vivid in my mind is a demonstration given by my teacher of psychiatry and neurology while I was a student in medical school. Incidentally, my teacher was an excellent neurologist whose name is prominently mentioned even in present-day textbooks. In the field of psychiatry, where he also had a vast theoretical knowledge, he practiced a typical kraepelinian approach. In the lesson I am referring to he was presenting to the class a catatonic patient who was in a statuesque position except for an "incongruous" smile which occasionally appeared and a movement of an arm repeated rhythmically from time to time. After demonstrating the classic catatonic features, including waxy flexibility, my teacher said to the patient, "Giuseppe, I have just received a telegram announcing that your mother has suddenly passed away." The patient did not wince. He continued to have his incongruous smile periodically and to move his arm from time to time. "Do you see," said the teacher, "how insensitive he is? He is not even affected by the news of the death of his mother." The whole class, myself included, was spellbound. What was so astound-

72

ing at that time was not so much the callousness with which the news of the alleged death of one's own mother was announced, but the fact that a son would remain impassive at such news. How was that possible? Was the patient still a human being? Was he able to experience sorrow, anxiety?

Of course, we know better now. In spite of the catatonic withdrawal the patient knew that the teacher was demonstrating a point, was not reporting a true piece of information. The patient knew much more: He was not unfeeling; he was sensitive and anxious to the point that he had to cut almost all the ties with a world which, in practically all communications, caused him so much fear, pain, was so callous and cruel. Now, almost four decades later, the greatest cruelty in this episode seems to me to reside in the fact that the professor did not know he was cruel. On the contrary, he wanted to help, he was motivated by his usual didactic fervor. As I have already mentioned, he was an excellent neurologist, a good man personally, but he lived and taught at a time when professors of psychiatry knew very little about psychodynamics.

Now, almost four decades later, it seems to me that the catatonic patient was very eloquent in his catatonic mutism. He was saying, "If you people are so cruel as to even be able to do this experiment on me, it is better for me to remove myself entirely from all of you." But he did not remove himself entirely. He smiled at us, from time to time, not incongruously, but at the incongruity of the world he was experiencing. And the rhythmic movement of his arm reminded us that he was alive, very much alive, in fact. Inside of him was volcanic anxiety, but an anxiety which cannot be expressed and which petrifies people in statuesque positions.

I do not imply that the patient was not to be considered sick, as some people who today deny the existence of schizophrenia would think. Obviously he was very sick. His sickness consisted of his inability to integrate or to cope with the negative influences of the world, also because the negative influences, past and present, were experienced in an intensified, extremely painful manner.

It is true that the anxiety of the schizophrenic is often so great that he has to withdraw not only from the activities of life, but also from his own feeling, thus giving the clinical picture, at a manifest level, of blunting of affect. In many cases we do not have withdrawal, but a typical paranoid delusional structure, which can also be interpreted as a defense against or a transformation of anxiety. As a matter of fact, the whole schizophrenic symptomatology can be viewed as a mechanism used to transform or diminish anxiety.

This statement may appear strange to the beginner in the field of psychiatry. If the patient feels persecuted, accused of being a spy, a murderer, a prostitute, if he believes his wife puts poison in his food, or that a bad odor emanates from his body, how can we think that his anxiety is decreased? Are not these delusions sufficient to cause a great deal of anxiety? They are: but they cause an anxiety which is not so traumatic or devastating as the previous anxiety which led him to schizophrenia. The anxiety now is experienced as coming from the external world. People accuse the patient of being a prostitute, a spy, but the patient knows better. He is innocent. He does not accuse himself any more. His self-esteem is not very high now; but better than before, when he used to consider himself worthless, unlovable, a failure, a disgrace to himself, sorry to have been born, sorry to be alive, hopeless about his future, extremely anxious about whether he would make it or not in life. All the conceptions which led to a devastating self-image and the feelings connected with these conceptions gave origin to the schizophrenogenic anxiety, the anxiety which shakes, disintegrates, or even destroys the inner self (1, 2).

But now the psychosis permits the patient to experience a type of anxiety which does not undermine the inner self. Instead of thinking that his wife poisons his life and that he is hurt inside by the failure of his marital relation, failure which he is partially responsible for, he believes his wife puts poison in his food. Instead of believing that he has a rotten personality, he thinks he has a rotten body which emanates a bad odor; instead of believing that she is worthless as a woman, she believes people think she is a worthless prostitute.

It is the anxiety about the self-image, about what one thinks or feels about oneself, that is the most dangerous. This anxiety is unjustified, especially to the degree to which it is experienced, but is very real as an experiential phenomenon. Anxiety about realistic dangers or external dangers is not schizophrenogenic. We know, for instance, that in cases of enemy invasion, defeat in war, adversity of all sorts, collective calamities, the incidence of schizophrenia does not increase. We have thus a paradoxical situation: In order to eliminate the schizophrenogenic anxiety or to transform it in one which is not schizophrenogenic, the patient becomes schizophrenic. To be falsely accused, as Sacco and Vanzetti were, let us say, does not produce schizophrenogenic anxiety, although it causes indescribable suffering. If you believe that you, too, are accused like Sacco and Venzetti, although you are not, and there is no evidence for such accusation, you are schizophrenic.

Now, all this has extremely important implications for the psychotherapy of the paranoid type of schizophrenia. In our therapeutic effort we want to help the patient do an enormously difficult thing. We want him to reconvert his present anxiety into the original one. In other words, he must no longer feel accused or persecuted by others; he must lose this type of anxiety. Now he should recognize that he accuses himself; he must come to grips with what he thinks and feels about himself. But this is the crux of the matter: This self-image is unacceptable, unbearable, causes so much anxiety. He cannot do what we want him to do. Of course we could give the patient phenothiazines, and he will lose the capacity to experience anxiety, and he may consequently lose symptoms. But the psychodynamic background for the symptoms has not changed. The patient is potentially the same. I am not a priori against drug therapy; I am using it myself with several patients when it is important to decrease immediately the intensity of the symptoms. However, I do not use massive doses which bring about a state of depersonalization. The treatment of choice in my opinion is psychotherapy.

In other writings I have described my method of helping the patient to reconvert externalized anxiety into the inner one (3). In this paper I shall mention only one aspect of this difficult procedure. The patient will be willing to reaccept an unbearable self-image, and the devastating anxiety which goes with it, if he feels the therapist is willing to share his anxiety. The burden of what to do with this anxiety now will be also the therapist's burden. Unless the patient has established a relatedness of basic trust with the therapist, and nourishes the feeling that the therapist will share his hidden, private, secret pain as a good mother would do, he is not going to relinquish the psychotic structure, is not going to change the type of anxiety (3).

If good relatedness is established, the patient will be more than willing to share with the therapist the anxiety of his own unbearable self-image. As a matter of fact, he will soon discover that the therapist is the best person with whom to look into this self-image. The therapist will help the patient to recognize that this very self-image is unrealistically bad because of historical events which occurred in childhood and because of an accumulation of consequent and interrelated distortions. It is with the help of the therapist that the patient will learn to see himself acceptable to himself and to others. This new way of looking at oneself does not imply that the patient has always been blameless, flawless, or the victim of others. On the other hand, if he is not afraid, he will recognize that he has to improve a great deal, has a moral responsibility to do his share toward his improvement. The patient must learn to choose, must learn to will, must learn to assert himself and his point of view.

In my book *The Will To Be Human* (4), I ask the question: What is the message, the personal value that the schizophrenic tries to express before it is distorted, first by his extreme anxiety and then by the psychosis? It is the basic value of every human being. He wants to be the sovereign of his will; he wants to will to be human. He wants to be totally himself, but he does not know how. Until he recovers, he finds sovereigns all over to which he attributes hostile intents, but not in himself.

So far I have referred to patients who transformed anxiety in psychotic structures. Nowadays, however, we see many patients in whom anxiety remains manifest anxiety. They show no blunting of affect or even paranoid structures, but obvious anxiety exuding from all parts, a pananxiety, as Hoch and Polatin (5) described it in the picture of pseudoneurotic schizophrenia.

Several clinical developments may occur. At times the anxiety is again externalized. The pseudoneurotic schizophrenic or the incipient schizophrenic may focus their anxiety upon things or facts which obviously are not related to the problems which affect their souls. They may be phobic about eating certain foods, wearing certain dresses, going to certain places, or presentments about certain accidents happening and so on. At other times the patient all of a sudden has a massive anxiety seemingly coming from nowhere. He is not yet psychotic, but he does not feel well, and he does not know what to do. He cannot even verbalize his anxiety, although at times he says he feels like breaking into pieces. This state of prepsychotic anxiety is dangerous; it may actually become a preschizophrenic panic, followed by a full-fledged psychosis. At times it occurs in particular situations, engendered by external factors; for instance, in youngsters who have been away to college, or in women who give birth to babies, or in strange and unusual circumstances, like meeting the spouse after a long absence.

Obviously in all these cases the patient has to face a challenge; however, it is a challenge that the majority of people are able to meet without disastrous results. What happens here is not just fear of failure or fear of not being able to cope with the difficult situation. The fear is that the failure will reveal once and for all the total defeat in the process of living which the patient has suspected one day will occur and which includes the past life as well as one's envisioned future. The promise of life will not be fulfilled. The patient now understands he was waiting for Godot.

In post-partum schizophrenic psychosis this fear manifests itself in connection with being a mother and with a double identification on the part of the patient with her own mother and with the child, who will be as badly treated as she was once (6).

In these moments of prepsychotic panic the important role of the therapist is detecting the overpowering anxiety and helping the patient to verbalize it, because most of the time the patient is not able to do so. He experiences only a diffuse, vague feeling, coming from obscure sources. Eventually the therapist will have to explain to the patient that this feeling is not based predominantly on the anxiety of the moment, as it seems, but on the old self-image that he conceived early in life. However, this is not the immediate role of the therapist. As I said before, at this stage the role of the therapist must be that of recognizing the anxiety, of helping the patient to express it, and of giving the patient the feeling that the therapist is there to share the burden of such anxiety and willing to do what he can to dissolve it.

Unfortunately many of these cases are not recognized. Anxiety-loaded telephone calls from youngsters in college are ignored by parents or interpreted as homesickness or momentary discouragement. In other circumstances in life the change in the patient is interpreted as a recurring variation in mood. Thus the anxiety is allowed to go beyond bounds and to undergo the schizophrenic transformation.

Now there are some therapists, fortunately a small minority, who believe it is good for the patient to become schizophrenic. The preschizophrenic patient is seen as a person who must go through a schizophrenic psychosis in order to solve his conflicts and eventually reach normality. I have never contributed to such apotheosis of schizophrenia, just as I have not supported other recent apotheoses of the disorder by those who see in schizophrenic cognition the supreme truth. Obviously there are many truths that we learn from schizophrenia, truths which have to do either with the bizarreness of the human spirit or its creativity, the loneliness of the human soul or its capacity for communion with fellow men, the petrifying catatonic loss of will or the ability to make free choices, the capacity for blaming, projecting, and hating and the tendency toward self-effacement. In other words, it is true that the student of schizophrenia and the person suffering from schizophrenia may enlarge their views or their experiences of human possibilities as well as of the human predicament, but this acknowledgment does not imply that we recommend schizophrenia or that we should not try to prevent its occurrence.

In my opinion it is not true that it is necessary for certain people to become schizophrenic in order to become normal. It is true only if unless he became schizophrenic the patient would not have the possibility of undergoing treatment and would have to go through life without knowing himself: a life impoverished by the measures adopted to fight the schizophrenogenic anxiety. It is much better instead to catch the patient when his anxiety has not gone beyond anxiety. Although I have been successful in treating many full-fledged schizophrenics, I have not been successful with some of them, fortunately a minority. I always remember this unsuccessful minority as an indication that once the anxiety has undergone the schizophrenic transformation, there is always a certain margin of uncertainty and the possibility of no *restitutio ad integrum*.

Schizophrenia is not the only condition presenting a stage which could be defined as being beyond the level of anxiety. Psychotic depression is another one. Needless to say, in many depressions, neurotic or psychotic, we also find a great deal of anxiety; but in the typical, deep, psychotic depression there is no longer anxiety. Whereas in schizophrenia the inner anxiety has been transformed by means of elaborate cognitive processes like delusions, hallucinations, and ideas of reference, in depression the predominant emotion has gone beyond anxiety and has become depression. Now the battle of life seems lost; the patient has not been true to himself. He has tried either to placate or please others and has negated himself. He either has devoted himself to an unworthy love or the person who was there to give him praise or a meaning to his life has died or gone away. A trauma of loss that he may have sustained early in his life is repeated: He will never obtain what he wanted; he will be deprived forever; forever he will mourn the irreparable loss.

When the patient is very depressed, he is not even aware of the negative ideas and negative appreciation of himself and of his life which led to his condition. The deep psychotic melancholia is a feeling which often drowns all ideas, all other feelings. The patient is aware only of his feeling of depression. At times he tries to justify his depression by stating that he is guilty, sinful, or incapable. Here again the job of the therapist is gigantic. Again he could prescribe antidepressant drugs which make the patient less sensitive to his depression, but the background for the depression would remain.

The patient must be helped first to recapture the ideas which led to a depressive attitude and eventually again helped to change depressive ideas into others which cause anxiety. The patient may not obtain what he wants; he may never repair the loss sustained early in life, but he may find a substitution. The person who recently died and was so important, perhaps by acting like a parental surrogate, was so important only because of some roles that the patient had attributed to him. Certainly sadness is a normal feeling when a person dear to us dies or disconnects himself from our life, but the feeling of hopelessness and inability to accept the loss, with consequent feeling of melancholia, is a pathologic outcome. Could it be that the patient relied on the departed person for sustenance, for narcissistic supplies, for approval? If he finds a substitute, is he afraid to lose him, too? But, most important, why does he depend so desperately on others in order not to be depressed? (7). Is the knowledge of such dependence making him anxious?

It is not an easy job to eliminate the depression. First of all, the recent ideas which acted as precipitating events, or all the old ideas connected with childhood losses and complexes, have become unconscious or experienced at the periphery of consciousness. The depression, when it has reached a psychotic stage, acts as repression does in other psychiatric conditions. The patient is aware only of the overpowering feeling of depression and has forgotten or repressed all the ideas or cognitive components. If, with our help there is a spirit of relatedness and a therapeutic attitude, we succeed in decreasing the repression, and the patient will become aware again of the unhappy ideas. The rediscovered ideas will bring about anxiety if not again depression. The patient who has become used to being depressed is more prone or more willing to be depressed than anxious, just as the paranoid is more likely or willing to be paranoid than anxious.

In simple words, we want to give hope to a hopeless person. But the psychotic hopeless person does not want hope because the other side of the coin of hope is anxiety. Hope is not certainty; it is a possibility. A possibility may not be actualized. One of the ways to remove anxiety is to remove hope; that is, to bring about hopelessness; that is, despair; that is, depression.

Why is the depressed person so unable to hope or so prone to change hope into anxiety? Because of the circumstances of his early life, which I have described elsewhere (8, 9), he has developed certain patterns of living by which he tries to attain what he wants: love, appreciation, recognition. These early patterns have been established generally in relation with his parents and strengthened or reactivated later in relation with the spouse, or another important person, or even an organization.

The patient tries to obtain love, approval, appreciation, recognition from parents, parent substitutes, or their symbolic equivalents. He expects from himself what he believes other people expect from him. But the ways by which he tries to attain his aims are rigid, not elastic. Sometimes he expects everything from others; at other times he indulges in aimless hypomanic activity; at other times he works hard, motivated only by duty and obligation. He has learned these patterns; he is anxious about abandoning the beaten path. Then he becomes fearful that he will not obtain what he wants by using the patterns to which he is accustomed, and he experiences despair. We have to help him to retrace all these steps in reverse.

I cannot possibly deal with these procedures, and the readers are referred to other writings (8, 9). This paper is aimed only at clarifying the role of anxiety in those severe conditions that proceed to a stage beyond anxiety. Anxiety stands out as the main psychiatric concern, whether it remains anxiety or has undergone the schizophrenic or depressed transformation.

REFERENCES

1. ARIETI, S.: New views on the psychodynamics of schizophrenia. *Amer. J. Psychiat.*, 124:453, 1967.
2. ARIETI, S.: The psychodynamics of schizophrenia. *Amer. J. Psychother.*, 22:366, 1968.
3. ARIETI, S.: The schizophrenic patient in office treatment. In *Psychotherapy of Schizophrenia*. Edited by C. Muller and G. Benedetti. Basel: Karger, 1963.
4. ARIETI, S.: *The Will to Be Human*. New York: Quadrangle Books, 1972.
5. HOCH, P. and POLATIN, P.: Psychoneurotic forms of schizophrenia. *Psychiat. Quart.*, 23:248, 1949.
6. ARIETI, S.: Introductory notes on the psychoanalytic therapy of schizophrenia. In *Psychotherapy of the Psychoses*. Edited by A. Burton. New York: Basic Books, 1961.
7. BEMPORAD, J. R.: New views on the psychodynamics of the depressive character. In *The World Biennial of Psychiatry and Psychotherapy*, Vol. 1. Edited by S. Arieti. New York: Basic Books, 1970.
8. ARIETI, S.: Manic-depressive psychosis. In *American Handbook of Psychiatry*, Vol. 1. Edited by S. Arieti. New York: Basic Books, 1959.
9. ARIETI, S.: The psychotherapeutic approach to depression. *Amer. J. Psychother.*, 16:397, 1962.

6

The Parents of the Schizophrenic
Patient: A Reconsideration

Published in 1977, this paper* returns to one of the major themes discussed in Chapter 1: the psychodynamics of family interrelations. It points out that although the influence of the family is very important in the psychogenesis of schizophrenia, it is not the only factor. Moreover, even when the impact of the family has been studied as a partial factor, this type of research has often been carried out with simplistic methods, biases, and disregard of the distortions made by the patient himself.

GENETICS HAVE BEEN ABLE TO OFFER presumptive evidence that a hereditary factor exists in schizophrenia. When different studies, carried out in different countries and with different methodologies, disclose that if schizophrenia occurs in a monozygotic twin, in at least 35% of cases it will develop sooner or later in the other member of the pair, even if the twins were reared apart, the evidence is persuasive. In fact, the incidence of schizophrenia in the general population is calculated to be only 0.85%.

This evidence, however, is not sufficient to explain the whole etiology of schizophrenia. First of all, it is inferred from statistics, but not proved. No Mendelian law acting in families of schizophrenics has been found. No distribution of schizophrenia resembling that of such hereditary diseases as Huntington's chorea, hemophilia, or muscular dystrophy has been observed. Moreover, if monozygotic twins are genetically equivalent, the concordance in relation to schizophrenia should be 100% in these cases; but it is not. These considerations and others suggest that although the

---

* Presented at the 20th Winter Meeting of the American Academy of Psychoanalysis, Atlanta, Georgia, December 5, 1976.

genetic factor is important, it provides only a potentiality, but other factors are necessary to change a potentiality into a clinical entity. The writer is one of the numerous authors who have searched for the missing etiological links in the environment of the patient. Like many other authors, he has found not even a single case, among the patients studied psychodynamically, who did not come from a disturbed milieu and did not present a very revealing psychodynamic history. It is thus plausible to assume that the combination or the causal encounter of the genetic and environmental factors, or the absence of compensatory opportunities, have a great deal to do with the disorder.

When we refer to the environment, of course we include everything other than the patient himself, but it is especially the role that the patient's mother and father have played in the psychogenesis of the disorder that has received the focus of attention. There is no doubt that the roles of the family as a whole, and especially of the parents, are very important. The aim of this paper, however, is to point out that many authors have exaggerated some features of these roles, transformed some others, and greatly minimized or totally ignored some aspects of this complex problem.

I think that now, almost three decades since the study of the family started to make a profound impact on modern psychiatry, we must reevaluate the field of family psychodynamics. We must recognize the mistakes that we have made in order to retain and stress only what is valuable and has passed the test of time. I believe that a reconsideration of the role of the family in the psychodynamics of schizophrenia is extremely useful also for the understanding of milder psychiatric conditions. In fact, once we have become well acquainted with the gross psychodynamic pathology of psychoses, we become better equipped to recognize milder forms of the same psychopathology in psychoneuroses and in character disorders. Similarly, if we recognize the theoretical misconceptions that we held and the therapeutic mistakes that we have made in our dealings with the psychotic, we can become more apt to spot less visible misconceptions and mistakes made in our dealings with less severe psychiatric conditions.

It was in the field of schizophrenia that the works of Harry Stack Sullivan, Frieda Fromm-Reichman, John Rosen, and other pioneers disclosed that the family had played a definite etiological role. And now it may be in the same field of schizophrenia that we can start to detect the errors made in such studies.

The fundamental error in my opinion is that of conceiving the patient as a being completely molded by external circumstances. The geneticist sees the origin of the disorder in the genetic code, hidden in the chromosomes of the patient; the family therapist sees it in the effect of the family and especially of mother and father. But geneticists and a large group of psychodynamic psychiatrists are closer than they think to one another's conceptions when they see the patient as entirely shaped by circumstances alien to his being or at the mercy of obscure forces or as a passive entity that has to accept ineluctably his chromosomic or familial destiny.

Obviously the patient is influenced very much by his family, but he is not just in a state of passive receptivity. Inasmuch as every human being is strongly influenced by his environment, we must acknowledge in him a fundamental state of *receptivity*. But he is not to be defined only in terms of a state of receptivity. Every human being, even in early childhood, has another basic function which we, following the French sociologist Lucien Goldmann (5), can call *integrative activity*. Just as the transactions with the world not only inform but transform the individual, with his integrative activity the individual transforms these transactions and in his turn he is transformed by these transformations. *No* influence is received like a direct and immutable message. Multiple processes involving interpersonal and intrapsychic dimensions go back and forth. According to the philosopher Giambattista Vico:

> "the being of man cannot be enclosed within a determinate structure of possibilities . . . but it moves, rather, among *indeterminable alternatives,* and even further, but its own movement generates these alternatives" (4) (italics mine).

Thus to depict the mother of the schizophrenic as a schizophrenogenic mother is a primitive simplification. The mother is schizophrenogenic if her negative qualities are also processed by the future patient in a schizophrenogenic way.

In other words, the patient makes his own contribution to his pathology. He picks up what he receives from the family, and he deforms it. The person who becomes schizophrenic deforms in a different way and more than the average person and the nonpsychotic. To use an analogy, the deformation of the patient may be compared to the deformation of a sound produced by an echo if the echo in its turn is echoed several times. The repeated and increasing deformation of the echo leads to a huge and unpredictable sound which, as we can hear in some ancient European buildings, at times is very harmonious, at other times cacophonic.

If we accept this possibility, the psychiatric disorder may still be viewed as related to a considerable extent to the pathogenic relationships in the family, but the intrapsychic role of the patient has to be included, too.

Many authors have been quite critical of the patient's parents, even of the parents' manifest behavior. Some authors have described the mother of the patient as malevolent, and one of them spoke of her perverse sense of motherhood (8). From reading some authors, one gets the impression that the parents of the schizophrenic are inhuman, cruel, perverse creatures. Other authors portray them as transmitting irrationality to the patient directly, just as they would transmit to him the language that they speak. Let us take some examples. A prominent author described a girl whose mother wished her to become a good writer like Virginia Woolf, even if that would imply committing suicide (7). Eventually the patient did commit suicide. In the same article the author, who wanted to report typical examples of parents of schizophrenics, mentioned a mother who, referring to her son, said to the doctor, "You must cure him—he is all of my life—when he started to become sick, I slept with him just like man and wife." Other thought provoking examples were given in the same article. A schizophrenic woman who was hospitalized used to have her genitalia examined by her physician father each time she returned home from a date in order to make certain she was still a virgin. The case is also reported of a female patient who not only spilled food all over herself, but blew her nose in the napkin. The patient did not know that it was wrong to do so because her father, an eminent professor, used to blow his nose in his napkin. In another case reported in the same article, the mother of a patient told her that she was afraid the father would seduce the patient's pubescent sister. The father had also confided that the mother was a lesbian and a menace to the three daughters. Another prominent author (6) reported the following example as a typical transmission of irrationality from the parents to the schizophrenic patient. A young paranoid patient, who was examined in connection with the Veterans Administration, made very few statements; however, he repeatedly said, "It's all a matter of chemistry and physics." The examiner then asked the parents what they thought about their son's illness. There was a long silence and finally the mother said, "Well, we don't know anything about it. It's just a matter of chemistry and physics to us." The father and the patient joined in a mild chuckle, both repeating in a low tone, "Yeah, just a matter of chemistry and physics."

If time would permit, I would quote many similar examples from articles of authors who have studied the father and mother of the schizophrenic. What I want to indicate instead is that although very dramatic and impressive, these examples are misleading. I do not deny that parents as those reported in the above examples exist. I have observed some of them myself, both in families of schizophrenics and of nonschizophrenics. However, if in articles and books on the family of the schizophrenic we report exclusively or almost exclusively parents as those that I have quoted, the reader will easily infer that these parents are the typical parents of the schizophrenic. I think we perpetrate an injustice on these unfortunate parents. But let us examine more accurately some of the reported examples. They are not internalization occurring through complicated intrapsychic mechanisms. Some of them are examples of obedience, like in the case of the girl who committed suicide as the mother had requested. Other examples portray pure and simple imitation, like the girl who blew her nose with a napkin as her father had done, or the patient, examined in the Veterans Administration, who thought it is all a matter of chemistry and physics. These are not examples of schizophrenic irrationality. What is transmitted by imitation, indoctrination, conditioning, etc., whether considered desirable or undesirable, is not schizophrenic per se. These types of transmission occur in schizophrenia, but *much more* so in neurotics and in the general population. In relation to the patient who was examined in the Veterans Administration, I must say with some regret that not only schizophrenics and their families, but also some of our colleagues believe that schizophrenia is all a matter of chemistry and physics.

Both the family and the culture in general may transmit irrationality through phenomena called psychological habituation, indoctrination, imitation, acceptance on faith, etc. But with the exception of rare cases of folie à deux, transmitted irrationality and transmitted peculiar behavior are not schizophrenic, delusional, or regressive per se. They may be unacceptable on a moral, medical, pedagogic or orthopsychiatric basis, but not as directly schizophrenogenic. The schizophrenic gives his own autistic, or primary process form to whatever has previously disturbed him with nonpsychotic psychodynamic mechanisms. It is the *transformation* and not the *imitation* that constitutes the schizophrenic essence of symptoms or habits. And that transformation is implemented through primary process cognition.

In the last 18 years I have compiled some private statistics, and although personal biases cannot be excluded and the overall figures are too small to be of definite value, I have reached different conclusions. In relation in particular to sexual assault, seduction, or rape, between parent and child, I have found these events much more frequently in the history of depressed, psychopathic, and hysterical patients than in the history of schizophrenics. I have also found that in 75% of cases of schizophrenia, the mother did not fit the image of the schizophrenogenic mother. I have found prevailing nonmaternal characteristics in only about 25% of the mothers of schizophrenics, and I do not know what percentage of mothers of nonschizophrenics have been nonmaternal. I have found the mother and father of the patient quite often disturbed, anxious, or hostile and detached, but only exceptionally to the degree described in some psychiatric literature. In the largest majority of cases I recognized in the mother a person who had been overcome by the difficulties of living. These difficulties had become enormous not only because of her unhappy marriage but, most of all, because of her neurosis and the neurotic defenses she built up in interacting with her children.

Another important point has been neglected in the literature. These studies of the patient's mother, starting from those of Fromm-Reichman and Rosen, were made at a time during which drastic changes in the sociological role of women were in a state of incubation. It was a period that immediately preceded the women's liberation era. It was the beginning of a time when a woman had to contend fully, tacitly, with her newly emerged need to assert equality. She could not longer accept submission, yet she strove to fulfill her traditional role. These social factors entered into the intimacy of family life and complicated the parental roles of both mothers and fathers.

I wish to add that this was the time when the "nuclear family," an invention of urban industrial society, came into its full existence. The nuclear family is destructive not only for the children, but also for the parents, and especially for the woman of the house. The home is often greatly deprived of educational, vocational, and religious values. It consists of a small number of people who live in little space, compete for room and for material and emotional possession, and are ridden by hostility and rivalry.

We can thus become aware of another dimension. Not only the negative characteristics of the mother are magnified and distorted by the future patient, but that seemingly original negative characteristics of the mother are in their turn a deformation, magnification, and rejection, conscious or unconscious, of roles that the mother believes society has inflicted on her. Now the family must be seen also as a pathogenetic culture carrier. What I am trying to say is that some of the traits of the mother which may seem schizophrenogenic may be a derivation of cultural influences, which also could then be called schizophrenogenic.

If what I have so far expressed is correct, we must investigate why many therapists, myself included, came to believe in the reality of the schizophrenogenic mother and less frequently of the schizophrenogenetic father. I believe that in the majority of cases we have fallen into a serious error (1). Schizophrenics who are at a relatively advanced stage of psychoanalytically oriented psychotherapy often describe their parents, especially the mother, in these negative terms, the terms used in a part of the psychiatric literature. We therapists have believed what our patients have told us. Inasmuch as approximately 25% of the mothers have proved to be that way, it was easier for us to make an unwarranted generalization that included all the mothers of the schizophrenics. We have made a mistake reminiscent of the one made by Freud when he came to believe that his neurotic patients had been assaulted sexually by their parents. Later Freud realized that what he had believed to be true was, in by far the majority of cases, only the product of the patient's fantasy.

It is true that some of the authors who have made these negative reports about the parents of the schizophrenic have studied only the family of the patients, and not the patients. But it is likely that they have been influenced by previous studies made exclusively on patients. From the late 40's to the early 60's the climate of opinion in psychodynamically oriented circles was to stress the "perverse sense of motherhood" of the mother of the schizophrenic. Many psychiatrists were influenced by this climate. I certainly was, and took for typical the characteristics that belonged to a minority. When I finally recognized my error and detected the half-truth which had become a myth, I hastened to express my reevaluation (1, 2, 3).

If my interpretation is correct, we must find out why or how many patients have transformed the image of the mother or of both parents into one that is much worse than the real one. In the second edition of my book *Interpretation of Schizophrenia* (3), I have reported in detail my own explanation of this phenomenon, which I am going to summarize here. In my opinion, what happens in the majority of cases is the following: The mother has definite negative characteristics—excessive anxiety, hostility, or detachment. The future patient becomes particularly sensitized to these characteristics. He becomes aware only of them because they are the parts of his mother that hurt, and to which he responds deeply. He ignores the others. His use of primary process cognition makes possible and perpetuates this partial awareness—this original part-object relationship. The patient who responds mainly to the negative parts of his mother will try to make a whole out of these negative parts, and the resulting whole will be a monstrous transformation of the mother.

In later stages this negative image may attract other negative aspects of the other members of the family or of the family constellation, so that her image will be intensified in her negative aspect. This vision of the mother is somewhat understood by the mother, who responds to the child with more anxiety and hostility. A vicious circle is thus organized that produces progressive and intense distortions and maladaptations. Two tendencies thus develop. One is to repress from consciousness the reality of the mother-patient relationship, but this is not a task that can be fully achieved. The other tendency is to displace or project to some parts of the external world this state of affairs. But this tendency also is not actualizable unless a psychosis occurs in childhood, and for the time being it remains only a potentiality. What I have said in relation to the mother could, in a smaller number of patients, be more appropriately said in reference to the father. In the majority of cases, the full extent of the negative image of the mother (and/or father) is repressed. It reappears in psychotherapy when the usual defenses are lost.

Why do schizophrenic patients who, in the course of treatment, become aware of the negative image of their parents, continue during a long stage of psychotherapy to see them in a negative way? Why in childhood did they focus on the negative aspects? We can give only hypothetical answers to this problem. The genetic vulnerability that I have referred to, or other particular contingencies occurring early in life, make the future patient experience more intensely a phenomenon that occurs to some degree in every living animal organism. Inasmuch as painful characteristics or negative parts of complex stimuli generally hinder adaptation, they are as a rule more dangerous from the point of view of survival. Evolution has thus probably favored a stronger response to them. We react more vigorously to pain than to pleasure, and to sorrow than to joy. Psychoanalytically oriented psychotherapy must help to put back the previous components in their proper proportion.

The therapist's knowledge that the patient transforms his experiences drastically is very important in psychotherapy. Until recently the therapist and the patient established a so-called therapeutic alliance based mainly on recrimination for what the parents had allegedly done in engendering the patient's misery. The therapist does not want to deny that the parents have played an important role, but he does not want also to magnify that role. That would be tantamount to altering the truth and hindering the progress of psychotherapy beyond the initial stages. The therapist must indicate also the contribution made by the patient to his own pathology. Unfortunately, quite a large number of authors who have studied the effect of the family on the schizophrenic patient have done so in a crude way, as if they were describing a rapport of simple linear causality. It would be like studying the intake of food, but not the functions of the digestive system and the metabolic processes of the body. Most of the time the autonomy, individuality, or even creativity of the patient have been neglected and have not been summoned to reestablish in the patient a willingness to reacquire mastery of his own life.

Between the conflict, which may have originated in the relationship with the parents, and the patient's unusual or bizarre overt behavior, many intermediary displacements and transformations—affective, cognitive, and conative—take place. Typical are cases like the following: the patient who believes he is Jesus Christ and wants to act and to be treated as if he were Jesus Christ; the patient who believes that people put poison in his food; the patient who receives messages from other planets; the patient who thinks he is powerful enough to control the world, to have the human race exterminated and replaced by a population of dogs. It is hard to believe that the parents transmitted literally these irrationalities to the patients. Had they done that, they too would have been schizophrenics.

Lest I be misunderstood, I want to clarify that the schizophrenic irrationality is certainly related to the influence of others, especially parents, but in a much more subtle way than described in some psychiatric literature. Let us take the example of the patient who believed that he could control the world, make the human race perish, and have it replaced by a population of dogs. This patient lost his mother at the age of three. He was brought up by two older sisters, who resented having to take care of him, and by a father who was a perfectionist. Because of his frustrations, the father was unhappy and hard to please. In order to stimulate the patient toward constant improvement, the father provoked great anxiety in his son, who came to believe he would never succeed in anything he tried. When the father remarried, the patient saw the stepmother as a caring person at first, but as hostile later and as a source of sexual stimulation from which he could not escape. The poor communication, the inability to properly ventilate the problems, and the resulting anxiety predisposed the patient to think that his father would always find fault with him and would never love him. And yet love from his father was what the patient wanted most; nothing could be more precious or more difficult to attain. Was there in the world a creature toward whom his father was lenient and not demanding, and on whom he bestowed love? Yes, the dog of the family, or rather the series of dogs that succeeded one another.

Only the adoption of primary process thinking made the patient change from a state of hopelessness and worthlessness into a position from which he felt he had the power to control or transform the world. The new world would be populated not by people, who withdraw from love, but by those who could obtain love—the dogs. When the acute phase of the episode was over and the patient was able to give a detailed personal history, he was easily helped to trace back the origin of his delusions. It was also explained to him that his original relations with his father, although unhappy and unhealthy, were already unrealistically transformed in childhood and made worse by poor communication, inability to see the totality of the picture, difficulty in finding compensations, and especially by the tendency to experience the rapport with his father in a restricted and unfavorable way. As we have already mentioned, the patient's relationship with his stepmother proved to be a difficult one and in its turn made the relationship with his father even more complicated because of a new and rather late oedipal situation.

Easy to understand is the case of a patient, a 22-year-old girl, who believed a famous actor was in love with her, although there was no evidence for it. She also believed that God had destined her for a great mission. There were hallucinatory episodes and ideas of reference. When she improved from the schizophrenic symptoms, she became depressed and attempted suicide. A few months after her suicidal attempt she improved from the depression and was discharged from the hospital. However, delusional ideas returned and she started psychotherapy on an ambulatory basis. She was seeing herself as an inconspicuous, infinitesimal entity in a family where her parents towered like giants. Since the time of her puberty she saw herself as unable to compete with her mother, a very successful woman who had found a very successful husband. Oedipal rivalry increased the distance between mother and daughter. Although it is true that mother and father were seemingly strong and secure people, they were not tyrannical or cruel. Because the patient felt so inferior to them, she magnified the strength of the parents as well as her own weaknesses and inferiority. This inferiority had eventually to be compensated by her grandiose delusions. Although it is true that the parents never understood fully the patient's sensitivity and her feeling of unworthiness and thus were unable to offer adequate comfort or compensation, it is also true that the patient transformed the parental images and transformed them into two insensitive rocks of Gibraltar, always there, purportedly to remind her of her inferiority. Her feeling of unworthiness was thus determined not just by the personalities of the parents, but by the way she reacted to those personalities and by what she added to them. Moreover, the patient's delusional ideas did not derive from any conception the parents had, but were her own private way of responding to the feeling of unworthiness. At a certain stage of treatment she thought her parents had provoked the state of unworthiness. Perhaps her interpretation had validity, but only inasmuch as she had added her own misconception to the attitude of her parents.

Thus the more we plunge into the psychodynamics, the more we discover how complicated are the interconnections of the various factors. Mother and father, or the family as a whole, are not just what they are. Their psychodynamic significance is the result of a combination of many interpersonal and intrapsychic processes which only now we begin to discover and disentangle.

REFERENCES

1. ARIETI, S.: The psychodynamics of schizophrenia: A reconsideration. *Amer. J. Psychother.*, 22:366-381, 1968.
2. ARIETI, S.: An overview of schizophrenia from a predominantly psychological approach. *Amer. J. Psychiatry*, 131:241-249, 1974.
3. ARIETI, S.: *Interpretation of Schizophrenia*, second ed. (completely revised and expanded), Basic Books, New York, 1974.
4. CAPONIGRI, A. R.: *Time and Idea. The Theory of History in Giambattista Vico.* Regnery, Chicago, 1953.
5. GOLDMANN, L.: *La Création Culturelle dans La Société Moderne.* Denoel-Gonthier, Paris, 1971.
6. JACKSON, D. D.: The transactional viewpoint. *Int. J. Psychiatry*, 4:543-544, 1967.
7. LIDZ, T.: The influence of family studies in the treatment of schizophrenia. *Psychiatry*, 32:237-251, 1969.
8. ROSEN, J. N.: *The Concept of Early Maternal Environment in Direct Psychoanalysis.* The Doylestown Foundation, Doylestown, Pa., 1963.

7

Recent Conceptions and Misconceptions of Schizophrenia

This paper, published in 1960, was read before the Association for the Advancement of Psychotherapy in 1958. That was a time when Thomas Szasz started to attack the concept of schizophrenia, when Bateson's double-bind theory was embraced enthusiastically and uncritically as an easy solution to the complex etiology of schizophrenia, and when existentialistic tenets coming from Europe were replacing psychodynamic concepts in some milieus.

Today the double-bind theory is moribund, Szasz continues to utter his lonely position, and the existentialist approach has received a modest place in the study of the psyche.

LIKE THE PENDULUM which swings back and forth, or the tides of the sea which advance and recede, so do our conceptions and misconceptions of schizophrenia. The theories in which we believed yesterday are discarded today, to be reaccepted tomorrow. This instability could be viewed simply as an expression of our ignorance or of the still prescientific level of psychiatry today. Many undoubtedly think that when the real theory of schizophrenia will be found, to such theory we shall all adhere.

I too share this expectation, to a certain extent, but not entirely. There is no doubt that our knowledge of schizophrenia is far from complete, and that advancements and discoveries are to be anticipated. But they will not necessarily bring stability, partly because of the particular place occupied by psychiatry as a science and partly because of the nature of schizophrenia. A complete theory of schizophrenia implies a complete theory of human nature—a theory that comprehends not only our biologic self, but that part of the self that is also subject to nonbiologic laws. And as long as that part of the self is subject to the pendulous course of our philosophic, social, and historic conceptions, the theory of schizophrenia will also undergo such pendulous course. These remarks do not intend to deny the less conspicuous but more enduring spiral course of progress which hides under these periodic oscillations.

Perhaps my comments may sound unduly critical and my attitude may appear iconoclastic. Such, however, is not my intention. Although fundamentally I criticize the theories which I shall review, I must also emphasize that I recognize that many of us have learned a great deal from them. I think all of these theories are valuable. It is because they tower so high that we can hit them so easily.

I intend to discuss: *first,* theories concerning the general concept and delimitation of schizophrenia; *second,* specific psychologic theories, such as Bateson's double-bind theory and Szasz's theory of deficiency of objects. Finally, in the third and main part of the paper, I shall discuss the existentialist approach to schizophrenia.

I shall not discuss the organic theories of this mental disorders, primarily because I do not subscribe to them. I feel that organic theories arise from misplacement of emphasis—from ascribing the cause to the effect. It is true that biochemical alterations exist in many cases of schizophrenia, but they may be considered psychosomatic in nature, the expressions of a disequilibrium which, although originally mediated principally by the neopallium, later involves functionally archipallic, diencephalic, and hypothalamic centers. I shall limit myself thus to the examination of psychologic theories.

THE CONCEPT OF SCHIZOPHRENIA

As I said before, several authors recently have tried to demolish the Kraepelinian concept of dementia praecox-schizophrenia. One of the most vigorous attempts is that of Thomas Szasz (1). Szasz calls the word "schizophrenia" a *panchreston*—a term coined by Hardin to denote dangerous words which are purported to explain everything, but which actually obscure matters. Szasz writes:

> . . . categories such as "schizophrenia" may be doubly harmful: first, such categories are unsatisfactory as readily validatable concepts for purposes of classification, and secondly, they give rise to the misleading impression that there "exists" a more-or-less homogeneous group of phenomena which are designated by the word in question. If this line of thought is correct—as I believe it is—[Szasz adds] it leads to the realization that the "problem of schizophrenia," which many consider to be the core-problem of psychiatry today, may be

truly akin to the "problem of the ether." To put it simply: there is no such problem.

Szasz adds that

> A better comprehension of the "real facts" . . . will probably lead to the gradual disappearance of this word, whose function, like that of all panchrestons, is to fill a scientific void.

Such an attack against the concept of schizophrenia was not prepared on the spur of the moment but has ramifying historic roots. It may even be remotely connected with Adolph Meyer's studies which taught that the schizophrenic syndrome is only one chapter of a long, longitudinal series of events and that the schizophrenic symptoms are only modifications of intensifications of the faulty habits in living which the patient disclosed prior to the psychosis.

Psychoanalytic and psychodynamic studies went much further than the psychobiologic, so that it became easy to see that the psychopathology of the schizophrenic did not start with the onset of the manifest symptomatology, but was subsequent to such factors as the unhappy marriage of the parents, the particular constitution of the family, the personality of the mother and father, a childhood characterized by exposures to early and excessive manifestations of anxiety and hostility, and so on. Additional studies revealed that, although a particular cluster of these factors is to be found much more frequently among schizophrenics than other people, actually, no psychodynamic mechanisms exist which are found exclusively in schizophrenia.

Further complication came, perhaps as an aftermath of Hoch and Polatin's concept of pseudoneurotic schizophrenia—that is, of a schizophrenic syndrome without typical schizophrenic symptoms. If we then go into the field of child psychiatry, the situation is even more confusing than in adult psychiatry. Today in many psychiatric centers every seriously disturbed child is considered *ipso facto* a schizophrenic, because of the dynamics and in relative disregard of the symptomatology of the case.

When we emphasize the similarity of psychodynamics in many psychiatric syndromes, we then tend either to expand the concept of schizophrenia to include all these conditions or to abolish it completely and to reach the conclusion that Szasz is right in calling schizophrenia a panchreston.

Now, it seems to me that we make two errors in following this procedure. The first one consists in the assumption that it is in the psychodynamic mechanisms that we must find the specificity of schizophrenia.

As long as we make that assumption we are on the wrong track. I do not want to be misunderstood on this point. The psychodynamic factors, including parental attitudes, childhood situations, and development of particular personality traits, are extremely important. Nevertheless, although it is true that without them there would be no schizophrenia, they do not in themselves constitute schizophrenia; they may, or may not, lead to the disorder.

We have schizophrenia only when the pre-existing dynamic factors lead to that particular form of progressive teleologic regression which generally, but not always, assumes the kraepelinian aspect. At times this type of regression is minimal and detected with great difficulty even by the expert; at other times it shows very easily in the escape from the abstract, the logical, the interpersonal and the plunging into the concrete, the paleologic, and the autistic. It seems to me then that we should not enlarge the use of the word schizophrenia, but rather restrict it to those cases where we have at least minimal signs of regressive mechanisms. If we look at the problem in this way, we shall find that, although in the schizophrenic syndrome there is much which is indefinite, variable, inconstant, accessory, and common to other conditions, there is nevertheless a particular schizophrenic core. The fact that the nature of this core has not been fully determined points to the incompleteness of our present concept of schizophrenia, but does not prove its fallacy.

The second mistake, which is becoming more and more fashionable, was already implied in what I said. Many people emphasize the fact that there is only a quantitative difference between the schizophrenic, the neurotic, and the normal. This statement is true in a literal sense; as I shall explain shortly. It also has a great deal of pragmatic therapeutic value. In the spirit of this pragmatic value Frieda Fromm-Reichmann often repeated this statement. Her genuine identification with the patient, as well as her feelings of moral equality with and respect for every member of the human community, made her emphasize with Sullivan the importance of what is common to the physician and the patient over what is dissimilar.

Nevertheless, I think this statement is only "literally" true. All differences in nature are basically quantitative differences, but it is the difference in quantity that produces the qualitative difference. A normal tired person may have hypnagogic hallucinations before he goes to sleep, a suspicious spouse may have a transient fit of paranoid jealousy, an anxious employee may think that his boss is talking about him behind his back, but as long as these abnormal mechanisms are quantitatively so minimal as to be checked and recognized, the person is not schizophrenic. It is only when the quantity of the symptoms is such that they acquire the upper hand, it is only when the way of living of the patient expresses itself not in contrast to, but in accordance with, the symptoms that the person will be schizophrenic. To use a metaphor, there is only a quantitative difference between a 39% and a 41% water solution of a substance, but if the dissolved substance precipitates when the concentration is 40%, the two solutions will no longer be only quantitatively different. They will become qualitatively different also, because one has a precipitation and the other has not. Once having reached the precipitating point, we have not only two solutions, but also a solution of continuity. There is only a minimal quantitative difference between the results obtained by the party that on election day gets 49% of the votes and those of the party that gets 51% of the votes, but the party that gets 51% wins and the other loses.

At different quantitative levels we have different confluence, integration, and reorganization of parts, so that the total picture acquires a true qualitatively different aspect and is ruled by different mechanisms. This applies not only to psychiatric syndromes but to anything in nature, from waves of light and chemical elements to new emerging traits in evolution. To emphasize that in schizophrenia there is only a quantitative difference has, however, as I said before, a pragmatic value. For instance, at times, in states of acute panic, one has only to reduce the anxiety of the patient slightly in order to see all the symptoms rapidly dissolve and the normal processes reacquire the upper hand.

THE DOUBLE-BIND THEORY

I shall start now to analyze specific theories of schizophrenia and I shall begin with Bateson's theory of the double bind. I assume that some of you have not yet come across an account of this theory and therefore I take the liberty of summarizing it.

Bateson (2, 3), an anthropologist who has worked a great deal in the field of human communication, thinks that the child who is later to become schizophrenic has been exposed repeatedly to double binds, that is, to a particular type of message which involves a double bind. For instance, the mother tells the child, "Pull up your socks." At the same time, her gesture implies, "Don't be so obedient." In this situation the child received the message, "Pull up your socks," but, if he does so, he is too obedient. The other message says, "Don't be so obedient," but if he does not obey he will incur mother's disapproval. In other words, he is damned if he does it, and he is damned if he doesn't. To use Bateson's own words, "If he solves a problem of human relationship at the level at which it is apparently offered, he will find himself in the wrong at some other level."

Another example taken from Powdermaker (4) and used by Bateson is the following: An aunt comes to visit and the little niece sees her. This aunt could not tolerate children, but mother has told the child, "Aunty loves you." The child is thus exposed to a double bind. Should she be bound by the message coming from mother, which says, "Aunt is a loving creature," or by the message coming directly from the aunt which seems to declare in an obvious manner, "I detest children"?

These are two different external binds, or at least an internal and an external one. The child has an external message which tells her she should respond with kindness to aunt and an inner message which tells her that she should respond with anger to the aunt.

A third and last example. A rejecting mother is awakened by the crying of the baby. She has an impulse to kill the child, but she controls herself and shows some kind of artificial kindness. The child perceives both messages and is confused.

Now, Bateson states that double-bind situations provoke helplessness, fear, exasperation and anxiety in the individual. According to him, the schizophrenic was exposed to a great many double-bind situations. The psychosis may be viewed as a way of dealing with double-bind situations. At times the psychotic masters the situation by shifting to the metaphoric field; more often he himself becomes an expert in setting double-bind situations. Bateson admits that the double-bind situation may be seen as ambivalence, in Bleuler's sense, but as a special ambivalence inasmuch as it is not merely indecision between possible alternatives but a circular process, or a feed-back mechanism. For instance, in the above given example the resolution of being kind to the aunt brings about in the child an automatic negative impulse which may also lead to the expression of anger. But the expression of anger also brings about its negative impulse, which will compel the child to be kind. And so, back and forth.

Now, let us examine the three postulates of Bateson: 1) that schizophrenia may be the result of excessive double-bind situations in childhood; 2) that the psychosis is a way of dealing with the environmental double-bind situations; 3) that the schizophrenic himself learns to use a large number of double-bind situations.

I think all of us would agree that our schizophrenic patients have been repeatedly exposed to this double-bind situation. But I think we would also agree that many neurotics were exposed, and many normal people, and we, too. In my own experience, I consider myself to have been almost always involved in a double bind. As a matter of fact, in this very lecture I am in a double-bind situation with every author I am discussing, including Bateson. I think that Bateson must be congratulated for having emphasized the frequency and the importance of this characteristic life situation, but this is a situation characteristic of man, not of schizophrenia.

If we were called upon to react not to double binds but only to single messages, in a sort of reflex or conditioned reflex manner, life undoubtedly would be much simpler and would offer much less anxiety, but it would not deserve to be called human; it would be a unidimensional life.

Double-bind situations represent not necessarily pathology but reflect the complexity of human existence. Culture itself exposes the individual to many double-bind situations, or, if we want to use the traditional terminology, to conflictual situations. For instance, it teaches us to be honest, sincere, and truthful at the same time that we have to respect the dignity of the individual, including that of an undesired relative who comes to visit us. It is not always easy to do so. The human being, however, is generally equipped to face highly complicated processes. He has been amply provided by nature with alternative neuronal patterns for this purpose. It is a long time since we stopped to believe that every psychologic function could be explained in accordance with the simple formula Stimulus-Response.

It is true that many pathologic situations involve double binds but it is also true that they may involve other highly complicated mental mechanisms. To mention another possibility: the ability to anticipate the future, which has the normal purpose of protecting us from danger, may actually become the source of anxiety, despair, and suicide. These high functions are mediated predominantly in the prefrontal and to some extent in the temporal cortex.

The healthy child learns to use these processes and apply them to those difficult situations which are part of his human life, including those similar to the one set up by the visiting aunt. But for the child who is to become schizophrenic, the double bind is not only a double bind; it is also one of the many carriers of hostility and anxiety from the general environmental situation. Being exposed to an atmosphere of excessive anxiety or hostility and not an atmosphere of basic trust, he is ill equipped to handle many situations, including double-bind situations. It is this general atmosphere to which he is exposed that is the primal source of his difficulties. Undoubtedly his consequent inability to handle these complicated situations increases his anxiety and hastens the breakdown. In other words it is not the double-bind mechanism per se which is pathogenetic but the use of it in a pathogenetic environment.

Many non-schizophrenogenetic stress situations involve a double bind. For instance, the situation of divided loyalty, like that of the soldier during the Civil War who had to fight in the Confederate Army and yet believed in the ideals of the Union Army. But we find the double-bind situation in many constructive areas. Without going too deeply into the fields of esthetics, we may say that there is no artistic production in the literary or the fine arts which does not resort to double or to multiple binds. At the first example that comes to my mind is Dante, the poet who gives life to the dead, who transports an earthy quality to the underworld and manifests the greatest pity and admiration for people whom he condemns to eternal damnation. And what about art itself? Is not art fiction from which we expect truth? And is not mathematics, according to some thinkers, in the same way a very artificial device which gives the greatest exactitude? And what about Hegel's thesis and antithesis?

The second assertion of Bateson is that the psychosis equips the patient to handle double-bind situations by escaping into metaphoric language. But the truth is that the language of the patient is not metaphoric for the patient himself. For instance, if a patient makes the statement that he smells a bad odor emanating from his body, his language is metaphoric or symbolic for us, because we interpret, and rightly so, that the patient feels that he is a rotten person, that he stinks in a metaphoric sense. The fact, however, is that the patient has an olfactory hallucination and he really smells a bad odor. What appears to us as a metaphoric expression is only a regressive phenomenon based on a concretization of perceptualization of an anxiety-laden concept about himself. By regressing to concrete, perceptual methods, the patient actually blots out highly symbolic multiple binds. On the other hand, he himself seems to be proficient in creating double-bind situations. This is true, not because he has learned this technique in childhood, as Bateson intimates, but because the schizophrenic uses and condenses several levels of mental integration at the same time, so that his statements have several concomitant meanings, just as the dreams of every person do.

THE THEORY OF DEFICIENCY OF INTERNAL OBJECTS

I am now going to discuss Thomas Szasz's view of schizophrenia (5). Whereas I could not accept the above-mentioned views of Szasz on the concept of schizophrenia, my response to his pathogenetic theory is a different one. Szasz is one of the most talented theoreticians of the new generation in the field of psychiatry and his contributions deserve deep study and high respect. Szasz's theory about schizophrenia is simply that the disorder is to a large extent caused by deficiency of internal objects. This theory is an original derivation of concepts already advanced in psychoanalysis, namely those of Melanie Klein and Fairbairn.

It is well known that Melanie Klein gives great importance to the so-called internal objects, that is, to psychologic experiences which are introjected into ourselves, but which originate from others.

Fairbairn and Szasz do not believe, as Freud does, that only the super-ego is composed of introjected objects; they feel that the ego, too, is so composed. It seems to me that this is an advance over the original Freudian theory. Although these three authors use a different terminology, they are actually not far away from the interpersonal school of psychiatry. Szasz, following Fairbairn, speaks of object-relationships in the process of growing up, but to a great extent object-relationships actually correspond to interpersonal relationships.

Szasz believes that schizophrenia is largely the result of a deficiency in internal objects, or deficiency of incorporated objects. Having incorporated so few objects, the patient has no models to use in his life. He is awkward and inadequate; no wonder that, when he leaves home and goes to college for the first time, he may develop a schizophrenic break.

First of all, let us ask ourselves: what are these internal objects? They are obviously not external objects which have been incorporated in their physical entities, but symbolic representations of them. What the child introjects from others are only social symbols and organizations of these symbols into higher constructs. The self is actually made up to a great extent of these symbols received from others. Thus, Szasz's hypothesis would mean that the preschizophrenic has a deficiency of social symbols and of organizations of these symbols and that it is this deficiency which leads to the psychosis.

In my opinion, this concept approximates the truth perhaps only in the simple type of schizophrenia and in child schizophrenia. But I consider it impossible to corroborate this assertion in the majority of cases. The preschizophrenic is not deficient in symbols; obviously, he is not deficient in private, individualistic symbols or paleosymbols, equivalent to the Freudian symbols. He is also not deficient in social symbols and in the organization of these symbols. He has acquired the language of the others, the symbols of the others, and has been able to indulge in the most complicated uses of abstract thinking prior to the psychosis. The important difference from the normal is that his organizations of symbols into higher constructs are not stable, are ready to be fragmented and rejected; they have never been fully accepted or assimilated, because they carried within themselves the anxiety of the early interpersonal relations. Thus in hallucinations and delusions, for instance, these internal objects or symbols are returned or projected to the external world after undergoing autistic modifications. Finally, when very advanced regression occurs, they are not even projected; then, there is a real deficiency of them. Summarizing, it is difficult to accept Szasz's theory that in the majority of patients who will develop schizophrenia there is a poverty of internal objects, because the history of the prepsychotic denies such poverty. What seems to exist instead is a vulnerability or fragility of the organizations of social symbols and internal objects, which is due to the emotional conditions under which early assimilations and organizations of these symbols took place.

THE EXISTENTIAL APPROACH TO SCHIZOPHRENIA

I come now to the evaluation of the contributions of the existentialist school of psychiatry to the understanding of schizophrenia, and I shall consider the works of the major representative of this school: Binswanger. As you know, existentialist psychiatry, following Heidegger's philosophy, is particularly concerned with the patient's way of being in the world, with the given; that is, with what is given here and now, in immediate experience, in a certain way as Zen Buddhism does. Thus, in writing about a patient to whom he gave the name Suzanne Urban, Binswanger (6) makes it clear that he is not going to discuss the constitution of the patient or the organic etiologic possibilities, or even the prepsychotic personality or the previous life experiences; no dynamic, no characterologic studies at all. His purpose is to analyze the patient's lived experience, what was immediately given to her in the structure of her existence, of her being in the world. There is no doubt that these existentialist writings exert a strong fascination, not only for the beauty of their style but also for the object of their study. The emphasis on the given, immediately increases the importance of the senses, of the sensory perceptions, as we find in fine art and music, and therefore confers to the study an esthetic quality and search, as we shall see in more detail in a few minutes.

Even the lack of consideration for what is psychodynamic may appear refreshing to some of us in America, who have been trained to consider important and relevant in psychiatry only what is dynamic. Dynamics means movement and therefore genesis, or ontogenetic development, movement of forces. The existentialist emphasizes what is not dynamic, what does not need to move, move toward or away, because it is already all there, to be experienced immediately in its entirety and depth, as you would experience a poem or a beautiful lake hidden in the mountains, without thinking of its geologic origin or of the botany of the surrounding flora. All this is beautiful and fascinating, but let us see its practical application in the treatment of a patient. I shall take as an example the already mentioned Binswanger's study of Suzanne Urban, which I am going to summarize.

Suzanne was admitted to the hospital at the age of 48. She was the third of four children in a Jewish family. A sister of the patient had committed suicide at the age of 29 by cutting her throat with a razor during an attack of melancholia with ideas of guilt and poverty. Another sister had an attack of depression during menopause. The father of the patient was a lawyer. Very little additional information is given about the parents.

Suzanne was a precocious child, for whom everyone had great expectations, and was rather stubborn, egotistical, and authoritarian. According to Binswanger, the parents were very affectionate and loving and professed a great deal of affection for the patient. In her turn, the patient idolized her parents, trying to satisfy all their wishes and desires. The onset of puberty caused Suzanne feelings of embarrassment. She attended high school and college. When she was 18 or 19 she started to read romantic novels. During these readings she would masturbate—not in the usual way but by rubbing one thigh against the other. Later she explained that this erotic pleasure was superior to that experienced during her married life from regular intercourse.

The family is described as what we would call ingrown. A real "cult" of the family, a strong feeling of loyalty and solidarity reigned between the members. Because of this feeling and of the fact that at 21 she was told that she was getting old, Binswanger thinks Suzanne decided to marry her cousin. Except for the suicide of the sister, the life of the patient is described as devoid of unpleasant experiences. The husband kept from her all worries connected with his business and loved her with an exalted sense of love. He never refused anything she wanted. In the beginning of their marriage she did not want to have children, but later she was sorry she did not have any. Fourteen months before she was admitted to the hospital, the husband noticed that he had trouble with his urination, probably a cystitis. Suzanne accompanied her husband to a physician, who told her that he had a very malignant type of cancer of the bladder and that the result of even an immediate operation would be doubtful. She became extremely upset and depressed, and decided to accompany her husband to a specialist in Paris. At first she wanted to know every detail about the operation, the results of the cystoscopy, of the urine examination, but then she became more and more depressed. She could not sleep; she refused to talk about anything except her husband's illness. She anticipated a long agony for him. She said she would prefer to kill him and then to kill herself. She prayed to God that He would make both of them die in an accident. Later she started to refuse food and to think that people around her were bad; that the servants were walking noiselessly in order to spy on her. She was then admitted into a private sanitarium where she stayed four weeks. There she felt she was constantly watched, persecuted, radiographed; that her property had been confiscated; that electric wires had been hidden around her to register all her steps and words. She had also been contaminated with syphilis, had cancer and every other disease conceivable. Voices were telling her that everything she would say was wrong. Small cameras had been hidden in the bathroom to photograph her when she was nude in the bathtub.

After four weeks she was discharged in care of her family, but her symptoms became more pronounced. Now she was not so worried about her husband's illness. Now she believed that the police persecuted her whole family. Some relatives have already been executed, others were being tortured. She had no insight at all into her illness and claimed she was perfectly well.

She was finally admitted to the sanitarium of Bellevue in Kreuzlingen, Switzerland. Nine months after her admission she was persuaded by her doctor to write, in a form of diary, an account of the beginning and development of her illness.

Binswanger read this diary and his existentialist analysis consists largely of the study of this diary. This is a procedure that Binswanger has adopted before; for instance, in the case of Ellen West (7). One gets the impression that he relies much more on these writings of the patient than on the therapeutic sessions.

In this diary Susanne described in a detailed and vivid way her subjective experiences from the time she went with her husband to consult the first doctor for what was thought to be a cystitis, to her first manifestations and distortions which culminated later in a paranoid framework.

In the second part of the book Binswanger makes an analysis of the illness so far described. He asks himself the usual existentialist question: What is the world of the patient? He feels that it is a world that shows the frightening ruin of a whole family, something similar to what occurs in ancient myths and in tragedies of every era. "It is a world in which a disquieting demoniac, powerful force holds all the strings, a world where nothing is due to chance but where everything is ruled by the laws of this demoniac force." This force wills evil inexorably. It has the aspect of an ancient curse, or avenger, which fights against a strong feeling of kinship and family cult, and reciprocal parent-child and husband-wife idolatry.

The so-called original scene, the consultation with the doctor who made the diagnosis of cancer, receives as much consideration by Binswanger as the so-called primal scene received in early orthodox Freudian literature. It is like the first act of a play in what he calls a "theater of terror." Binswanger seems to see the development of the psychosis as the progression of a well written play which has a consistent unity, and in which what happens in the second and final acts is only a natural, ineluctable development of what happened in the first act. The original scene of the first act consists of the complaints of the husband during the original cystoscopy, the anxiety of Suzanne waiting for the diagnosis, finally the face of the doctor when he makes the fatidic announcement, the expressions of despair of the surrounding persons, then the frightening pantomime of the doctor who holds her hand tightly to make her understand that she should not by her expression reveal the situation to the husband.

It is a scene of terror. According to Binswanger, this feeling of terror expands to the whole world. In what may be viewed as the second act, it becomes the atmosphere of the world of the patient, her being in the world. It is a global affective tonality. Finally, in what may be seen as the third act, this theme of terror is transformed into a delusional world. The police, the physicians, the neighbors, the existing diseases, everything around her becomes part of this world of terror. The patient who was at first prisoner of her own terror, now becomes prisoner in a world of terror.

Binswanger undoubtedly does a painstaking job in showing how the whole psychosis is consistent with this world design in which terror is the theme, the all-embracing feeling. He carefully describes all the transitions to demonstrate the consistency of the overall design and gives a vivid account of the uniqueness of the subjective experiences of the patient.

At this point we would like to know what happened to the patient as a result of the treatment, but this is not reported. Apparently the whole book is devoted to an existentialist analysis of the symptomatology of the patient. But there are many other things which are left out, or which we would like to know or to understand better. Here are some of them: Although we empathize with the feelings of the patient when she learned the diagnosis of the husband's illness, we cannot understand why such news, painful as it was, should lead to a psychosis. In this long report we find nothing about the background which made the psychosis possible after the so-called original scene. Except for the repeated allusion to this family cult, we cannot find any dynamic interpretation. All the members of the family loved each other with intense, devout love. The facts that the marriage was not a love marriage but determined only by the family cult and that Susanne was sexually frigid receive no consideration. No connection is made between the way the patient felt consciously or unconsciously toward her husband, and the way she felt after she heard about his fatal illness. We are led to accept the statements of the patient and the other members of the family at their face value. I confess that I asked myself the question, "Can Binswanger really be so naive, or am I naive in attributing to Binswanger such a naiveté?"

Reading other existentialist books and discussing this matter with some friends who are students of existentialism, I found out that I myself have a sort of naiveté. My naiveté consists mostly in asking the question, "Why?" Why did the patient become psychotic? Why did she develop this paranoid system? The existentialist psychiatrist does not ask "Why?" He only asks "How?" "How did the patient become psychotic?"

Of course, there is nothing wrong in asking "How?" Perhaps we must give credit to the existentialists for emphasizing this point and recognize that we underestimated the importance of the how, but on the other hand we should not, as they do, stop at the how.

Following the lead of Kierkegaard, they do not try to prove anything, but only to express an attitude, a "How?" Following Kierkegaard, they also believe that, especially in the state of extreme emotional crisis one sees the significance of one's life. In other words, they feel that anxiety increases one's awareness, and to this increased awareness they devote so much study. Now, it is very true that in moments of crises and anxiety one's awareness increases, but only in certain respects. It is also true that anxiety decreases, or restricts, or distorts, our awareness of things, as psychoanalysis teaches. Our awareness, as a matter of fact, may decrease to such a point that we have huge repressions. Although the existentialists may be correct in reminding us of the manifest, conscious anguish, we should by no means neglect the rest—to use Freud's beautiful metaphor, the rest of the iceberg which is under water. How can we study the human psyche without trying to reach the not-given from what is given, without inferring and explaining, without expanding our awareness by understanding the symbols?

For instance, important as it is to grasp the anguish of Suzanne Urban in her world of terror, which we know is very real to her, is it not even more important to understand another terror of which we know nothing, but which perhaps always was in a state of potentiality in her? Is not the illness really the expression of another terror which consists of obscure threats and derives from obscure origins? And is not the illness perhaps a peculiar way to deny or to solve this other obscure inner terror (8)?

In reading Binswanger's works and those of other existentialists, I am reminded of works on esthetics, especially on poetry or on the theater. Now I myself like poetry and the theater very much, and furthermore I feel that we psychotherapists have unduly neglected the field of esthetics. But I also feel that esthetics alone is not enough. The person who studies a poem or a work of art tries to understand the work of art as intensely as he can, but he does not want to change it. One has the same feeling in reading these existentialist reports—the feeling that no attempt is made to change the patient. On the contrary, what occurs in the last stage of the illness is seen as the inevitable occurrence, like the last stanza of a poem, the last motive of a song, or the final act of a play. Everything is seen as fitting the world design, a superior symmetry. It is true that the existentialist tries to understand the uniqueness of the subjective experience of the patient, the so-called *Erlebnis*, but this uniqueness, like the uniqueness of the artistic expression, is not changed and cannot be changed without asking ourselves why; why is that in this way? If we do not ask why, but remain at this esthetic contemplation when we deal with psychiatric patients, we often really misplace our esthetic sense. With due regard to some exceptions, the symptom of the patient is at best pseudo-esthetic. It is true that it may be unique, but it is never univocal. It may reflect the particular anguish of the patient, but lacks the cosmic resonance of the real work of art, and may be compared to a mediocre work of art which reflects not a message but only the subjective expression of the neurosis of the artist.

I say this not to disparage the patient, but in order to help him, because, although I respect his need for uniqueness, I must help him to liberate himself from his progressive and devastating desocialization. In his need for uniqueness the artist may need to be alone, and is capable of being alone, but the patient apparently could not be so alone and unique without becoming psychotic.

Reading reports like the one I have summarized, one gets the feeling that the patient remains alone, in spite of the attempt made to understand the uniqueness of his experiences. We do not find in this report the caring endeavor of Frieda Fromm-Reichmann, who tries to help the patient to see why the therapist and he experience things in different ways. We do not recognize the attempts of Mme. Sechehaye to adapt herself to the psychotic world in order to trace back the deceitful meanders of the patient's symbolism; we do not detect Sullivan's attitude of the participant observer. As a matter of fact, we have the feeling that the existentialist psychiatrist does not participate at all. Like a spectator in the theater, he is not apathetic; he feels, admires, and suffers, but does not participate. He remains in the audience.

Believing that he must let himself be guided by the nature of things themselves, by the natural process of metamorphosis, the existentialist psychiatrist does not go on the stage to dismantle the paranoid scenery. If, instead, he becomes too enchanted by the scenery, in which he sees not only destruction but also the harmony of a world design, he may be at a loss in retrieving the little me in the patient, lost in all these flourishing stage settings. He may not be able to help the sufferer to reacquire his inner harmony, the real harmony.

Perhaps, one could say, with this attitude the existentialist tries to recapture a sense of tragedy, that tragic sense which many modern men have lost, with consequent trivialization and flattening of life. I concede to the existentialist that the tragic aspect is very important in the human condition, but I have a specification to make: There are two kinds of tragedies. One type follows the Greek paradigm, where we men are the ineluctable victims of destiny, predestined to suffer and die. And there is nothing we can do. Ananke, necessity of fate, is the cruel puppeteer which pulls the strings of us puppets. This is the tragedy Binswanger sees in Suzanne Urban.

But there is a second type of tragedy, the tragedy of the Judeo-Christian tradition: the tragedy of Joseph, sold into slavery by his own brothers, the tragedy of Job, the tragedy of Christ, where the tragedy leads to the triumph of man, the tragedy where the heroes are not *les petites marionettes*, but where they themselves pull the strings which at times may move the world.

As therapists we must find inspiration for our work in this second type of tragedy. If tragic failure is seen not as a possibility but as the ineluctable aspect of man, how can we not fail in our therapeutic endeavor?

We must also add that although Binswanger describes how the atmospheric quality of terror becomes transformed into the delusional world, he does not explain how this is made possible by the adoption of certain formal mechanisms (9), like the concretization and perceptualization of the experiences, and adoption of a special type of thinking as described by Kurt Goldstein (10), Vygotsky (11) and von Domarus (12). The basic forms of existence that he borrows from Heidegger cannot properly fit the schizophrenic transformation.

An additional point needs to be mentioned also. The cases reported by Binswanger are those of well organized, not regressed, paranoid patients. In America, some of them would be classified not as schizophrenics, but as paranoid states or similar diagnoses, because of their well organized systematization of their delusions. Now it is relatively easy to see the world design in these paranoid systems. Actually the world design is the paranoid work itself. Had Binswanger selected more disintegrated or more regressed patients, he would not have been able to differentiate a world design, unless by the world design he were to mean the picture of progressive disintegration itself.

REFERENCES

1. SZASZ, T.: The problem of psychiatric nosology. A contribution to a situational analysis of psychiatric operations. *Amer. J. Psychiat.*, 114:405, 1957.
2. BATESON, G., JACKSON, D. D., HALEY, J., and WEAKLAND, J.: Toward a theory of schizophrenia. *Behavioral Sci.*, 1:251, 1956.
3. BATESON, G.: Schizophrenic distortions of communication. In *Psychotherapy of Schizophrenic Patients*. Edited by C. A. Whitaker. Boston: Little, Brown, 1958.
4. POWDERMAKER, F.: Concepts found useful in treatment of schizoid and ambulatory schizophrenic patients. *Psychiatry*, 15:61, 1952.
5. SZASZ, T.: A contribution to the psychology of schizophrenia. *Arch. Neurol. Psychiat.*, 77:420, 1957.
6. BINSWANGER, L.: *Le Cas Suzanne Urban.* Paris: Desclee de Brouwer, 1957.
7. BINSWANGER, L.: The case of Ellen West. In *Existence.* Edited by R. May, E. Engel, and H. F. Ellenberger. New York: Basic Books, 1958.
8. ARIETI, S.: Schizophrenic thought. *Amer. J. Psychother.*, 13:537, 1959.
9. ARIETI, S.: *Interpretation of Schizophrenia.* New York: Brunner, 1955.
10. GOLDSTEIN, K.: The significance of psychological research in schizophrenia. *J. Nerv. & Ment. Dis.*, 97:261, 1943.
11. VYGOTSKY, L. S.: Thought in schizophrenia. *Arch. Neurol. Psychiat.*, 31:1030, 1934.
12. VON DOMARUS, E.: The specific laws of logic in schizophrenia. In *Language and Thought in Schizophrenia; Collected Papers.* Edited by J. S. Kasanin. University of California Press, 1944.

8

Volition and Value: A Study Based on Catatonic Schizophrenia

Catatonic schizophrenia is studied not only in its psychodyna-mics and special symptomatology, but as a phenomenon which may help us to clarify the larger concepts of will and value. The ideas expressed in this paper started a trend of thought which will lead me, approximately 10 years later, to write the book The Will To Be Human.

I HOPE I shall be permitted to begin presentation with a personal memory, which goes back to more than twenty years ago, when I first arrived in this country.

Among the many things that came to my attention was the fact that undoubtedly Dante's *Divine Comedy* was the best known work of Italian literature in America. For the second place, however, two books were actively competing: one was *Decameron* by Boccaccio; the other *Pinocchio*, a little book for children, written by an otherwise obscure author named Collodi.

That *Decameron* should enjoy such popularity in America I was not surprised, being not completely unaware of the universal appeal of its subject matter. But that Pinocchio should be so well known, that was amazing!

What was so fascinating about the story of this wooden puppet? Pinocchio was a puppet, but unlike his sibling puppets, did not need a puppeteer to move his strings. He was capable of motions on his own, of willed acts. But what was the result? From the very first moment that his father, carpenter Geppetto, finishes making him, he gets into trouble. As soon as Geppetto gives the last touch to his legs, the legs start to move

109

and kick Geppetto. And from that moment on it is one naughty thing after another. Pinocchio is a real psychopath.

In a leap of artistic imagination Collodi overlooked the great evolutionary process of billions of years, which first gives autonomous movement to organic matter, then coordinated motion, finally voluntary acts and moral deeds.

Collodi's intuition created a paradoxical situation; while Pinocchio must act as a moral human being, he cannot. As the story evolves in the book he becomes tamed, socialized, industrious and acquires a conscience. When this gradual transformation is completed, he has miraculously changed into a child of flesh and blood, a regular member of the human race.

I do not have the time to go into the many fascinating allegorical implications of Pinocchio, nor do I have the time to give even a succinct summary of that evolutionary process, which starting with the most elementary movement ends with those highest moral deeds that Western man exemplifies in accordance with the paradigms of the various roots of our civilization: as *areté*, or the harmonious action of the Greeks; as *mitzva*, or the good deed of the Jews; as *virtus*, or the way of man, according to the Romans.

In the first part of this paper I shall present some of the highlights of this phylogenetic and ontogenetic process, and some of the psychopathological arrests and deviations. Lest I am misunderstood, my references to phylogenetic mechanisms are not attempts to explain, in Jungian fashion, the dynamics of psychopathological conditions occurring today. Phylogenetic studies are important in studying the structural or formal mechanisms, but not content or motivation. In the second part of this paper I shall make an attempt to show how catatonic schizophrenia represents the most dramatic disintegration of this development. This will be illustrated with a case report.

The first movements that we must study in relation to motor actions are no longer the reflexes, as we did until a few years ago, but the so-called autorhythmic movements (12, 16), spontaneous movements of the organism from which eventually reflexes or fixed patterns of responses emerge in evolution. But neither autorhythmic movements nor reflexes can be called real volitional acts.

The first real volitional act is an inhibition, or at least an inhibition of a reflex response. For instance, during toilet training, the baby has the impulse to defecate when the rectum is distended by the passage of feces. The child, however, learns not to yield to the impulse and to postpone defecation in spite of the fact that it would be more pleasant to do so. He learns to control his sphincters because his ability to do so will affect his relation with mother. Obviously he has the neurophysiologic potentiality for sphincter control, but such control, inasmuch as it affects the people in his environment, is not purely a physiological act; it is also a social one. Furthermore in order to control himself, he must inhibit the still available simpler and more pleasant physiological mechanisms of immediate defecation.

His first act of will is thus at the same time an inhibition and a compliance to the will of others. It seems almost a paradoxical contradiction, just as paradoxical as negativism is a little later as an assertion of the emerging will (5). But will is a very complicated and portentous function, and like many other complicated functions appears to originate from what at first seems its opposite, just as logical thought originates from what at first seems its opposite: irrational thought. But somebody could object: Are acts of inhibition and compliance, as they occur, for instance, in toilet training, really the first voluntary acts? What about those actions of the baby, who toward the fifth or sixth month of life grabs rattles and other objects? Certainly these acts of the baby, like grabbing a rattle, must be included under the large category of conative acts, but actually they are not volitional in a mature sense; they are protovolitional. The baby responds to the stimulus rattle and enjoys the pleasure of the response which later on he seeks again. But there is no choice, not even a minimum of conflict, as there is between pleasing mother and defecating. If the action is a reflex response or, though conative, has the purpose only of maintaining the homeostasis or of producing immediate pleasure, without alternative possibilities, we do not yet have volition, but protovolition.

Inasmuch as these alternative possibilities are at first created by the exposure to the interpersonal situation, the act of will becomes, so to say, socialized. The action loses its primitive characteristic of a purely motor or physiologic mechanism because its outcome is anticipated in relation to the interpersonal world. As Parsons (13, 14) writes, action is not concerned only with the internal structure or processes of the organism, but with the organism in a sort of relationship. Action has additional dimensions, which may be called at the same time the social and the moral dimensions.

At this early ontogenetic level, volition is not only inhibition but also, as I said before, extreme submission. It is more than submission: it is enormous receptivity to the interpersonal world. This enormous receptivity is necessary for the development of the social self, or as Erikson (8) would say, for the epigenesis of the ego. It has some hypnotic qualities and may be related to the phenomenon of hypnosis. Hypnosis may be a more acute artificial reproduction of this stage of life when the child is extremely receptive to the will of others and does not remember who gave the instructions or suggestions. Later on he may rationalize his unconsciously introjected attitudes. The transference is also a repetition of attitudes generally acquired during this period of high receptivity. The origin of the transference is repressed and the phenomenon is rationalized. We have thus that triad of characteristics that Spiegel (15) considers inherent in the hypnotic situation.

This transient period of suggestibility has more manifest sequels in primitive cultures, where mass hypnosis, voodoo phenomena, and latah are relatively common (6). It is perhaps not too difficult to understand the importance of suggestibility in primitive society. As Kelsen (10) has described, in primitive societies *to do* and *to be guilty* are approximately the same thing. To do is at least potentially to be guilty because often one does not know the event that will follow one's action. The event might even have an effect on the whole tribe, such as an epidemic or drought. When the prevailing way of thinking is ruled not by deterministic or scientific causality, but by what is considered the will of animate things, the will becomes a portentous and frightening weapon. Its possession is liable to make one feel very guilty. But one will not feel very guilty if one accepts the will of others, of the gods, or the collective will of the tribe in a form of almost automatic obedience.

Automatic obedience is not the only way primitive men free themselves from guilt and fear. They also refrain from acting freely; they perform only those acts which are sanctioned by the tribe. For any desired effect, the tribe teaches the individual what act to perform. The life of primitive man is completely regulated by a tremendous number of norms and restrictions. The individual has to follow the ritual for practically everything he does. By performing the act according to the ritual, the primitive believes that he will avoid guilt for the act. These rituals are found again at an ontogenetic level as compulsive acts. The individual, who has not been able to develop his potentiality of acting freely without anxiety or guilt may resort to obsessive-compulsive mechanisms to obviate this anxiety and guilt.

In normal development we find a minimal quantity of compulsive behavior, just as we find traces of autism and of automatic obedience, etc. But in persons whose development was accompanied by excessive anxiety, obsessive-compulsive behavior may remain more pronounced than normal, and later on, when the individual is confronted by difficulties, obsessive-compulsive patterns may be resorted to again.

The psychopathic person does not resort to obsessive behavior. His attempt to remove anxiety will consist in allowing his actions to follow his desires without consideration of the interpersonal world, or of the rightness or wrongness of the act.

The patient who is to become catatonic is generally a person given to fits of overpowering anxiety, especially anxiety connected with the carrying out of some action. He generally does not resort to hypnotic or autohypnotic mechanisms, nor to psychopathic denial of responsibility. When in his life he is confronted with an important challenge or decision which causes him excessive anxiety, he fabricates many obsessive-compulsive mechanisms. But the anxiety may overpower him acutely, and he may not have time to manufacture compulsions. The anxiety will then be experienced as fear and guilt connected with any action and will be generalized to every action, to every movement determined by the will. He has a last resort to avoid these feelings: to fall into catatonic immobility. In stupor the immobility is complete, but in other less pronounced catatonic conditions it is not. The patient follows orders given by others not because he is in a state of automatic obedience or hypnosis, but because these orders are willed by others, and therefore he does not have the responsibility for them. In the state called waxy flexibility he retains the positions imposed by others, even if uncomfortable, because he cannot will to change position.

Most of these acute catatonic episodes are forgotten by the patient when he recovers, so that there is a scarcity of reports in the literature about these experiences and their interpretation. I have been able to collect a few rare cases in which full memory was retained, and I have reported some of them elsewhere (3, 5).

I am now going to report the case of John, which bears striking similarities to others reported by me, but which also bears some important differences that, in my opinion, may increase our understanding somewhat of the pathology of volition and value.

CASE REPORT

John is an intelligent professional man in his thirties, Catholic, who was referred to me because of his rapidly increasing anxiety— anxiety which reminded him of the one he experienced about ten years previously, when he developed a full catatonic episode. Wanting to prevent a recurrence of the event, he sought treatment.

The following is not a complete report but only a brief history of the patient and a description and interpretation of his catatonic episode as it was reconstructed and analyzed during the treatment.

The patient is one of four children. The father is described as a bad husband, an adventurer who, although a good provider, always caused trouble and home instability. The mother is a somewhat inadequate person, distant from the patient. John was raised more or less by a maternal aunt who lived in the family and acted as a housekeeper.

Early childhood memories are mostly unpleasant for John. He recollects attacks of anxiety going back to his early childhood. He also remembers how he needed to cling to his aunt; how painful it always was to separate from her. The aunt also had the habit of undressing in his presence, causing him mixed feelings of sexual excitement and guilt. Between 9 and 10 there was an attempted homosexual relation with his best friend. During his prepuberal period he remembers his desire to look at pictures of naked women, and how occasionally he would surreptitiously borrow some pornographic books or magazines from his father's collection and look at them. Fleeting homosexual desires would also occur occasionally. He masturbated with fantasies of women, but he had to stimulate his rectum with his fingers in order to experience, he says, "a greater pleasure." Among the things that he remembers from his early life are also obsessive preoccupations with feces of animals and excretions in general of human beings. He had a special admiration for horses, because "They excreted such beautiful feces coming from such statuesque bodies."

In spite of all these circumstances, John managed to grow more or less adequately, was not too disturbed by the death of his aunt, and did well in school. There were practically no dates with girls until much later in life. After puberty he became very interested in religion, especially in order to find a method to control his sexual impulses. Anything connected with sex was evil and had to be eliminated. This attitude was in a certain way the opposite of that of one of his sisters who was leading a very promiscuous life. John considered the possibility of becoming a monk several times; however, he was discouraged from doing so by a priest he had consulted. When he finished college at the age of 20, he decided to make a complete attempt to remove sex from his life. He also decided to go for a rest and summer vacation at a farm for young men where he would cut trees, enjoy the country, and be far away from the temptations of the city. On this farm, however, he soon became anxious and depressed. He found out that he resented the other fellows more and more. They were rough guys. They used profane language. He felt as if he were going to pieces progressively. He remembers that one night he was saying to himself, "I cannot stand it any more. Why am I this way, so anxious for no reason? I have done no wrong in my whole life. Perhaps I should become a priest or get married." When he was feeling very badly he would console himself by thinking that perhaps what he was experiencing was in accordance with the will of God.

Obsessions and compulsions acquired more and more prominence. The campers had to go chopping wood. This practice became an ordeal for John because he was possessed by doubts. He would think, for instance: "Maybe I should not cut this tree because it is too small. Next year it will be bigger. But if I don't cut this tree another fellow will. Maybe it is better if he cuts it, or maybe that I do so." As he expressed himself, he found himself "doubting and doubting his doubts, and doubting the doubting of his doubts." It was an overwhelming, spreading anxiety. The anxiety gradually extended to every act he had to perform. He was literally possessed by intense terror. One day, while he was in this predicament, he observed another phenomenon which he could not understand. There was a discrepancy between the act he wanted to perform and the action that he really carried out. For instance, when he was undressing he wanted to drop a shoe, and instead he dropped a big log; he wanted to put something in a drawer and instead he threw a stone away. However, there was a similarity between the act that he had wanted and anticipated and the act he actually performed. The same phenomenon appeared in talking. He would utter words, which were not the ones he meant to say, but related to them. Later, however, his actions became more and more disconnected. He was mentally lucid and able to perceive what was happening but he realized he had no control over his actions. He thought he could commit crimes, even kill somebody and became even more afraid. He was saying to himself: "I don't want to be damned in this world as well as in the other. I am trying to be good and I can't. It is not fair. I may kill somebody when I want a piece of bread." At other times he had different feelings. He felt as if some movement or action he would make could produce disaster not only to himself but to the whole camp. By not acting or moving he was protecting the whole group. He felt that he had become his brothers' keeper.

Fear soon became connected with any possible movement. The fear was so intense as to actually inhibit any movement. He was almost literally petrified. To use his own words, he "saw himself solidifying, assuming statuesque positions." However, he was not always in this condition. As a matter of fact, the following day he could move again and go to chop wood. He had one purpose in mind: to kill himself. He remembers that he was very capable of observing himself, and of deciding that it would be better for him to die than to commit crimes. He climbed a big tree and jumped down in an attempt to kill himself but received only minor contusions. The other men, who ran to help him, realized that he was mentally ill, and he was soon sent to a psychiatric hospital. He remembers understanding that he was taken to the hospital and being happy about it; at least he was considered sick and not a criminal.

But in the hospital he found that he could not move at all. He was like a statue of stone.

There were some actions, however, which could escape this otherwise complete immobility: the actions needed for the purpose of committing suicide. In fact he was sure that he had to die to avoid the terror of becoming a murderer. He had to kill himself before that could happen.

During his hospitalization, John made 71 suicidal attempts. Although he was generally in a state of catatonia he would occasionally make impulsive acts such as tearing his strait jacket to pieces and making a rope of it to hang himself. Another time he broke a dish in order to cut the veins of his wrist. Other times he swallowed stones. He was always put under restraint after a suicidal attempt. He remembers, however, understanding everything that was going on. As a matter of fact, his acuity in devising methods for committing suicide seemed sharpened.

When I questioned him further about this long series of suicidal attempts, John added that the most drastic attempts were actually the first ten or twelve. Only these could really have killed him. Later, the suicidal attempts were not very dangerous. He performed such acts as swallowing a small object or inflicting a small injury on himself with a sharp object. When I asked him whether he knew why he had to repeat these token suicidal attempts, he gave me two reasons. The first was to relieve his feeling of guilt and fulfill his duty of preventing himself from committing crimes. But the second reason, which he discovered during the present treatment, is even stranger. To commit suicide was the only act which he could perform, the only act which would get beyond the barrier of immobility. Thus, to commit suicide was to live; the only act of life left to him.

The patient was given a course of electric shock treatment. The exact number could not be ascertained. He improved for about two weeks, but then he relapsed into catatonic stupor interrupted only by additional suicidal attempts. While he was in stupor he remembered a young psychiatrist saying to a nurse, "Poor fellow, so young and so sick. He will continue to deteriorate for the rest of his life." After five or six months of hospitalization his catatonic state became somewhat less rigid and he was able to walk and to utter a few words. At this time he had noticed that a new doctor seemed to take some interest in him. One day this doctor told him, "You want to kill yourself. Isn't there anything at all in life that you want?" With great effort the patient mumbled, "Eat, to eat." In fact, he really was hungry as his immobility prevented him from eating properly, and he was inefficiently spoon fed. The doctor took him to the patients' cafeteria and told him, "You may eat anything you want." John immediately grabbed a large quantity of food and ate in a ravenous manner. The doctor noticed that John liked soup and told him to take even more soup. From that day on John lived only for the sake of eating. He gained about sixty pounds in a few weeks. When I asked him if he ate so much because he was really hungry, he said, "No, that was only at the beginning. The pleasure in eating consisted partially in grabbing food and putting it into my mouth." Later it was discovered by the attendants that John would not only eat a lot but he would also hoard food in his drawers and under his mattress.

I cannot go into detail about many other interesting episodes which occurred in the course of his illness. John continued to improve and in a few months he was able to leave the hospital. He was able to make a satisfactory adjustment, to work, and later to go to a professional school and obtain his Ph.D degree. On the whole he has managed fairly well until shortly before he decided to come for psychoanalytic treatment.

I shall now attempt an interpretation of these phenomena. It is obvious that John underwent an overpowering increase in anxiety when he went to the camp and was exposed to close homosexual stimulation. His early interpersonal relations had subjected him to great instability and insecurity and had made him very vulnerable to many sources of anxiety. This anxiety, however, retained a propensity to be aroused by or be channeled in the pattern of sexual stimulation and inhibition. His personality defenses and cultural background made the situation worse. John was not like Pinocchio, i.e., deprived of that part of the self called social self, conscience or superego; nor could he go against his cultural-religious background as his philandering father and promiscuous sister. Sex was evil for him, and homosexuality much more so. As a matter of fact, homosexual desires were not even permitted to become fully conscious.

When he was about to be overwhelmed by the anxiety, he at first resorted to some of the defenses commonly found in precatatonics. He found refuge in religious feelings. God or religion gave him the order of eliminating sex from his life and of becoming a monk. This may be considered a form of autohypnosis, but as we have already mentioned at the beginning of this paper, hypnosis and autohypnosis do not work well with catatonics. He resorted, then, to obsessive-compulsive mechanisms. The anxiety which presumably was at first connected with any action that had something to do with sexual feelings became extended to practically every action. Incidentally, Ferenzi (9) has reported similar feelings in one patient. Every action became loaded with a sense of responsibility. Every willed movement came to be seen not as a function but as a moral issue. Every motion was not considered as a fact but as a value. This primitive generalization of his responsibility extended to what he could cause to the whole community. By moving he could produce havoc not only to himself but to the whole camp. His feelings were reminiscent of the feelings of cosmic power or negative omnipotence experienced by other catatonics who believe that by acting they may cause the destruction of the universe (5).

To protect himself at first, John resorted to obsessive thinking and compulsions, as, for instance, when he was cutting trees. But even this defense was not sufficient to dam his anxiety; as a matter of fact, it made the situation worse and gave rise to other symptoms. The first one was the unrelatedness between the act, as anticipated and willed, and the action which followed. But, and this is a point of great importance, at first the actions were not completely unrelated from their anticipation. They were analogic. In other words, two actions, like dropping a shoe and dropping a log, had become psychologically equivalent, i.e., they were identified just because they were similar or had something in common. This fact is, in my opinion, of theoretical importance because it extends to the area of volition or of willed mobility those characteristics which have already been described in paleologic or analogic thinking of schizophrenics (4). It would seem to indicate that the same basic formal psychopathological mechanisms apply to every area of the psyche. It may also be connected with neurological studies of motor integration, as recently outlined by Denny-Brown (7). The analogic movement may be viewed as a "release" or "dedifferentation or loss of restriction to specific attributes of adequate stimulus."

The reason that this phenomenon of generalized analogic movement escapes notice and has not been reported in the literature so far, is to be found in the fact that it is of very transient occurrence. In most patients the symptomatology proceeds rapidly to following stages, e.g., the stage where the actions are completely unrelated to the will, as in catatonic excitement, or the stage in which the actions are all eliminated, as in catatonic stupor. The catatonic excitement may be the result of two facts. In some cases the patient senses that he is sinking into stupor because he is afraid to act and tries to prevent this occurrence by becoming overactive and submerging himself in a rapid sequence of aimless acts. In other instances the opposite is true and the patient acts, but his actions are so unrelated to the conceived or willed actions as to result in a real movement-salad, the motor equivalent of word-salad. The patient then has no other resort but to sink into the immobility of the stupor.

In many cases the barrier of immobility is not completely closed. In a very selective way it may allow passage to actions of obedience to the will of others or to some special actions of the patient himself.

In the case of John the actions necessary for the suicidal attempts were allowed to go through. Incidentally, these suicidal attempts in catatonics, accompanied by religious feelings and eventually by stupor, have often led to the wrong diagnosis of the depressed form of manic-depressive psychosis. Kraepelin (11) himself described suicidal attempts and ideas of sin in catatonics, but did not give to them any psychodynamic significance. What is of particular interest in our case is the fact that the suicidal act eventually became for John the only act of living. It is not possible here to examine in greater detail the therapeutic effect of the encounter of John with the doctor in the hospital. Important is the fact that the doctor gave John permission to eat as much as he wanted. Thus the only previously possible act (of killing oneself) was replaced with one of the most primitive acts of life, nourishing oneself. I have described the placing-into-mouth habit in very regressed schizophrenics (1). In slightly less regressed patients we find the hoarding habit (2), a stage John went through in his progress toward recovery. In acute cases of catatonia we often find, in very acute form, symptoms appearing in other types of schizophrenia after many years of regression.

Many other aspects of the interesting case of John cannot be examined for lack of space. However, I feel that adding what we have learned from John to what has been reported about other cases (3-5), some conclusions may be drawn:

1) Catatonia is predominantly a disorder of the will. It is not a disorder of the motor apparatus.

2) Contrary to appearance, the state of catatonia is not that of an ivory tower. It is a state where volition is connected with a pathologically intensified sense of value, so that torturing responsibility spreads like fire to every possible act. Such pathological sense of responsibility reaches the acme of intensity when a little movement of the patient is considered capable of destroying the world. Alas! This conception of the psychotic mind reminds us of its possible actuality today, when the pushing of a button may have such cosmic effects! Only the oceanic responsibility of the catatonic could include this up-to-now unconceived possibility.

3) The passivity to the suggestion of others found in some catatonics is not an acceptance of power from others, as in hypnosis, but a relief from responsibility.

4) Only those actions may go through the catatonic barrier which may compensate or atone for the intensified responsibility. This selectivity is dramatically exemplified in our case report, where only the movements necessary for self-inflicted death penalty could be carried out, but even

more than that—where self-inflicted death penalty became the only voluntary movement, thus life itself.

5) Catatonia may present certain phenomena such as the analogic movement which may be related to the general pathological functioning of the psyche as well as to principles of neurological disorganization.

6) The recognition that the catatonic patient is not an ivory tower but, on the contrary, a volcano of not at all petrified feelings, lends itself to possible therapeutic maneuvers, already in course in other cases, which will be reported elsewhere.

REFERENCES

1. ARIETI, S.: The "placing-into-mouth" and coprophagic habits. *J. Nerv. &. Ment. Dis.*, 102:307, 1945.
2. ARIETI, S.: Primitive habits in the preterminal stage of schizophrenia. *J. Nerv. & Ment. Dis.*, 102:367, 1945.
3. ARIETI, S.: *Interpretation of Schizophrenia.* New York: Brunner, 1955, pp. 109-120.
4. ARIETI, S.: *Interpretation of Schizophrenia.* New York: Brunner, 1955, pp. 194-209.
5. ARIETI, S.: *Interpretation of Schizophrenia.* New York: Brunner, 1955, pp. 219-238.
6. ARIETI, S. and METH, J.: Rare, unclassifiable, collective and exotic psychotic syndromes. In *American Handbook of Psychiatry*, Vol. 1. Edited by S. Arieti. New York: Basic Books, 1959, chapter 27, p. 546.
7. DENNY-BROWN, D.: Motor mechanisms-introduction: The general principles of motor integration. In *Handbook of Physiology.* Edited by J. Field. Washington: American Physiological Society, 1960, 2:781.
8. ERIKSON, E. H.: Identity and the life cycle. *Psychological Issues*, Vol. 2. New York: International University Press, 1959.
9. FERENCZI, S.: Some clinical observations on paranoia and paraphrenia. In *Sex in Psychoanalysis.* New York: Basic Books, 1950.
10. KELSEN, H.: *Society and Nature—A Sociological Inquiry.* Chicago: University of Chicago Press, 1943.
11. KRAEPELIN, E.: *Dementia Praecox and Paraphrenia.* Edinburgh: Livingston, 1925.
12. LORENZ, K. Z.: Comparative behaviorology. In *Discussion on Child Development.* Vol. 1. New York: International University Press, 1954.
13. PARSONS, I.: *The Social System.* Glencoe: The Free Press, 1951.
14. PARSONS, I. and SHIES, E. A.: *Toward a General Theory of Action.* Cambridge: Harvard University Press, 1951.
15. SPIEGEL, H.: Hypnosis and transference: A theoretical formulation. *A.M.A. Arch. Gen. Psychiat.*, 1:634, 1959.
16. VON HOLST, E.: Von Dualismus der motorischen und der automatischrhythmischen Funktion im Ruckenmark und von Wesen des automatischen Rhythmus Pflug. *Arch. ges. Physiol.*, 237:356, 1936.

9

The "Placing-Into-Mouth" and
Coprophagic Habits

Written after a series of papers devoted exclusively or pre-
dominantly to neuropathological subjects, this is my first paper
in clinical psychiatry, published in 1944. This paper, which
deals with the most regressed schizophrenic patients, led to my
interest in seeking out correlations between psychotic symptoms
and cerebral dysfunctions, perhaps psychosomatic in origin.

IN THE WARDS of psychiatric hospitals, where cases are treated in the most advanced stages of their illness, it is a common observation to see patients picking up from the floor and putting into their mouth inedible objects found in their immediate environment and within easy reach (the placing-into-mouth habit). These objects are grasped indiscriminately, put into the mouth, gnawed, chewed, licked, sucked, often eaten and not seldom swallowed with great risk.

On the autopsy table of Pilgrim State Hospital it is a relatively common experience to find in the stomach or intestines of patients who were affected by the most advanced stages of dementia praecox, spoons, stones, pieces of scrap iron, wood, paper, cores, etc.

As a typical example, will be mentioned briefly the case of A.R. (Hospital No. 5562). This patient entered Pilgrim in October 1933 at the age of 32. On admission he had delusions and hallucinations, but was fairly well preserved. The diagnosis of dementia praecox, paranoid type, was then made. Subsequently he showed a steady downhill progression in his mental condition. He became negativistic, mute, manneristic and idle. He had the habit of wetting and soiling, and required a great deal of supervision. On frequent occasions it was necessary to tube-feed him. He did not show any interest in his surroundings, appearing completely with-

121

drawn and living an almost vegetative existence. In the dining room, however, he showed some interest, grabbing food and eating in a ravenous manner. On December 31, 1939 he died of acute intestinal obstruction. At autopsy 14 spoon handles were found in the colon, 2 spoon handles and a suspender clasp were found in the stomach. In the terminal ileum was a rolled piece of shirt collar which was the cause of the obstruction.

The grasping and ingestion of the objects may be accomplished by a quick movement, as a prompt reaction to a visual stimulus, or by a slow movement, apparently not accompanied by any emotional coloring. If the patients are under some mechanical restraint, they may try to reach the objects directly with their mouth.

Among demented patients in advanced stages of their illness, most commonly schizophrenic in nature (1), it is not rare to see some of them grasp their own feces, chew them and eat them often with great pleasure and satisfaction (coprophagia). These coprophagic patients may put into their mouth everything indiscriminately and incidentally their own feces, but this is rather exceptional. As a rule, they show a marked discrimination in putting into their mouth specifically their own feces. Other patients often smear themselves with their own excrements.

Are these habits only manifestations of a silly, purposeless behavior of demented patients or are they determined by deeper causes, perhaps being a manifestation of released mechanisms which belong to lower levels of integration?

The writer agrees with the latter point of view. Reported observations in the fields of comparative psychology, child psychology and psychiatry, experimental neurology, anthropology and psychoanalysis may be interpreted as corroborating such a belief.

Let us first examine the ingestion habit or "oral tendency," if we wish to use a term successfully employed by other authors (6-8) for different observations.

This habit of regressed psychotics has some points in common with what is generally observed in children about the end of the first year of age. When confronted by objects of a certain size, children of one to two years of age grasp these objects and attempt to put them into their mouth. There is no discrimination made between edible and nonedible objects; the baby places in his mouth anything that comes within his reach and licks, sucks or eats it.

"If the object is too heavy or cannot be grasped with the hand . . . the infant brings his mouth close to the object and licks or, in the case of clothing or bibs or blankets, sucks at it" (5). Rugs, cotton, leaves, worms, wool, wood, stones and paper are eaten or at least put into the mouth. "The objects eaten are the objects accessible; accessibility and not 'craving' or 'appetite' governs their selection" (5). All parents have observed this particular behavior when their children have reached this age and attribute it erroneously to various causes. Most of the time they attribute it to incipient teething or to increased appetite. Generally the people who have charge of the child remove the object from the child's mouth with their own hands, fearing it may be swallowed. But the child, if let alone, will test the object and often reject it if it is not edible or if it has an unpleasant taste. Only relatively seldom is the object swallowed, with serious consequences. It seems almost as if taste discrimination, or at least oral discrimination by means of the sensory properties of the oral cavity, supersedes the visual one. In pathological conditions this habit persists up to the third and even fourth year and is erroneously called perverted appetite or pica.

In a series of papers issued in 1937, 1938 and 1939, Klüver and Bucy (6-8) described interesting observations on trained monkeys after the extirpation of both temporal lobes. The extirpation included Brodmann's areas, 22, 21, 20, the area 19 being left untouched. The removal of both lobes constantly caused typical manifestations, whereas the ablation of only one lobe or of an entire lobe and a part of the other did not bring about characteristic results.

The authors found that the monkeys, after this surgical treatment, showed an irresistible tendency to grasp anything within reach. They placed the grasped object in their mouth, bit it, touched it to their lips and finally would eat it, if edible. If inedible, the object was rejected. All objects, edible or not, were grasped indiscriminately. Every operated monkey manifested this particular type of reaction, environmental changes having apparently no influence at all. It seemed as if all previous learning had no influence whatsoever on their behavior. As a matter of fact, the established reactions to visual and weight differences were superseded by the constant grasping and putting-in-mouth reaction (called, by the authors, oral tendencies). In addition, it seemed to the observers as if the animal were "acting under the influence of some compulsory or irresistible impulse. The monkey behaves as if it were forced to react to objects . . . in the environmental stimulus constellation." It seemed to be dominated by only one tendency, namely, the tendency to contact every object as quickly as possible, any visual object immediately leading, whenever possible, to a motor response.

A different kind of forced ingestion of inedible objects is reported in another field of investigation. Members of savage tribes are in the habit of eating some inedible substances (geophagy). They are almost forced to eat these objects since they cannot prevent eating them when they see them. This habit is highly discriminatory for a certain substance in a given tribe but retains almost a compulsory characteristic.

The above-mentioned examples taken from different fields of investigation have some features in common, namely, the picking up of objects from the immediate environment and placing them into the oral cavity, no discrimination being made concerning their nature or no consideration being paid to the fact that they are not edible. These actions have in all the cited instances a more or less compulsory characteristic.

It could be objected that such similarities are only apparent or very superficial and the differences could be emphasized. But the differences may be due to various factors acting contemporaneously with the common factor which may be an expression of a certain level of development. The differences could be explained without difficulty. The precise execution of movements of the monkey and the lower and less accurate movements of the child may be attributed to the fact that voluntary movements have not yet been well acquired by the child, whose central nervous system is not yet completely myelinized, while they have been acquired by the monkey.

Unlike the child, the bitemporal monkey of Klüver and Bucy can indefatigably continue to grasp every object, to react repetitiously in this way to every visual stimulus. This is probably because the damage or the lack of cerebral areas causes the animal's hyperactivity or that state of "being forced by the stimulus," similar to what is observed in human cases with extensive cerebral defects (3). The highly discriminatory geophagic habit of savages may be one of few vestiges of a much more primitive level. The fact that deteriorated schizophrenics presenting the described behavior, grasp objects not in such number and rapidity as the Klüver and Bucy monkey or at every opportunity as the child, may be explained if we take into consideration the other aspects of the schizophrenic picture. The volitional and emotional impairment of the schizophrenic may be responsible for such difference. It must also not be forgotten that, as Storch pointed out (11), the archaic primitive formations in schizophrenics "break in" only here and there through the psychic superstructure and not continuously.

Klüver and Bucy give an interesting preliminary interpretation of some behavior characteristics of their bitemporal monkeys in considering the latter as "psychically blind" (6). Since in their tendency to approach and place in their mouth "without hesitation" all objects, the animals show no discrimination, no preference for food nor for learned reactions and no ability to concentrate on particular objects, the authors consider these monkeys to be psychically blind. The writer has not the advantage of the valuable direct observations of the authors, but if he has understood correctly Klüver and Bucy come to the "psychic blindness" or visual agnosia conclusion in view of the fact that the animal which has undergone the removal of both temporal lobes, grasps and uses each object indiscriminately, even though it had learned before the operation to distinguish the objects and use them discriminately. But is that behavior really due to "psychic blindness" or to that "compulsory or irresistible impulse" which forces the monkey, as well as the child, and at times the regressed schizophrenic, to grasp any object within reach? We must direct our attention also to the fact that the ability to appreciate differences in lightness, size, shape, distance, position and movement is not reported impaired in these monkeys. Therefore, we can reach the conclusion that the only bodies which are not "recognized" are the bodies with a definite sharp three-dimensional shape. Although it does not seem possible to explain the forced placing-into-mouth reaction of these monkeys on account of some visual agnosia, it could not be disproved that they are really in a certain way psychically blind. As a matter of fact, in a certain sense even the child of one to two years of age may be considered partially psychically blind. The visual stimuli often do not lead the child to recognize the objects, his visual perceptions are still partially agnostic. By means of the mouth, more than by his eyes, the one-year-old child explores what is still unkown to him. Werner states (12): "The mouth is the primitive means of knowing objects, that is, in a literal sense, through the grasping of the objects. The spatial knowledge of an object results from a sucking in of the thing through the mouth and a consequent tactual discovery and incorporation." However, the child apparently does not grasp and put into its mouth the objects in order to know them, but under a certain kind of primitive impulse. It happens that in doing so he starts to know the objects and this behavior has beneficial results for him. The demented schizophrenic in advanced stages of regression may also be considered, in a certain way, as partially psychically blind because the visual stimuli of the objects do not elicit cognitive and affective associations concerning their inedibility and the relative danger of putting them into his mouth and eating them. However, the possibility must be taken into consideration that he is conscious of the inedible qualities of these objects, but that he cannot inhibit the impulse to grasp them. Such possibility cannot be ruled out. We may, however, advance the hypothesis that this behavior of children, bitemporal monkeys and regressed schizophrenics is a primitive way of reacting, which is characteristic of a certain level of development and is inhibited or transformed by higher centers. In other words, we may deal with one of those responses in which a short-circuiting takes place between the functions of reception and those of reaction instead of the usual way with participation of the higher centers. These reactions are intermediate between reflexes and voluntary acts, having some characteristics of compulsory acts. The "placing-into-mouth" reaction seems to belong to a much lower level than the archaic forms of inner experiences described by Storch in schizophrenics but at a higher level than for instance the grasp reflex, found in infants of one to three months and in adults with lesions of the frontal lobes, although the grasp reflex does not always appear as a true reflex but frequently as a prehension attitude implying some voluntary action. Schilder, however, considers the taking of objects into the mouth "at least as primitive as grasping" (10). This placing-into-mouth reaction is apparently not caused by any agnosia but seems to belong coincidentally to a level at which high apperceptions elaborating visual stimuli are not yet possible. This primitive reaction may have its early origins even in low vertebrates. It may have some connection with the feeding response of amphibians, reptiles and birds, animals in which the temporal lobe is represented only by the hippocampal area. Although its main purpose in phylogenesis is to contact food, it certainly is also a means of recognizing objects, especially for those animals whose visual centers have not reached a high degree of development.

It is also interesting at this point to recall that psychoanalysis describes an oral stage of development. This stage, at which mental patients may be fixed or to which they may regress, is characterized by the paramount importance of the oral cavity and its sensory properties. It seems, therefore, that we have here a typical illustration of the inter-relations, emphasized by Grinker (4) and others, of psychiatry, psychoanalysis and neurology, even in its experimental part.

Taking into consideration the coprophagic habit, the fact is worthy of mention, that such behavior is usual in healthy apes. To my knowledge this fact has not yet been reported in relation to psychiatric implications. In the Laboratory of Primate Biology of Yale University, directed by Dr. Yerkes, the writer had opportunity to observe how frequent was such a habit in the chimpanzees kept in captivity. In one of his recent publications, Dr. Yerkes states (13): "Causes, controls and prevention [of coprophagy among captive chimpanzees] have been sought diligently, but with discouraging results. The hypothesis that coprophagy is induced by dietary deficiency, as for examples in mineral, vitamin, or roughage, insufficient food, or overlong intervals between feedings, finds no support in the inquiries conducted in our laboratories. We suspect, therefore, that the factors underlying the behavior are complex."

Köhler (9) had previously described such peculiar behavior of primates. He reported that out of many chimpanzees studied by him only one did not indulge in coprophagy. He states that the habit of smearing themselves with excrements is also frequent among chimpanzees. Such habits have not been observed in healthy monkeys. In mental patients this behavior is observed especially among catatonics and hebephrenics. Although it is a sign of advanced regression, it is not as malignant as the "oral tendency" here described, belonging probably to a less primitive level. As a matter of fact, catatonics, who have eaten feces or smeared themselves, occasionally gain a temporary remission (2) or even an apparently complete recovery (personal observations). It is interesting to observe here too that psychoanalysis considers the coprophagic habit as an expression of the anal character which is described as being formed after the oral stage.

REFERENCES

1. BLEULER, E.: *Textbook of Psychiatry*. New York: Macmillan Company, 1924.
2. CHRZANOWSKI, G.: Contrasting responses to electric shock therapy in clinically similar catatonics. *Psychiat. Quar.*, 17:282, 1943.
3. GOLDSTEIN, K.: The modification of behavior consequent to cerebral lesions. *Psychiat. Quart.*, 10:586, 1936.
4. GRINKER, R. R.: The inter-relation of neurology, psychiatry and psychoanalysis. *J.A.M.A.*, 116:2236, 1941.
5. KANNER, L.: *Child Psychiatry*. Springfield, Ill.: Charles C Thomas, 1935.
6. KLÜVER, H. and BUCY, P. C.: "Psychic blindness" and other symptoms following bilateral temporal lobectomy in rhesus monkeys. *Amer. J. Physiol.*, 119:352, 1937.
7. ———: An analysis of certain effects of bilateral temporal lobectomy in the rhesus monkey with special reference to "psychic blindness." *J. Psychol.*, 5:33, 1938.
8. ———: Preliminary analysis of functions of the temporal lobes in monkeys. *Arch. Neurol. & Psychiat.*, 42:972, 1939.
9. KÖHLER, W.: *The Mentality of Apes*. New York: Harcourt, Brace & Co., 1925.
10. SCHILDER, P.: *Brain and Personality*. New York: Nervous and Mental Disease Publishing Company, 1931.
11. STORCH, A.: *The Primitive Archaic Forms of Inner Experiences and Thought in Schizophrenia*. New York: Nervous and Mental Disease Publishing Company, 1924.
12. WERNER, H.: *Comparative Psychology of Mental Development*. New York: Harper & Bros., 1940.
13. YERKES, R. M.: Personal communication.
14. ———: *Chimpanzees. A Laboratory Colony*. New Haven: Yale University Press, 1943.

10

Primitive Habits and Perceptual Alterations in the Terminal Stage of Schizophrenia

If early cases of schizophrenia lend themselves better to psychodynamic formulations, the cases at the terminal stage of schizophrenia show a state of regression which presents similarities to the Klüver and Bucy syndrome and definite perceptual alterations. A psychosomatic involvement of the central nervous system in schizophrenia is considered again in this paper, in 1945.

IN THE LAST DECADE the main interest in the study of schizophrenia has been concentrated on cases of the early stage of this illness, which are the most suitable for dynamic psychologic investigations and in which a better response to the newly devised shock treatments is obtained. The study of cases of chronic schizophrenia has, on the other hand, been rather neglected except for statistical purposes. I am in accord with the numerous other workers who think that even the study of patients in the most advanced stages of this illness may eventually reveal important information on the nature of this condition. This point of view led to the present investigation of peculiar habits and of quasineurologic (or neurologic?) phenomena noted in the terminal stages of dementia praecox. The word habit is employed here for want of a better term. It is used to mean a certain type of behavior intermediate between reflexes and voluntary acts but always definitely reactive in nature. Goldstein's (1) term "performance" could be used except for the fact that the behavior discussed here is a special kind of performance, being spontaneous and habitual. The term "automatic act" is also discarded because by this term is often meant an act which has become such through repetition or training. The study on the coprophagic habit has already been reported (2). The habit of "placing into mouth" has also been discussed (2) but will be reconsidered here in relation to broader implications. The phenomenon of negativism will not be included in this report because it is not found exclusively in the terminal stage of dementia praecox but is more characteristic of less advanced stages. Other habits which belong to preterminal stages of dementia praecox will be discussed in later contributions.

This study was carried out on 250 female patients with the chronic form of schizophrenia who had been hospitalized in institutions for mental disease from seven to forty-seven years.

OBSERVATIONS

It is well known to all observers that decreased activity is one of the most common, though not a constant, characteristic of progressing schizophrenia. This motor reduction often interferes with the dietary requirements of the patient to such a point as to bring about a state of malnutrition, anemia and, occasionally, avitaminosis. This inactivity, which is a part of the psychic isolation of schizophrenia, is noted throughout the long years of progressing regression, interrupted only by occasional and transitory partial remissions. In patients, however, who continue to regress indefinitely, a more or less sudden increase in motor activity is noted at a certain moment. As a rule such an increase is not transitory but lasts for the lifetime of the patient, or until a physical illness neutralizes its effects. It is when this partial increase of motor activity takes place that what I call the terminal stage of dementia praecox begins. In the patients whom I observed and whose clinical records I studied, such a stage started any time from seven to forty years after the onset of the illness, but it probably may start even sooner, or later. This increase in activity is only relative, since the patients remain somehow underactive in comparison with normal subjects. Their actions, which are now more numerous, appear sharply reactive or impulsive: They are reactive to certain habitual situations, which will be taken in consideration shortly, or impulsive, inasmuch as they appear to be due to sudden internal stimulation. The patients may be impulsively destructive, assaultive and much more violent than previously. At this stage of the illness they do not seem able any longer to experience hallucinations or to elaborate delusions, although it may be that since they are no longer capable of expressing themselves verbally, such symptoms cannot be elicited. In fact, their verbal expressions are either completely absent or reduced to a few disconnected utterances.

The most striking changes, however, are noted in the dining room. The patients who had always eaten so little as to have reduced themselves to a state of malnutrition now seem to have a voracious appetite (bulimia) and often gain a considerable amount of weight. The nurses often report that these patients have the habit of stealing food. In reality, closer observation reveals that the concept of stealing is not implied in the actions of these patients. They cannot prevent themselves from grabbing food at the sight of it, so that they are better termed food grabbers. Observations in the dining room reveal other interesting habits. A few of these patients show preference for certain foods. No matter how many kinds of food are in their dish, they always grasp first and eat the preferred food. They do not alternate the various kinds, as normal adults do, but only when they have entirely finished the preferred food do they start to eat the others. Similarly, if they show several degrees of preference, they first eat the food which is the first choice; when this is finished, they eat the second choice, and so on. If there are desserts, they are generally eaten before anything else. It seems that the patients are obliged to react first to stronger stimuli. The preference for a certain food is not shown by all patients who are food grabbers. On the other hand, such preference is maintained only for a brief period after the acquisition of the food-grabbing habit. After this period the patients seem to eat with avidity any kind of food. Whatever belongs to the category of edibility is equally and promptly reacted to. Another characteristic which is often observed is the extreme rapidity with which these patients eat (tachyphagia). In a few minutes these food grabbers may finish the rations of several patients, if not prevented. Often they do not leave in the dish any remnant of food but clean the plate with their tongue.

The patients may remain indefinitely at this stage characterized by the food-grabbing habit, but the majority progress more or less rapidly to a more advanced stage, characterized chiefly by what I have termed the habit of "placing into mouth." At this stage the category of edibility is no longer respected. Whereas the patients had previously distinguished themselves for grabbing food and food only, now they manifest the habit of grabbing every small object and putting it into the mouth, paying no attention at all to the edible or nonedible nature of it. If not prevented, these patients pick up from the floor crumbs, cockroaches, stones, rags, paper, wood, clothes, pencils and leaves and put them into the mouth. Generally they eat these things; occasionally they swallow them, with great risk. Many patients, however, limit themselves to chewing these nonedible objects and finally reject them. When they eat or swallow dangerous materials, such as an ink well or a teaspoon, they are erroneously considered as suicidal. Closer observation reveals, however, that the idea of suicide is not implied in their action. They simply react to a visual stimulus by grasping the object and putting it into the mouth. They act as if they were coerced to react in this way. It is as though they were especially attracted by small three dimensional stimuli, which seem to be distinguished more distinctly than usual from the background.

The patient may remain indefinitely at this stage, but some of them progress to a more advanced phase, which is characterized by apparent sensory alterations. On account of the lack of cooperation and communicability of these patients, such alterations cannot be studied with the usual neurologic technic, but much stronger stimuli, not ordinarily used, or observation of the patient's reactions in certain special situations must be employed. Therefore only gross alterations are reported here, and no claim to accuracy is made.

It seems as though the patients who have reached this stage are insensitive to pain. They appear analgesic not only to pinprick but to much more painful stimuli. When they are in need of surgical intervention and have to have sutures in such sensitive regions as the lips, face, skull or hands, they act as though they could not feel anything, even in the absence of any anesthetic procedure. I have many times sutured wounds caused by their violent and assaultive behavior without eliciting any sign of pain or resistance. Other patients seem to feel some pain, but far less than normal persons would. Only exceptionally is there a local withdrawal. The same anesthesia is noted for temperature. The patient may hold in his hands a piece of ice without showing any reaction. Pieces of ice may also be placed over the breast, abdomen or other sensitive regions without eliciting any reaction or defensive movement. Such patients also appear insensitive when the flame of a candle is passed rapidly over the skin. They may sit near the radiator, and if they are not removed, they may continue to stay there even when, as a result of close contact, they are burned. This state of insensitivity is in my opinion one of the chief causes of the large number of burns occurring in wards in which deteriorated schizophrenic patients live.

One may be induced to interpret this lack of responsiveness to pain and temperature stimuli not as true anesthesia but as an expression either of catatonic inactivity or of a certain kind of "inner negativism." Repeated observations have, however, led me to the conclusion that such an interpretation is not valid. The patients who show anesthesia for pain or temperature stimuli are not as a rule inactive; on the other hand, they show the aforementioned relative increase in activity which, together with the apparent anesthesia, is responsible for numerous accidents. The possibility that these patients do not react to dangerous sensations on account of inner negativism is, in my opinion, also untenable because many such patients do not show other signs of negativism. As I have already mentioned, the phenomenon of negativism, although not absent at this stage of the illness, is much more commonly observed in patients who have reached a less advanced stage. On the other hand, the possibility that pain and temperature sensations are perceived, but that only the affective components of such perceptions are lost, must be taken into consideration and will be discussed later. In a small number of patients this apparent anesthesia or hypesthesia for pain and temperature stimuli is only transitory. Even patients who have been insensitive to heat for several months may to some extent reacquire capacity to perceive pain or temperature sensations or both. Occasionally striking changes occur at brief intervals. However, I have the impression that some degree of hypesthesia is always retained. Partial hypesthesia is also found in many patients who have not yet reached what is here called the terminal stage. Tactile perception does not seem impaired in these patients. Tendon and superficial reflexes are not only present but often increased. The corneal reflexes are also present. On the other hand, many, but not all of the patients who present anesthesia for pain and temperature stimuli seem also to have lost the sensation of taste. When they are given bitter radishes or teaspoons of sugar, salt, pepper or quinine, they do not show any pleasant or unpleasant reaction. They do not spit out the unpleasant substances as quickly as possible, as do control mental defective persons or deteriorated patients with organic disease, but continue to eat the entire dose without hesitation. Some of them seem to recognize salt but do not object to pepper or quinine. Others react mildly to quinine but not to pepper or salt.

In contrast to this lack of reactivity to pain, temperature and taste stimuli is the normal reaction to strong olfactory stimuli. Patients who did not react at all to such stimuli as flames, pieces of ice and suturing react in a normal way when they smell such things as ammonia and strong vinegar. They withdraw quickly from the stimulus, with manifest displeasure. Such a reaction strikes the observer, inasmuch as many other strong stimuli from other sensory fields do not bring about any response, or only a mild reaction. It seems as though the phylogenetically ancient olfactory sense could better resist the schizophrenic process. However, the schizophrenic patient does not seem to make use of these olfactory sensations as he could, probably on account of that lack of initiative which more or less characterizes the entire course of his illness.

The aforementioned phases of the terminal stage of dementia precox (phases characterized by the food-grabbing habit, the "placing into mouth" habit and apparent anesthesia for pain, temperature and taste sensations and preponderance of the olfactory sense, respectively) do not always occur in the order given. A large number of patients, especially, but not exclusively, those of the paranoid type, remain indefinitely at a less advanced stage. In others two stages of the illness overlap. For instance, a few patients who have the food-grabbing habit may retain the capacity to hallucinate. Other food grabbers may already have anesthesia for pain and temperature stimuli, and so on. However, the order described is the one in which I have most commonly observed appearance of the symptoms. Occasionally a patient may improve and return to a less advanced stage. Intravenous injections of sodium amytal do not produce any perceptible change in the picture of the terminal stage of schizophrenia.

INTERPRETATION

A genetic approach may help in explaining some of the habits described. In fact, it is possible to interpret them not as newly acquired habits but as behavior manifestations of lower levels of integration.

The food-grabbing habit reminds one of what is generally observed in cats, dogs, monkeys and other animals. The animal is coerced to react to the food, at the sight of it. The food does not stand for itself but is what Werner (3) calls a "thing of action." It is a "signal thing," the sight of which leads immediately to a fixed action. The animal cannot delay the reaction or channel the impulse into longer integrative circuits. Similarly, others of the habits previously described disclosed the same syncretic characteristics encountered in more primitive organizations. It is well known that when monkeys, dogs, cats and other animals are given at the same time different items of food, they eat first the preferred food (for instance, meat in case of the dog, or banana in case of the monkeys), and only when the entire portion of the preferred food is finished do they start to eat the other foods. They cannot alternate the various kinds but are coerced to react first to the strongest stimulus. Also, a $3\frac{1}{2}$ to 4 year old child, if not prevented, eats first the preferred food, and only when he has finished it does he eat the others.

When the patients become even sicker, this integration of the stimuli is seen as more primitive so that they react to edible and nonedible objects in the same way by grasping them and putting them into the mouth. The category of edibility is no longer respected. This "placing into mouth" habit was discussed in a previous report (2). It was there emphasized that a similar behavior is noted in children approximately 1 to 2 years of age. The similarity of this behavior to that observed by Klüver and Bucy (4) in monkeys which underwent removal of both temporal lobes was also discussed. There is one chief difference, however: Whereas the monkeys are described as smelling the grasped object before placing it into the mouth, children and deteriorated schizophrenic patients do not smell the object but put it immediately into the mouth. However, if the olfactory tracts of the monkeys were cut previous to removing both temporal lobes, no smelling was observed. Klüver and Bucy considered the monkeys with both temporal lobes removed as psychically blind (being unable to recognize the edible or nonedible nature of the objects in spite of the fact that they were trained before the operation to make this differentiation). I am inclined to consider the "placing into mouth" habit in deteriorated schizophrenic patients as a primitive response in the mechanism of which a short-circuiting takes place between the functions of reception and those of reaction, with exclusion of usual normal paths which involve higher centers. It may be that instead of the normal path a circuit is used similar to that involved in the relatively primitive physiologic complex which Edinger (5) called "oral sense." As happens in all other short-circuit reactions, an impulse or coercion to react, and not asymbolia, may be responsible for the "placing into mouth" habit. Klüver and Bucy considered as hopeless any attempt to reduce to one basic defect the polysymptomatic picture presented by their monkeys with bitemporal lobectomy. Although any comparison is hypothetic, it may be that these monkeys have this oral habit because after the surgical operation they are coerced to react to tridemensional visual stimuli and have to use short circuits. This consideration, however, does not deny the possibility that these monkeys are, at least partially, psychically blind. On the other hand, they probably are psychically blind, as considerations to be discussed later will indicate. The same inability to distinguish between edible and nonedible objects was also noted by Langworthy (6) in cats which underwent removal of both frontal poles. The tendency to grasp every object and to put it into the mouth was also reported by von Braunmühl and Leonhard (7) in cases of Pick's disease. It may be of some importance to mention also that I have noted the sudden occurrence of bulimia, tachyphagia and the "placing in mouth" habit after bilateral prefrontal lobotomy in a catatonic patient who had been sick for more than ten years.

The analgesia observed in some of the deteriorated patients may now be considered. Several authors have reported altered perception of pain in cases of early catatonia, and Bender and Schilder (8) discussed this subject in relation to the capacity to acquire conditioned reflexes. In my experience the hypesthesia found in patients with early catatonia is generally not so severe as that observed in patients who have reached the terminal stage, and often is not detected if, instead of pinprick, one uses stronger stimuli. Anesthesia for temperature and taste stimuli is even more rare in patients with early catatonia and is not comparable to that encountered in my patients, with conditions originally diagnosed as various types of dementia praecox. However, the possibility is not denied that the nature of the phenomenon may be the same. In many of the common textbooks on psychiatry no mention is made of this analgesia encountered in some deteriorated schizophrenic patients. Bleuler (9), however, described this phenomenon as follows:

> Worthy of note is an analgesia which occurs in schizophrenia not too rarely and which is sometimes quite complete. It is responsible for the fact that the patients readily injure themselves purposely or accidentally.

In agreement with the observations of Bender and Schilder on patients with early catatonia, I am inclined to believe that the real sensation of pain and temperature is not lost in my patients. The fact that the corneal reflexes are always retained may be a proof of it. However, these patients seem to be unaware of the painful and thermic stimuli and do not show any emotional reaction to them. They seem to be unable to perceive the stimuli. In other words, the rough sensation may be present but remains isolated and is not elaborated to the perception level. The patients are unable to recognize the emotional and cognitive value of the thermic and painful stimuli and therefore are unaware of the possible dangers which they at times imply. That is the reason that they often hurt themselves. These patients for all practical purposes have agnosia and may be compared to persons with sensorial aphasia who hear a spoken language without understanding it.

Is this loss of nociceptive perception only an exaggeration of the general schizophrenic emotional indifference? Probably the cause of these psychophysiologic derangements is the same, but for all practical purposes these patients are better described as having agnosia and may be termed "psychically analgesic," and not apathetic only. They fail to perceive pain and temperature sensation, not only from an emotional but from a cognitive point of view. That is the reason that they so often hurt themselves if they are not under constant supervision. The problem whether these phenomena are due to loss of emotional capacity or to loss of perception of pain and temperature sensation is probably only academic at present, when so little is known about emotivity and its relation to perception of pleasant and painful sensations. Herrick (10), who took into consideration this relation, stated: "Pain, considered psychologically and neurologically, is a sensation, and a different neurological mechanism for unpleasantness and pleasantness must be sought." Pain, however, is in normal conditions always associated with unpleasantness. In the patients described it is not. The relation between emotional indifference and agnosia has also been taken into consideration by von Monakow and Mourgue (11), who observed impairment of emotions in aphasic persons. In other publications (12) the same authors considered the possibility that asymbolia may be due to disturbances in the affective sphere.

The fact that taste perception is often lost or impaired in these analgesic patients and that the olfactory perceptions are preserved instead is also thought stimulating. The association of taste and pain asymbolias points to the conclusions that taste should be included among the general somatic sensations, as investigations by the school of Fulton (13) and by Shenkin and Lewey (14) seem to prove. The striking survival of smell perceptions, which are phylogenetically very old, may induce one to think that the archipallium is more resistant than the neopallium to the schizophrenic process. The olfactory sense, which is the dominant sense in lower vertebrates, seems to reacquire in some deteriorated schizophrenic patients a position of predominance among the senses, not because of increased acuity but because of impairment of perceptions of stimuli coming from other sensory fields. However, contrary to what is found in lower vertebrates, these schizophrenic patients do not take advantage of the olfactory sense as they could, possibly on account of their general volitional impairment or general withdrawal. It is interesting to observe that the sense of smell in schizophrenic patients is not involved even in short-circuiting reactions, whereas it was involved in the monkeys of Klüver and Bucy. The fact that perception and emotional reactions connected with the sense of smell are not impaired in many patients in the terminal phases of schizophrenia may be due instead to the peculiarity that the olfactory stimuli are the only sensory stimuli which do not pass up to the thalamus.

The last consideration may induce one to examine the possibility of anatomic interpretations of the symptoms described. Any interpretation of this kind has of course to be considered preliminary at the present time, when so much remains to be learned about the schizophrenic process. Furthermore, any deduction concerning human beings made from experimental observations on animals may be advanced only in a hypothetic way.

If, on the basis of reported observations, one were to localize an alleged pathologic process responsible for the release of the primitive habits previously described, one would probably have to incriminate the prefrontal lobes (Langworthy) and the temporal lobes, (Klüver and Bucy, von Braunmühl and Leonhard), and the lesions would have to be bilateral and presumably symmetric. The problem of localizing the process responsible for the analgesia is even more difficult, after the work of Head, although there is again much evidence that the parietal lobes are the site of sensation and perception of pain. Schilder and Stengel (15) found asymbolia for pain in cases of lesions of the gyrus supramarginalis; Bender and Schilder expressed the belief that it is impossible to deny the presence of a dysfunction of the same areas in catatonic patients presenting pain asymbolia. Patterson and Stengel (16) reported "apperceptive blindness" and asymbolia for pain in a case of Lissauer's dementia paralytica in which lesions in the parastriatal areas were present. Since in my patients pain asymbolia is often associated with taste asymbolia, or "psychic ageusia," it may be that the perceptual centers for taste and pain are located near each other. It has already been mentioned that recent investigations seem to confirm a parietal localization of the taste centers (17). These anatomic considerations are not solidly founded. However, one deduction has a certain probability of being correct. If, on the basis of the reported observations, one were to localize an alleged pathologic process responsible for the symptoms occurring in the terminal stage of schizophrenia, one would have to place it in the so-called silent areas, or great association areas, and not in the recognized primary cortical centers. These areas would, also, be approximately those which, according to the investigations of Flechsig (18) and Vogt (19), are the last to myelinate and the last to appear phylogenetically. Bilateral impairment of these great association areas would make impossible those "long-circuiting processes" mentioned by Fulton (20) and reemphasized by Cobb (21), and would be responsible for the occurrence of short-circuit processes manifesting themselves as primitive habits.

The theories of Orton (22) seem also confirmed by my observations. According to this author, three levels of cortical elaborations may be distinguished (22a). The first elaborative level, consisting of the so-called projection areas, or the arrival platform cortex, is the first to receive

stimuli of external origin. The second level, consisting of the areas surrounding the projection zones, or the arrival platform cortex, registers
and interprets the material arrived at the first level. The third level, consisting of the great associative areas, which are the last to myelinate, correlates the data brought in by the various pathways. According to Orton,
impairment of a level causes "cross over" of impulses from a lower level
to the effectors, so that primitive patterns of reactions are produced. He
called this return of primitive patterns "resurgence by defect" (22b).
Orton stated the opinion that in catatonia there is an impairment of
the third level of elaboration (22a). In extremely deteriorated schizophrenic patients one may assume that the third, and partially the second,
levels of elaboration are impaired. In this way it is possible to explain
both certain asymbolias and the short-circuiting processes which resurge
by defect. It is now also possible to understand better the complex symptoms reported in the valuable contributions of Klüver and Bucy (4). The
monkeys deprived of both temporal lobes also present visual asymbolia
and primitive habits ("placing into mouth" or "oral tendency"). Since
the great association areas have undoubtedly thalamic connections (23), it
may be possible to find an anatomic interpretation of the emotional
impairment.

All the foregoing evidence suggests, but does not demonstrate, that the
schizophrenic process either is organic in nature or at a certain stage is
associated with organic changes. Goldstein's (24) position when he stated
"I am inclined to assume that equivalent functional changes can be produced by organic, i.e., structural or clinical as well as by psychological
derangement" may be maintained. He spoke also of "protective deterioration," after having described certain similarities between the impairment
of abstract thinking associated with schizophrenia and that accompanying
organic lesions.

The new psychosomatic concepts may also be resorted to. If Weiss and
English's (25) formula, "psychologic disturbances → functional impairment → cellular disease → structural alteration," is accepted to explain
the pathogenic mechanisms of cardiovascular and gastrointestinal conditions, why should it not be accepted to explain derangement of the
nervous system, which is more directly under the fire of psychologic
stimuli? The functions or structures which are phylogenetically more
recent may be the ones more easily impaired, even by psychologic stimuli,
so that when, after a long course, the impairment is complete or almost
complete, resemblance may be obtained to lower levels of integration
which have not yet acquired such functions or structures. Thus, the terms

"regression" and "deterioration" would have the same meaning when applied to schizophrenic patients, unless by deterioration one wants to specify only the irreversibility of the syndrome; and for both may be substituted Lewis' (26) term "deviation."

REFERENCES

1. GOLDSTEIN, K.: *The Organism: A Holistic Approach to Biology Derived from Pathological Data in Man.* New York: American Book Company, 1939.
2. ARIETI, S.: The "placing-into-mouth" and coprophagic habits, studied from a point of view of comparative developmental psychology. *J. Nerv. & Ment. Dis.,* 99:959, June 1944.
3. WERNER, H.: *Comparative Psychology of Mental Development.* New York: Harper & Brothers, 1940.
4. KLÜVER, H. and BUCY, P. C.: (a) "Psychic blindness" and other symptoms following bilateral temporal lobectomy in rhesus monkeys. *Amer. J. Physiol.,* 119: 352, June 1937; (b) An analysis of certain effects of bilateral temporal lobectomy in the rhesus monkey, with special reference to "psychic blindness." *J. Psychol.,* 5:33, 1938; (c) Preliminary analysis of functions of the temporal lobes in monkeys. *Arch. Neurol. & Psychiat.,* 42:972, Dec. 1939.
5. EDINGER, L.: Ueber die dem Oralsinne dienenden Apparate am Gehirn der Säuger. *Deutsche Ztschr. f. Nervenh.,* 36:151, 1908-1909.
6. LANGWORTHY, O. R.: Behavior disturbances related to decomposition of reflex activity caused by cerebral injury: An experimental study of the cat. *J. Neuropath. & Exper. Neurol.,* 3:87, Jan. 1944.
7. VON BRAUNMÜHL, A. and LEONHARD, K.: Ueber ein Schwesternpaar mit Pickscher Krankheit. *Ztschr. f. d. ges. Neurol. u. Psychiat.,* 150:209-241, 1934; cited by Klüver and Bucy, 4c.
8. BENDER, L. and SCHILDER, P.: Unconditioned and conditioned reactions to pain in schizophrenia. *Amer. J. Psychiat.,* 10:365, Nov. 1930.
9. BLEULER, E.: *Textbook of Psychiatry.* Translated by A. A. Brill. New York: The Macmillan Company, 1924.
10. HERRICK, C. J.: *An Introduction to Neurology,* Ed. 5. Philadelphia: W. B. Saunders Company, 1931.
11. VON MONAKOW, C. V. and MOURGUE, R.: Introduction biologique à l'étude de la neurologie et de la psychopathologie. Paris: Félix Alcan, 1928.
12. VON MONAKOW, C. V.: Die Lokalisation in Grosshirn und der Abbau der Funktionen durch korticale Herde, Wiesbaden: J. F. Bergmann, 1914. Mourgue, R.: Neurobiologie de l'hallucination: Essai sur une variété particulière de désintégration de la fonction. Brussels: Maurice Lamertin, 1932; cited by Klüver and Bucy, 4c.
13. The following works are cited by J. F. Fulton: *Physiology of the Nervous System,* ed. 5. New York: Oxford University Press, 1943. (a) W. S. Börnstein: Cortical representation of taste in man and monkey: I. Functional and anatomical relations of taste, olfaction and somatic sensibility. *Yale J. Biol. & Med.,* 12:719, July 1940; (b) II. The localization of the cortical taste area in man and a method for measuring impairment of taste in man, *ibid.,* 13:133, Oct. 1940; (c) H. O. Patton and T. C. Ruch: *Thalamic and Cortical Localization of Taste in Monkey and Chimpanzee,* to be published.
14. SHENKIN, H. A. and LEWEY, F. H.: Taste aura preceding convulsions in a lesion of the parietal operculum. *J. Nerv. & Ment. Dis.,* 100:352, Oct. 1944.

15. SCHILDER, P. and STENGEL, E.: Asymbolia for pain. *Arch. Neurol. & Psychiat.*, 25: 598, March 1931.
16. PATTERSON, M. T., and STENGEL, E.: Apperceptive blindness in Lissauer's dementia paralytica. *J. Neurol. & Psychiat.*, 6:83, July 1943.
17. v. Fulton (13) and Shenkin and Lewey (14) above.
18. FLECHSIG, P.: *Ueber die Lokalisation der geistigen Vorgange insbesondere der Sinnesemfindungen des Menschen*, Leipzig: Veit & Co., 1896.
19. VOGT, O.: Der wert der myelogenetischen felder der grosshirnrinde. *Anat. Anz.*, 29:273, 1906.
20. FULTON, J. F.: *Physiology of the Nervous System*, ed. 4. New York: Oxford University Press, 1938. Cited by Cobb (21).
21. COBB, S.: *Foundations of Neuropsychiatry*. Baltimore: Williams & Wilkins Company, 1941.
22. ORTON, S. T.: (a) The three levels of cortical elaboration in relation to certain psychiatric symptoms. *Amer. J. Psychiat.*, 8:647, Jan. 1929; (b) Neuropathology: Lecture notes. *Arch. Neurol. & Psychiat.*, 15:763, June 1926; (c) Some neurologic concepts applied to catatonia, *ibid.*, 23:116, Jan. 1930.
23. ARIËNS KAPPERS, C. U., HUBER, G. C., and CROSBY, E. C.s *The Comparative Anatomy of the Nervous System of Vertebrates, Including Man*. New York: The Macmillan Company, 1936. Vol. 2.
24. GOLDSTEIN, K.: The significance of psychological research in schizophrenia. *J. Nerv. & Ment. Dis.*, 97:261, March 1943.
25. WEISS, E. and ENGLISH, O. S.: *Psychosomatic Medicine: The Clinical Application of Psychopathology to General Medical Problems*. Philadelphia: W. B. Saunders Company, 1943.
26. LEWIS, N. D. C.: Personal communication to the author.

11

The Possibility of Psychosomatic
Involvement of the Central Nervous
System in Schizophrenia

This paper, published in 1956, reaffirms the importance of correlating psychological disorders with studies of cerebral functions and expands previously reported data about the psychosomatic involvement of the CNS in schizophrenia.

THREE FACTORS have greatly handicapped neurology in its effort toward an understanding of psychological and psychopathological problems. The first factor is shared with the rest of medical sciences. Physicians, trained in the scientific tradition, are reluctant to use any method which is not strictly empirical. Mental constructions, working hypotheses, are generally frowned upon as armchair speculations, more appropriate to the field of philosophy than to the field of medicine, and complete reliance has been put upon laboratory experiments and clinical observations. Obviously it would be absurd to minimize the tremendous accomplishments obtained through clinical and experimental research. Nevertheless, physicians should once more compare their research with those in the fields of physics and chemistry, where great progress has been made by a combination of experiments and a formulation of theoretical hypotheses. Such an eminent scientist as James B. Conant (11) thinks that "the history of science demonstrates beyond a doubt that the really revolutionary and significant advances come not from empiricism but from new theories." Obviously, sooner or later it is necessary to submit any new theory to the empirical test. In spite of the predominant antitheoretical trend, even in the field of neurology, theoretical concepts like those of Jackson (21) and Goldstein (17) and the more recent theory of emotion advanced by Papez (34) have been very fruitful in stimulating important work.

The second factor which has delayed neurological progress toward psychological understanding consists of the poor use of data offered by related fields. For instance, it is the belief of the writer that a more intense application of a genetic approach, such as the one followed by Werner (38) in the field of psychology, and a greater use of the findings of Cassirer (10) and Langer (26) in their studies on the symbolic functions of the mind, could enrich neurology very much.

The third factor is the relative disregard of neurology which dynamically-oriented psychiatrists (with a few outstanding exceptions, like those of Grinker, Kubie, David Rioch, Ostow and E. Weinstein) have recently acquired. Overreacting to previous positivistic approaches, most of them feel that neurology has not much to offer to the understanding of dynamic psychology, and they tend to ignore this field, whereas they maintain much closer relations with other branches of medicine, like internal allergy, dermatology, etc.

The present writer is one of the dynamically-oriented psychiatrists who believe that neurology has great contributions to make to psychology if its boundaries are enlarged. He fully subscribes to DeJong's point of view, expressed recently in an editorial (12) that "Neurology is an expanding discipline, and it must not be limited by arbitrary boundaries —it must reach out beyond its customary confines."

An area where further expansion is urgently needed is the study of the central nervous system itself in the field of psychosomatic medicine. Only an historically-determined trend toward disconnecting psychiatry entirely from neurology is responsible for the fact that whereas every organ or system of the body (such as skin, cardiovascular and gastrointestinal apparatuses, etc.) has been recognized as affected by many psychosomatic disorders, the central nervous system has been given only secondary consideration. And yet the central nervous system is the organ of highest functionality; it is the organ which is first affected by psychogenic stimuli before they are channeled toward the other organs of the body. Could it not be that under a certain psychological stress a more or less specific functional disintegration of habitual neuronal patterns takes place?

In the following pages the author will consider the possibility of a functional alteration of the nervous system in schizophrenia. A study of the primary psychogenic factors which lead to the condition is beyond the purpose of this article, and therefore a complete interpretation of the disorder will not be attempted.

Whereas those authors who have been interested in determining the role of the central nervous system in schizophrenia have chiefly investigated the possibility of organic pathology, although histologic evidence was lacking or controversial, we shall be concerned with another problem, that is, what parts of the central nervous system are functionally involved in the symptomatology of schizophrenia.

It seems beyond doubt that most of the symptoms of schizophrenia, at least in the initial stage of the illness, are *mediated* through the cerebral cortex. This statement does not exclude the theoretical possibility of an extracortical pathology in the etiology of schizophrenia. The author of this article does not believe so, but some researchers think that some pathology of the diencephalon or of the pituitary-adrenal system is responsible for the disorder. However, even if such hypotheses could be confirmed, symptoms like delusions, hallucinations, ideas of reference, word-salad, etc., would have to be recognized as cortical phenomena, which could occur only in the presence of an extracortical pathology.

These symptoms involve high symbolic processes and require the function of the cerebral cortex, regardless of whether the cortex is in a normal or pathological condition, and regardless of whether a pre-existing extracortical pathology is necessary to enhance the disorder.

The second step in our thinking consists in determining what cortical areas are involved in the pathological symptoms of schizophrenia. At this point we may make a general statement, already implied in the foregoing: all the cortical areas, whose function is well known today, do not seem to be *primarily* involved in the symptoms of early schizophrenia. For instance, it is obvious that the motor, sensory, extrapyramidal areas, etc. are not primarily involved in schizophrenia. If a patient, as a result of a delusion, commits an absurd action, many cortical areas, like the visual, pyramidal, extrapyramidal, are of course involved in the execution of this action, but the participation of these cortical areas is not pathological *per se*. It is the motivation, the symbolic meaning and lack of control of the absurd action which are pathological. If we exclude the sensory and motor areas and the language centers as directly or originally involved in the psychopathology of schizophrenia, only three cortical areas are left to be considered. One is an ill-defined area including most of the temporal lobe and very small parts of the occipital and parietal lobes. We shall call this area TOP area (from *T*emporal, *O*ccipital, *P*arietal) (Figure 1). The second important area occupies the whole

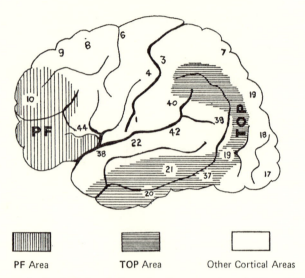

PF Area   TOP Area   Other Cortical Areas

FIGURE 1. Cerebral hemisphere showing extension of PF and TOP areas. Explanation in the text.

prefrontal area. We shall refer to this area with the abbreviation PF. The third area consists of the archipallium and mesopallium, including the rhinencephalon, the hippocampus, the cingulate gyrus and possibly the posterior orbital gyri. Part of this area borders on the TOP area. We shall take these three areas into consideration separately.

TOP AREA

Anatomically, this area includes a large part of the temporal lobe (Brodmann's areas 20, 21 and 37) and a small part of the parietal and occipital lobes, consisting of the most central parts of Brodmann's areas 7, 19, 39 and 40. The parietal part is crossed by the interparietal sulcus. Histologically in Nissl sections it resembles the structure of the sensory associative areas. It receives projections from the lateral thalamic nucleus and from the pulvinar. The part of area 19 which is included in the TOP area possibly belongs more to the parietal than to the occipital lobe. It also has projections from the pulvinar.

Much less is known anatomically of the temporal part of the TOP area. Krieg (25) calls this area one of the great *terrae incognitae* of the cortex. Thalamic connections to and from this part of the cortex have not been well established.

Phylogenetically the TOP area is one of the most recently evolved areas. Even such high species as Pithecanthropus Erectus and especially Homo Rhodesiensis had only a rudimentary development of this area, as may be deduced from Tilney's writings (36). Furthermore, together with other neopallic areas, it has no direct connections with the "reticular system" of the brain stem.

From a point of view of neuropathology, the TOP area is rather seldom involved in pathological conditions which could reveal its specific functions. Hemorrhages, softenings or neoplasms are generally unilateral. In addition they either do not involve the totality of this area or, if they do, they expand to surrounding regions.

In senile psychosis and cerebral arteriosclerosis the TOP area is involved less than the prefrontal area. Maybe this relative resistance to the senile or arteriosclerotic process is to be attributed to a different blood supply. Whereas the prefrontal area receives its supply mainly from the branches of the anterior cerebral arteries, the TOP area is irrigated by branches of all the three major arteries of the brain.

The TOP area is involved in Pick's disease, but this point will be taken into consideration later in this paper.

From a physiological point of view the TOP area may be considered as the center of functionality of a much larger area including the whole parietal, occipital and most of the temporal lobes. These three lobes form that part of the brain which receives stimuli from the external world and processes them into progressively higher constructs. We may divide this large part of the brain into four levels.

Before examining these four levels separately, however, we must make it clear that we do not consider them as sharply-defined physiological entities. Following the teaching of Jackson, when we attribute a function to a particular cortical area, we mean only that that function is represented predominantly but not exclusively in that area. The cortex is to be conceived not as a mosaic of distinct localizations, but as a pattern of overlapping representations, which are all more or less connected. These overlapping representations, however, have a relative concentration in certain areas. When we refer to levels, we refer only to these relative concentrations.

The first level consists of what Orton (33) called the arrival platforms. It includes the borders of the calcarine fissure, Heschl convolution, and the post-central gyrus (with other contiguous small areas of the parietal cortex and small portions of the pre-central gyrus). These are the areas where crude sensation occurs.

The second level is the level of perception or recognition. It consists of area 18 for vision, a portion of the first and maybe second temporal gyrus for hearing, and an undetermined area of the parietal lobe for general sensation. If lesion occurs at this level, the patient is not able to perceive, that is, to recognize what he experiences. He suffers from various forms of asymbolias like, for instance, psychic blindness. At this level conditioned reflexes occur. This is also the level at which the symbolic activity of the mind manifests itself in the form of *signs*. A sign is something which stands for something else which, however, is present or about to be present in the total situation of which the sign is a part (26). For instance, the ringing of the bell is the sign for the trained dog of the incoming food.

The third level (parts of Brodmann's areas 22, 39, 40, 19) is much more complicated. Although it may exist in a very rudimentary form even in some high infrahuman species, it is only in humans that it acquires prominence. The following are some of the functions of this complicated level:

As Nielsen (32) has described, voluntary recall of past sensations and experiences takes place at this level. This function implies some kind of primitive abstraction because in recalling one must separate or abstract a recognized experience from the other memories with which it was associated. The experience which was recognized at the second level is now abstracted from memories and voluntarily revisualized. In order to function in this way at this level, the subject must have the ability to reproduce mentally *the image* of the external stimulus. Images are not signs, but *symbols*, inasmuch as they stand for something which is *not present*. Since the images do not reproduce exactly the external objects, they are the most elementary creative functions of the individual. They retain an individual, private character and cannot be shared with any other human being.

At this level many other functions occur. Not only images, but external stimuli (caused or not caused by the individual) start to stand for something else which is not present, and, therefore, become *symbols*. Phylogenetically, symbols are preceded by *paleosymbols*, which are symbols valid only for the person who creates them. For instance, a person sees a connection between a sound and a situation or object, and that sound becomes the paleosymbol of the object or the situation. The paleosymbol becomes a symbol when its symbolic value has been accepted by at least a second person. The symbol produces in the person who pronounces it the same response that he produces in others (30). Verbal communication and socialization start at this level. For instance, if in a primordial human family one of the siblings happens to associate the sound ma-ma with the mother or with the image of the mother, and if a second sibling understands that the sound ma-ma refers to mother, language is originated. Language consists of *social* or *common symbols*. But at this level the sound ma-ma refers only to a particular mother, the mother of the two siblings, and not to any mother. In other words, the symbol ma-ma *denotes,* but does not possess much *connotation power* (1).

Lack of space does not permit a discussion of the connections of this third level with the frontal lobes, connections which permit an expansion of the faculty of speech. All the language centers belong to the third level although, as we shall see shortly, they would not have expanded without the influence of the fourth level.

Most authors follow Orton (33) in recognizing only the three mentioned levels of elaboration. According to the present author a fourth level must be differentiated, which anatomically consists of the TOP area (Brodmann's areas 20, 21, 37, parts of 7, 19, 39, and 40). This is the area where all the excitements coming from the lower levels are synthesized and elaborated into the highest mental constructs. Of course, as we have already mentioned, we must not consider this area as isolated or functioning by itself. First of all it is associated by fibers which pass through the corpus callosum, with the corresponding area of the opposite hemisphere. It is also connected with much lower structures through the archipallium. As we shall see shortly, it has important connections with the frontal lobes, without which it could not function at all. Furthermore, one should by no means think that only the TOP area is required for the highest mental processes. The neuronal network which mediates the highest mental processes extends to much lower levels. (See engram in Figure 2.) However, the highest engrams or esthesotypes, to use a very appropriate concept recently proposed by Mackay (29), need a place in the TOP area, almost as a center toward which all the associations of which they consist converge. The fact that the esthesotype extends to many lower levels has confused several researchers and has fallaciously led many to conclude that no cortical localization is possible and that what counts is only the extension of the cortical area.

But let us go back to the TOP area. In the opinion of the writer this area is needed for the highest processes of abstraction. These processes presuppose and require processes of socialization, which in simple forms have already started at the third level. As I have illustrated elsewhere, no high abstraction is possible if the individual in his development has

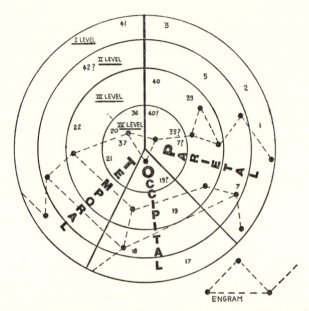

FIGURE 2. Diagram showing the four cortical levels of integration, represented schematically as four concentric areas in the temporal, occipital and parietal lobes. The numbers refer to Brodmann's areas. Explanation in the text.

not come into contact with other people (1). It is through contact with other human beings that verbal symbols continue to increase in number and that those previously acquired develop abstract meaning, that is, *connotation* or *categorical significance*. For instance, the term mother eventually refers not only to the mother of the individual or the mother of all the siblings, concept which is generally connected with one visual image, but to any mother, to mothers in general. In the TOP area, the thought processes become more and more elaborated and more distant from paleosymbols, images and perceptions. The TOP area also facilitates or permits the full expansion of the third level. In fact language would consist only of a few words, and only with *denoting* power, if processes mediated at the fourth level would not require a tremendous increase in vocabulary. This is another instance of the overlapping of levels which I have described elsewhere (1).

In Figure 2 the temporal (with the exception of the hippocampus and related structures), the occipital and the parietal lobes are represented in a circular diagram. The four concentric circles represent the four different levels of integration. At the center is located the TOP area toward which all the other levels of elaboration converge. Like all diagrams, this one is just intended as a didactical device and, as such, oversimplifies complicated neurological mechanisms. Among the important things which for sake of simplification are omitted in the diagram are: 1) The associations between the different parts of temporal, occipital and parietal lobes; 2) the associations with other cortical areas, like the frontal lobes; 3) the associations between the two hemispheres; 4) the cortico-subcortical associations. Furthermore, the spatial proportions of the different areas are not exactly respected.

In my opinion there is no doubt that the functions mediated in the TOP areas are altered in the schizophrenic syndrome. Coordinating the experiences of many authors with my own, I have described in detail elsewhere how in schizophrenia there is a gradual return from the abstract to the concrete, from a form of highly socialized symbolization to a form of symbolization which is decreasingly conceptual and social and more perceptual in character (1). Even the thought processes, deprived of abstract symbolization, abandon our common logic and become paleologic (2, 3, 4). At first the symbols lose the connotation power and denote only; then they become paleosymbols, that is, understood only by the patient; finally they become completely perceptualized or regressed to the levels of images or perceptions, as in the case of hallucinations. In other words, in schizophrenia there is a reluctance or inability to use engrams or esthesotypes which need neurons located in the TOP area. At first there is a tendency to lose only the functions of the neuronal patterns which include the central parts of the TOP areas; later, as the illness progresses, there is a tendency to avoid almost entirely the functions of neuronal patterns which require any part of the TOP areas, and there is an inclination to use only the functions mediated by the first, second and third levels. In other words, there is a reduction or simplification in the neopallic neuronal configurations of the highly symbolic mental processes.

The foregoing does not imply at all that the TOP areas of the two hemispheres are affected by some kind of organic pathology. The disintegration or loss of their functions may be viewed as psychogenic. Their functions, in fact, by permitting complicated interpersonal relations and human conflicts may engender the greatest anxiety in human beings.

With this partial or complete psychogenic elimination of the functions of the TOP areas, however, the schizophrenic does not obtain adjustment at a lower level of integration. In the process of evolution all the nervous areas readjust themselves, by means of new associations, every time a new area appears, changes or extends. The whole nervous system and especially the cortex is in a state of maladjustment when the TOP areas are in a state of decreased functionality, even if this decreased functionality is psychogenic in origin. In other words, the schizophrenic regresses but does not integrate at a lower level, just as an experimental animal of a species normally provided with the cortex does not integrate at a non-cortical level when the cortex is experimentally removed, because its whole organism is adjusted or attuned to the presence of the cerebral cortex. The schizophrenic's disintegration will continue. Furthermore, together with the eliminations of the functions of high levels (Jackson's negative symptoms), there is a resurgence of inhibited functions (Jackson's positive symptoms), such as paleologic thinking, perceptualization, etc.

In several patients whom I have examined after decades of illness and who were reduced to vegetative existence in back wards of state hospitals (5, 6), I have observed also agnosia to pain, temperature and taste, and a syndrome not too dissimilar from psychic blindness and primitive habits, reminiscent of the one described by Klüver and Bucy (22, 23, 24) in monkeys after bilateral removal of the temporal lobes. The crude sensations remained. It could be that in these patients the areas of functional impairment extended beyond the TOP areas and involved also the third level and part of the second.

PF OR PREFRONTAL AREA

For didactical purposes we have taken into consideration the TOP area first, but the prefrontal area is even more important in the psychogenesis of schizophrenia. The TOP areas elaborate the material coming from the external world, but it is the prefrontal areas which permit this elaboration to a degree where schizophrenogenic conflicts are possible.

Increasing evidence indicates that the functions of the PF areas are very important, even if these functions are hard to define and, to a certain extent, still obscure. In addition to control of some visceral functions, at least four psychological functions of the prefrontal lobes have so far been recognized. These four functions are certainly interrelated and possibly different manifestations or different degrees of the same basic process.

The first function is the ability to maintain a steadfastness of purpose against distracting impulses from the environment (28); in other words it is the function of focal attention. The importance of focal attention as a prerequisite for higher mental processes has been very well illustrated by Schachtel (36). As Schachtel writes, each act of focal attention does not consist just of one sustained approach to the object to which it is directed, but of several renewed approaches. Focal attention requires ability to suppress secondary stimuli and to delay the response.

It is obvious that the high elaborations of stimuli described in connection with the temporal, occipital and parietal lobes could not take place if this function of the prefrontal lobes would not permit it.

A second function of the prefrontal areas is the ability to anticipate the future. Whereas animals are able to anticipate events which occur only within a very short period of time (from a few seconds to a few minutes from the time the stimulus took place), man is able to anticipate mentally distant events. The importance of this faculty in the engendering of anxiety cannot be overestimated; in fact anxiety is based on *anticipation* of danger, as Freud has repeatedly shown. As I have written elsewhere in more detail, even without the faculty of distant anticipation, anxiety is possible, but only a short-circuited anxiety similar to that experienced by infrahuman animals (7). In animals, anxiety is experienced when the stimulus indicates a present danger, or a danger which will follow shortly after the stimulus, or when the animal is at the same time stimulated by two conflictful stimuli. In addition to this type of anxiety, human beings experience long-circuited anxiety, that is, an anxiety which is due to anticipation of distant danger. This anxiety persists even when the external stimulus has disappeared because the external stimulus is replaced by an internal one, that is, by a chain of mental processes which permit the anticipation of distant future. Anticipation of distant future would not be possible if the individual would not receive high forms of symbols from the third and fourth levels of the posterior brain. For instance, for the calf the mother cow exists only when he perceives her, that is, when the visual stimulus of the cow or another stimulus, which is simultaneously associated with the cow or follows at very brief interval, is perceived. But a man can think of his mother even when the mother is absent because he is able to substitute mother with the symbol "mother." The symbol "mother" places mother in the three temporal dimensions: past, present, future.

A third function of the prefrontal lobes is the ability to permit planned or seriatim functions. By seriatim functions is meant the organization or synthesis of skilled acts or thoughts into an orderly series (31). Although some high species, like monkeys and apes, are capable of simple seriatim series, this function expands very much in man. Seriatim functions imply ability 1) to anticipate a goal, and 2) to organize and synthesize acts or thoughts in a given temporal sequence for the purpose of reaching the anticipated goal (9).

The fourth function of the prefrontal lobe is the ability to make choices and to initiate the translation of the "mental" choice into a motor action.

Some experiments have proved that infra-human animals also learn to choose; that is, they learn what choice to make in certain experimental sets and what choice not to make (19, 39). These experiments are valuable in the study of "equivalent stimuli" and of a function of primitive abstraction, but do not really demonstrate the presence of the ability to choose as it exists in human beings. Long-circuited choice as it occurs in human beings implies: 1) inhibition of secondary stimuli, ranging from spurious stimuli to suggestions from other people (first function); 2) ability to anticipate the goal and the effect of a certain action as well as of other possible actions (second function); 3) planning the possible actions in a seriatim pattern (third function); 4) actually selecting one of the possible actions and initiating the movement, that is, translation of the plan into motor action.

These four steps actually include many substeps which cannot be taken into consideration here. We must emphasize once more, however, that these steps could not take place if the posterior brain would not provide high forms of symbolism.

Now there is no doubt that these functions of the prefrontal lobes are disturbed in schizophrenia. The one which comes first to our mind is the ability to anticipate the future. This function is an absolute prerequisite for long-circuited anxiety and is the basis of any complicated mental conflict. In schizophrenia it tends to be teleologically replaced by more primitive processes which require shorter circuits. The same thing could be repeated for seriatim thinking. Greenblatt and Solomon (18) feel also that the frontal lobe circuits sustain the emotional tension of the psychotic, and Freeman and Watts (14) have well described the importance of future anticipation in the engendering of psychoses. These functions do not seem to be very disturbed in well systematized paranoids, possibly because at the beginning of the illness these patients resort predominantly to the mechanism of projection in the attempt to remove anxiety. At a subsequent stage, however, these functions become impaired in paranoids too. The delusions change from the persecutory to the grandiose type and are more and more related to the present time: "I *am* a king."

The other prefrontal functions are also disturbed in schizophrenia. The ability to make choices or to translate thoughts into actions is particularly altered in catatonia, but this point will not be discussed here as the author plans to illustrate it in detail in another contribution. As to the ability for steadfastness or focal attention, we know that it is very much impaired in schizophrenics. Their span of attention is very limited.

ARCHIPALLIUM AND HYPOTHALAMUS

The archipallium and the hypothalamus may be thought of as playing an important role in schizophrenia. Since great importance is attributed today to these structures in the mechanism of emotions, we could even be inclined to think that an altered functionality of the archipallium could explain the affective impairment which is so pronounced in schizophrenia. One could even be induced to the hasty conclusion that the original cause of this mental condition is to be found in this part of the nervous system. At the present stage of our knowledge, such possibility cannot be denied categorically. However, to the author of this article such an interpretation seems improbable. The author, of course, is directed by the fundamental idea, which may prove wrong, that the first functions and structures to be affected in schizophrenia are the last to appear in phylogenesis. If a *primary* dysfunction of the archipallium, which is the most ancient part of the cortex, will be demonstrated, all the genetic theories which so far have proved so valuable in both the fields of neurology (Jackson) and of dynamic psychiatry (Freud) will collapse.

The author does not mean that the archipallium is not involved in schizophrenia. On the contrary, a neopallic dysfunction, even if functional, is bound to have important repercussions upon the archipallium too. If we follow again Jackson's principles, we may think that the hypofunctionality of neopallic areas must be accompanied by a release and hyperfunctionality of the archipallium. Since we know so little about the functions of the archipallium and of its single parts, we cannot explain how this release is manifested, or why, for instance, instead of increased emotionality we find decreased emotionality in schizophrenia. Of course, under the name archipallium many different structures are included whose interaction is almost completely obscure. The interesting study on cats by Bard and Mountcastle (8), however, may throw some light on this subject if their findings are valid for the human species too. These authors produced a state of placidity in cats by removing the neocortex. After this operation anger and sham rage could not occur, and nociceptive stimuli elicited only mild responses. However, if the same animals were subjected to removal of the gyrus cinguli or to other parts of the rhinencephalon, they became angry and ferocious. These interesting experiments seem to indicate that archipallic structures inhibit the hypothalamus. In other words the neocortex restrains the inhibitory functions of the rhinencephalon. If the neocortex does not function, the rhinencephalon increases its inhibitory function on the hypothalamus. This increased inhibition may explain also the impairment in the *expression* of emotion which we find in schizophrenia. It may, moreover, explain the defective homeostatic biochemical functions in schizophrenia which have been described by many authors (15, 20) and which are connected of course with the functions of the hypothalamus and of the visceral brain.

GENERAL INTERPRETATION

We shall recapitulate now what we have mentioned about the possibility of a psychosomatic involvement of the CNS in schizophrenia.

Whatever is the origin of the series of events which ultimately leads to the psychosis, the overwhelming anxiety, the difficult interpersonal conflicts, and the disturbing high forms of symbolism are predominantly mediated in those cortical areas which in this paper have been called the PF and the TOP areas. These areas are the highest in the evolutionary scale; they are the last to appear in phylogeny and the last to myelinize in ontogeny. They are probably the most vulnerable areas of the central nervous system from a functional point of view, at least in those people who have an hereditary predisposition to schizophrenia. This hereditary vulnerability may be direct, that is, immediately involving the functions of these two areas, or indirect, by disturbing another area whose normal functioning is a prerequisite for the good functioning of the PF and TOP areas. The impact of the psychological conflicts is too much to bear for a part of the central nervous system which is already genetically vulnerable. At times it may be too much to bear even if such hereditary predisposition does not exist. On the other hand, the hereditary vulnerability alone, without the psychogenetic factors, would not be enough to engender the disorder. A disintegration of the neuronal patterns which involve predominantly these two areas may take place, and a reintegration or formation of simpler circuits which use these high areas less, and eventually not at all, may follow.

This neuronal reintegration may thus be seen deterministically and also adaptationally or restitutionally. In fact, there seems to be a psychosomatic attempt to return to lower levels of integration, levels which do not permit complicated interpersonal symbolism and long-circuited anxiety. Orton (33) too thought that shorter circuits or cross-overs are used in schizophrenia and especially in catatonia, but he thought that the process involved was organic and affected specifically the centers connected with the longer circuits.*

In the writer's conception, at the same time that these cortical centers or parts of them are in a state of psychosomatic hypofunctionality, other centers or some other parts of them, or some lower neuronal configurations or patterns are released and cause characteristic symptoms. Hughlings Jackson's concepts are valid in relation to schizophrenia too. For instance, when logical thinking is impaired, paleological thinking comes to the surface. When social symbols disappear, paleosymbols replace them. Concepts become more and more perceptual, and anticipation of the future is replaced by thoughts concerning the present.

One could raise the objection that an organic condition affecting *bilaterally* the PF and the TOP areas should give a symptomatology similar to schizophrenia, but that so far this occurrence has not been reported. Actually the only organic disease which would approximate a bilateral involvement of these areas, and these areas exclusively, is Pick's disease. In Pick's disease the symptomatology is similar to that found in cases of very regressed schizophrenics, who have been sick for many years, but has very little in common with the symptomatology of early cases. In both Pick's disease and schizophrenia there is an impairment of the abstract attitude described by Goldstein, that is, there is occurrence of Jackson's negative symptoms. However, in schizophrenia there is also a resurgence of many positive symptoms (paleologic thought, hallucinations, etc.) which are not present in Pick's disease. This may be due to the fact that in Pick's disease, as well as in other organic conditions, several levels are affected at the same time, and therefore a release of inferior cortical processes is prevented. We know in fact from neuropathological studies how diffuse are the alterations. In Pick's disease they do not involve only association areas, but also primary centers and many subcortical structures (13). Even when the lesions are patchy, we can hardly believe that they selectively involve only some higher neu-

---

* The material in italics has been inserted for this volume.

ronal configurations and respect lower. This state of affairs explains why Jackson's positive symptoms are not so clearly seen in organic conditions which involve the cortex. Functional conditions involving the cortex are in my opinion a better demonstration of Jackson's concepts than the organic. For instance, Goldstein's studies, which concern predominantly organic cases, have emphasized the impairment of the abstract attitude but have not sufficiently studied the characteristics of the re-emerging concrete attitude, because these characteristics can hardly appear when several levels or sublevels are affected at the same time.

Re-emerging primitive functions as a rule are not useful to the patient although they include also those restitution symptoms studied by Freud (16). In fact, as we have already mentioned, the regressed patient does not become adjusted, but maladjusted at a level at which he cannot integrate. The hypofunctionality of the neopallic areas which we have examined must also alter associations with other areas, not only the neighboring one but also the distant, through long association bundles, commissures like the corpus callosum, the corticothalamic and thalamocortical tracts, etc. This is a process of functional diaschisis, similar to the organic diaschisis described by Von Monakow (37). Direct connections of these neopallic areas with the brain stem reticular system do not seem to exist (27). The brain stem reticular system is of ancient origin and seems more concerned with the basic physiological than with the symbolic functions of life. However, undoubtedly indirect connections exist through the archipallium.

We may visualize in schizophrenia also a process which may be called functional *dysencephalization,* in a certain way the opposite of *encephalization.* As it is well known, with the latter term some neurologists have called the shifting toward higher centers of the functions which in lower species are mediated by lower or more caudal centers. In schizophrenia the opposite takes place: not only is there a return of the functions of the released lower center but also a tendency of the function of the higher center to be mediated by the lower center. For instance, often abstract thought processes which take place in the highest centers are mediated instead at a perceptual level and become auditory hallucinations.

The three processes of the re-emergence of lower functions, of functional diaschisis and of dysencephalization determine a state of dysequilibrium and of psychological splitting, which is so characteristic of this mental disorder. How does the organism defend itself from this disorganization? With further regression. The process thus repeats itself in a vicious circle that leads to complete dilapidation. This circular process is one of the characteristics of functional regression which is lacking in organic conditions. In the latter we may have the phenomenon of diaschisis, but there is not complete disintegration because the resurgence of the functions of lower levels or sublevels is minimal in comparison to functional conditions. If further deterioration occurs, it is only because the organic process itself expands or produces other damages, like gliosis, hydrocephalus, hemorrhages, etc. Some intoxications, however, just as those caused by mescaline, may be selective enough in their physiological action to reproduce a specific cortical hypofunctionality, and subsequent subcortical dysfunctions, similar to the ones occurring in schizophrenia.

In conclusion the schizophrenic process may be viewed as a psychosomatic or teleologic attempt to integrate the patient at a lower level. With comparatively few exceptions, however, this attempt fails because the process engenders other self-perpetuating mechanisms which lead to regression. An artificial partial attempt to integrate the schizophrenic at a lower level is, of course, made by frontal leucotomy and other psychosurgical procedures. These procedures have scientific validity because they remove, at least partially, the functions of such areas as the PF and do not unchain progressive regression. However, whether one should change a psychosomatic disorder for one which, together with symptoms, removes permanently a great part of the essence of man and reduces him to an almost infrahuman state, appears questionable to those who today see an increasing hope in the psychotherapeutic approach.

SUMMARY

Two areas of the cerebral cortex are considered very important in mediating the symptomatology of schizophrenia. The first area includes a large part of the temporal lobe (Brodmann's areas 20, 21 and 37) and small parts of the parietal and occipital lobes (central sections of Brodmann's areas 7, 19, 39 and 40). The second area includes the prefrontal lobes. It is demonstrated how in schizophrenia there is a gradual impairment or decrease in the functions of these areas and a return of primitive mechanisms. A third area, which consists of the archipallium, is also considered very important in the symptomatology of schizophrenia, but only secondarily involved.

The described cortical impairment is considered psychogenic, aiming at a return to levels of organization where overwhelming anxiety, derived from high forms of symbolism, cannot be experienced. The process is thus seen as a teleologic regression which, however, fails inasmuch as it brings about nervous mechanisms which complicate rather than simplify the dysequilibrium.

REFERENCES

1. ARIETI, S.: *Interpretation of Schizophrenia.* New York: Brunner, 1955.
2. ARIETI, S.: Autistic thought. Its formal mechanisms and its relationship to schizophrenia. *J. Nerv. & Ment. Dis.,* 111:288, 1950.
3. ARIETI, S.: Special logic of schizophrenic and other types of autistic thought. *Psychiatry,* 11:325, 1948.
4. ARIETI, S.: Primitive intellectual mechanisms in psychopathological conditions. Study of the archaic ego. *Amer. J. Psychother.,* 4:4, 1950.
5. ARIETI, S.: The placing into mouth and coprophagic habits. *J. Nerv. & Ment. Dis.,* 99:959, 1944.
6. ARIETI, S.: Primitive habits and perceptual alterations in the terminal stage of schizophrenia. *Arch. Neurol. & Psychiat.,* 53:378, 1945.
7. ARIETI, S.: The processes of expectation and anticipation. Their genetic development, neural basis and role in psychopathology. *J. Nerv. & Ment. Dis.,* 102:367, 1947.
8. BARD, P. and MOUNTCASTLE, V. B.: Some forebrain mechanism involved in the expression of rage with special reference to suppression of angry behavior. *Res. Pub., A. Nerv. & Ment. Dis.,* 27:362, 1947.
9. BRICKNER, R. M.: *The Intellectual Functions of the Frontal Lobes; a Study Based upon Observation of a Man Following Partial Bilateral Frontal Lobectomy.* New York: Macmillan, 1936.
10. CASSIRER, E.: *The Philosophy of Symbolic Forms.* New Haven: Yale University Press, 1953.
11. CONANT, J. B.: *Modern Science and Modern Man.* New York: Columbia University Press, 1952.
12. DEJONG, R. N.: Editorial. *Neurology,* 5:353, 1955.
13. FERRARO, A. and JERVIS, G.: Pick's disease. Clinicopathologic study with report of two cases. *Arch. Neurol. & Psychiat.,* 36:739, 1936.
14. FREEMAN, W. and WATTS, J. W.: *Psychosurgery.* Springfield, Ill.: Charles C Thomas, 1942.
15. FREEMAN, H. and CARMICHAEL, H. T.: A pharmacodynamic investigation of the autonomic nervous system in schizophrenia. *Arch. Neurol. & Psychiat.,* 33:342, 1935.
16. FREUD, S.: Psychoanalytic notes upon an autobiographical account of a case of paranoia (dementia paranoides). *Collected Papers,* 111:387, 1946.
17. GOLDSTEIN, K.: *The Organism. A Holistic Approach to Biology Derived from Pathological Data in Man.* New York: American Book Company, 1939.
18. GREENBLATT, M., and SOLOMON, H. C.: *Frontal Lobes and Schizophrenia.* New York: Springer Publishing Co., 1953.
19. HAMILTON, G. V.: A study of trial and error reactions in mammals. *J. Anim. Behav.,* 1:33, 1911.
20. HOSKINS, R. G.: *The Biology of Schizophrenia.* New York: Norton, 1946.
21. JACKSON, J. H.: *Selected Writings.* London: Hoder and Stoughton, 1932.
22. KLÜVER, H. and BUCY, P. C.: "Psychic Blindness" and other symptoms following bilateral temporal lobectomy in rhesus monkeys. *Amer. J. Physiol.,* 119:352, 1937.

23. KLÜVER, H. and BUCY, P. C.: An analysis of certain effects of bilateral temporal lobectomy in the rhesus monkey with special reference to "psychic blindness." *J. Psychol.*, 5:33, 1938.
24. KLÜVER, H. and BUCY, P. C.: Preliminary analysis of functions of the temporal lobes in monkeys. *Arch. Neurol. & Psychiat.*, 42:972, 1939.
25. KRIEG, W. J. S.: *Functional Neuroanatomy.* Philadelphia: The Blakiston Co., 1947.
26. LANGER, S. K.: *Philosophy in a New Key.* Harvard University Press, 1942.
27. LIVINGSTON, R. B.: Some brain stem mechanisms relating to psychosomatic medicine. *Psychosom. Med.*, 17:347, 1955.
28. MALMO, R. B.: Interference factors in delayed response in monkeys after removal of frontal lobes. *J. Neurophysiol.*, 5:295, 1942.
29. MACKAY, R. P.: Toward a neurology of behavior. *Neurology*, 4:894, 1954.
30. MEAD, G. H.: *Mind Self and Society.* University of Chicago Press, 1934.
31. MORGAN, C. T.: *Physiological Psychology.* New York: McGraw-Hill, 1943.
32. NIELSEN, J. M.: *Agnosia, Apraxia, Aphasia. Their Value in Cerebral Localization.* New York: Hoeber, 1946.
33. ORTON, S. T.: The three levels of cortical elaboration in relation to certain psychiatric symptoms. *Amer. J. Psychiat.*, 8:647, 1929.
34. PAPEZ, J. W.: A proposed mechanism of emotion. *Arch. Neurol. & Psychiat.*, 38: 725, 1937.
35. SCHACHTEL, E. G.: The development of focal attention and the emergence of reality. *Psychiatry*, 17:309, 1954.
36. TILNEY, F.: *The Brain from Ape to Man.* New York: Hoeber, 1928.
37. VON MONAKOW, C. V.: *Die Lokalisation in Grosshirn und der Abbau der Functionen durch Korticale.* Wiesbaden: Bergman, Herde, 1919.
38. WERNER, H.: *Comparative Psychology of Mental Development.* Chicago: Follet, 1948.
39. YERKES, R. M.: Modes of behavioral adaptation in chimpanzees to multiple choice problems. *Comp. Psychol. Mono.*, 10, 1934.

Part II
OTHER PSYCHIATRIC ISSUES

12

The Present Status of Psychiatric Theory

The cogent issues in psychiatric theory as they appeared to me in 1968, are reviewed here. Biochemical and hereditary theories are not included in this review. The conclusion is reached that the mind-body split remains as an unsolved problem and a focus of discomfort for theoreticians. It is also concluded that while many concepts of classic and neo-Freudian psychoanalysis must be recognized as valuable and durable contributions, others are in need of revision. Cognition must be given a much larger role.

INSOFAR AS ALL sciences contain elements which are not observable or operationally definable, theories play a basic role. They are hypotheses or provisional interpretations of facts which make the facts easier to interpret, integrate, and unify. Also, they open up possibilities of further inquiry. However, when they are accepted on faith, as if their validity had already been proven, they may become straitjackets which prevent further growth.

Theory is of fundamental importance in psychiatry too. The present article cannot include all or most aspects of this vast subject but will be limited to a critical review of the main contemporary issues. Because it would require much more space than is available, one major issue— general psychiatry versus existentialism—will not be considered.

THE NEUROPSYCHIATRIC SPLITTING

The mind-body problem, of which man has been aware since early history, has been a source of discomfort to most thinkers, especially since Descartes. In our field it appears under the form of the neuropsychiatric splitting. Just as many philosophers have tried to explain that there is an underlying unity that comprehends both physical and mental phenomena, so there are a proportionally comparable number of psychiatrists who advocate neuropsychiatric unity. But at this stage of our knowledge this professed unity discloses a splitting.

Griesinger can be considered the founder of the neuropsychiatric school of thought, which still prevails in many countries. Shortly before his death he wrote: "Psychiatry and neurology are not merely two closely related fields; they are but one field in which only one language is spoken and the same laws rule" (42). Actually, Griesinger and many generations of neuropsychiatrists tried to subsume psychiatry under neurology (or neuropathology). For such an outstanding psychiatrist as Kraepelin, general paresis remained the paradigm of mental disease.

The cultural climate of the 19th and beginning of the 20th centuries predisposed one to view the realm of the mental under the larger category of the physical. As we shall see in greater detail in the next section, Freud himself, who, more than anybody else illustrated the importance of psychological factors, tried to interpret them as manifestations of a quantifiable, probably physical, energy.

The splitting persists in several forms, and psychiatrists of various orientations have tried to overcome it or bypass it in different ways. For instance, several authorities oppose the use of the words organic and functional to distinguish psychiatric disorders on the grounds that an organ must always be there to mediate a function. Cobb wrote: "Every symptom is both functional and organic" (14). As I wrote elsewhere (3), in the neuropsychiatric frame of reference, Cobb's statement is perfectly valid: Every symptom is functional inasmuch as it consists of a physiological function, and organic, inasmuch as it requires the organ that mediates it, either in its anatomical integrity or in its pathological alterations. The statement, however, carries the implicit admission that such states as the functional and the organic do exist. Even if we could find, to use Eccles' formulation (17), that some specific spatio-temporal patterns of neuronal activity evoke particular sensory experiences, we would ascertain only an empirical association but would not explain the transformation of a physical phenomenon into a mental one.

Recent works by neuroanatomists, neurophysiologists, and neurosurgeons have enlightened the biological aspect of human behavior and seem to point toward a materialistic or interactionist interpretation of the problem. It is relevant to mention here Papez's theory of emotion (31), which opened up paths of inquiry and recognized the role of the archipallium in mediating emotional experiences, MacLean's studies of what he called the visceral brain (28), Moruzzi's and Magoun's pioneer work on the reticular system (29), Penfield's stimulations of the cerebral cortex (32), Hebb's theory of cell-assembly as explanation of psychological phenomena (24), and Eccles' works on the physiology of nerve cells and membrane (16).

Psychosomatic medicine, by trying to explain how much the mind effects the body, perpetuates the dichotomy. However, as reported in a monograph edited by Felix Deutsch (15), the contributors almost unanimously adhered to a monistic orientation and felt that there is no longer need to talk, as Freud did, of a "mysterious leap" from the psychic to the physiologic, or vice versa. One of the contributors was again Cobb, who wrote:

> I maintain that there is no leap at all for one who believes that mind is not a supernatural phenomenon but is *the active integration of the billions of nerve cells and hundreds of cell masses of the living brain.* Mind is a function of the brain just as contraction is a function of muscle or as circulation is a function of the blood-vascular system. (Italics are Cobb's.)

A philosopher would not be satisfied with Cobb's statement. Even if we would know how the integration of the billions of nerve cells occurs, we could not explain how and why this integration would give origin to such completely different phenomena as the psychological processes. Putting into one category the functions of muscles, cardiovascular system, and subjective psychological phenomena means assuming as already solved the problem which still needs solution.

In an altogether different formulation, Szasz too manifests distaste for the dualistic mind-body conception (39). By insisting that mental illness is a myth and has only a vague resemblance to physical illness, by stressing that the practice of psychiatry deals "with personal, social and ethical problems in living," and by translating psychopathology into a frame of reference where the terminology of "sign-using, rule-following, social roles, and game-playing" is adopted, he seems to adhere to a mentalistic orientation. Perhaps future writings of this stimulating author will show how he tries to overcome the dichotomy.

Von Bertalanffy also has made a profound study of the mind-body problem. He writes that he does not believe that he will "arrive at final solutions dear to the heart of philosophers, but [that he] may make some progress relevant to psychological theory and psychiatric practice" (13). He postulates an isomorphism between the constructs of psychology and neurophysiology: not a naive isomorphism which implies a photographic similarity between psychological and brain processes but a correspondence between psychological events and special codes and programs which are mediated by the nervous system.

He believes that neurophysiology and psychology can be further unified. No attempt should be made to "reduce" the one to the other; rather, one should seek a generalized theory which could be applied to both. He believes that recent theoretical formulations, like those constructed in cybernetics, information theory, general system theory, game and decision theory, are applicable to both fields. I agree that general system theory and cybernetics have so far made the most convincing inroad into this obscure problem. However, I cannot see how these theories can explain the phenomenon of subjective or private experience.

In conclusion, the mind-body or neuropsychiatric split remains a focus of discomfort for by far the majority of psychiatrists who are concerned with theory. A monistic conception would appeal more to our sense of "theoretical elegance"; it would satisfy our need for consistency and would appear more congruous with prevailing scientific positions. However, we cannot, in a form of obstinate psychological denial, bluntly state that the problem does not exist; nor can we hide it under terminological screens or belittle it with semantic euphemisms. The truth is that we have not solved it and that we must live with it, until, or unless, an unforeseeable breakthrough—a superior synthesis—will eliminate it. Recent outstanding accomplishments in the field of molecular biology, such as the discovery of the cellular processes responsible for the acquisition and transmission of genetic information, may not only not fill but, on the contrary, widen the gap between the level of our knowledge of general biology and that of psychology.

CLASSIC PSYCHOANALYSIS AND GENERAL PSYCHIATRY

The problem of the relation between general psychiatry and classic psychoanalysis is at the present time the one which is receiving the most consideration from psychiatric theoreticians, and probably is second in importance only to the mind-body problem. In a historical review from antiquity to modern times, including all the great contributors from Aretaeus to Karl Menninger, no author could be picked who had greater impact in the field of psychiatry than Sigmund Freud.

In spite of Freud's towering position, psychiatry need not accept the whole Freudian theory. Every psychiatrist today uses such concepts or premises as the prominent role of early life; the psychodynamic denouement of psychological factors; the symbolic aspect of behavior and mental processes, including dreams; the existence of an inner psychological reality as important as the external; the unconscious state of a large part of our mental processes; a special relation or transference, to be used as a therapeutic tool. Other psychiatrists, myself included, would add the proposition that mental processes may be divided into primary and secondary.

Such a list of discoveries and/or theoretical formulations is so impressive that one of its items would have been enough to immortalize Freud. This list does not need to be enlarged. In my opinion, the following major tenets of classic psychoanalysis cannot, at this stage of our knowledge, be included in the body of general psychiatry:

a. The Libido Theory

This theory is based on the proposition that psychological phenomena, including neurotic and psychotic disorders, should be interpreted "in terms of the economics of the libido" (20). This libido, as a type of energy, was for a long time identified by the Freudian school with sexual tension, even if deviated from the proper genital patterns and directed toward oral and anal outlets or sublimated into other psychological phenomena.

Recently this energy has been viewed less as sexual and more as a psychic energy which is used in all mental functions. Arlow and Brenner (11) refer to it as a mental energy, which derives from the id. It could be free or bound, sublimated and neutralized. However, there is no evidence that such energy exists. A concept like that of force can be used metaphorically for connoting psychological factors which have the power to produce certain effects. The term should not be used literally, in the way it is generally applied to physical energies, like the hydraulic, thermic, or electric.

Motivation, as a tendency to seek pleasure and to avoid unpleasure, is certainly a fundamental psychological factor and is based on the feelings of the organism: that is, on sensation, emotion, and other physiological experiences. Physiologists have repeatedly stated that it is not necessary to postulate the existence of investments of special energy (cathexes) to explain the occurrence of motivation (27). Unconscious motivation is a more complicated phenomenon which requires the understanding of what occurs beyond awareness, and does not necessitate a cathectic interpretation.

The adoption of the libido theory is considered by some as deriving from Freud's need to remain in a biological frame of reference. Actually, the libido or drive-cathexis theory is not a biological theory; it is an application to the psyche of concepts borrowed from the inorganic field of physics. But concepts which are applicable to the inorganic world (at least, as it was seen by 19th-century physicists) are not necessarily relevant to biological levels of integration. In the libido theory, general biology and neurophysiology are bypassed. The leap is from inorganic physics to psychology.

Early in his professional life, Freud made strong efforts to interpret psychological phenomena in a quantitative system of reference. The principle of inertia, constancy, the notion of Q, are all attempts made by Freud, during his writing of the Project, to explain psychological phenomena in terms of physics and economics. All these attempts failed and he never published the Project (18). When shortly afterwards he minimized considerations of economics and physics and focused on psychological phenomena, he wrote that classic of all times, *The Interpretation of Dreams,* which remains his masterpiece (19). But the idea of giving a quantitative-energetic interpretation of psychological phenomena continued to prey on Freud's mind, so that in his subsequent writings, including his revisions of *The Interpretation of Dreams,* he had to return to the economic point of view.

b. The Concept of Id

When Freud abandoned the topographic theory and adopted the structural, he could no longer equate the unconscious with the most primitive part of the mind. This primitive part he called the id. It is from the id that the other parts of the psyche (ego and superego) would eventually differentiate. The concept of id has remained a nebulous one. Freud contradicted himself on this issue many times.

Most of the time the id is conceived as an unstructured reservoir of energy—the source of instincts (10). Freud referred to it as "a chaos, a cauldron of seething excitement" (21). Yet psychoanalytic literature very frequently refers to motivation, memories, symbols, mechanisms, and archaic processes which originate in the id. How is this possible, if the id has no structure whatsoever but is only a reservoir of energy and instincts? If the instincts have to be expressed in the forms of primitive wishes, where are the wishes formed? Where is the psychic representation of the wish mediated?

Many analysts of the Freudian school realize that it is increasingly difficult to accept the original formulation of the id. For some of them, for instance Schur (35) and Holt (25), it is impossible to conceive an id without structure. By structure, we must mean predominantly immature forms of cognition. For the last 20 years I have illustrated in several publications the various forms of immature cognition (1-9). These writings have been almost completely ignored by classic psychoanalysts.

A way to obviate the difficulty inherent in the concept of id is to eliminate altogether the division of the psyche into id, ego, and superego, and to assume in its place a hierarchy of levels of psychological integration. We may retain, after Freud, the designation of primary process for all forms of immature functioning and the designation of secondary process for all forms of mature, even if incorrect, functioning. These levels of integration may function harmoniously or disharmoniously, in conjunction or in partial autonomy. Under the influence of Darwin, many prominent authors of various orientations—Hughlings Jackson (26), Kurt Goldstein (23), Heinz Werner (41), and Jean Piaget (33)—have advocated a developmental hierarchical structure of the psyche.

c. The Genetic Fallacy

The proposition that initial conditions determine fully the subsequent course of psychological phenomena leads to the genetic fallacy. In fairness, we must specify that several psychoanalysts, for instance Rapaport (34), speak of overdetermination: that is, of the fact that more than one and often several causes determine given psychological events. However, the prevailing attitude in many psychoanalytic circles, at least until not too long ago, was that conditions occurring very early in life determine what will take place in subsequent ages. There is no doubt that childhood conditions are extremely important, much more so than conditions occurring in subsequent ages. Nevertheless, we should not make the error of considering them the *exclusive* determinants of psychological events.

In the terminology of general system theory, the psyche is not a closed system but an open system; that is, open to continuous influences from factors occurring outside the system (12). Psychopathological structures are also open systems. If they were closed systems they would follow psychological entropy and would soon disappear. Psychopathological conditions, too, are states of various degrees of improbability, which are maintained by negative psychological entropy coming from outside of the original system.

Also, motivation, conscious or unconscious, cannot be accepted in a Freudian sense as a tendency moving only toward the gratification of infantile strivings, wishes, etc. In one of his last formulations, Freud wrote: "The symptoms of neuroses are exclusively, it might be said, either a substitute satisfaction of some sexual impulse or measures to prevent such a satisfaction, and are as a rule compromise between the two" (22). In a large part of classic psychoanalytic literature, not only neurotic behavior but every kind of behavior, including creative activity, is interpreted as based on the satisfaction of sexual instincts or other simple emotional or psychological states, or on the displacement or sublimation of such states. Simple levels of physio-psychological organization, such as states of hunger, thirst, fatigue, need for sleep, sexual urges, or relatively simple emotions, such as fear about one's physical survival, are powerful dynamic forces and require many additional studies. However, they do not include the motivational factors which are possible only at higher levels of development where highly cognitive processes are possible.

Although motivation can be understood as a striving toward pleasure or avoidance of unpleasure, *gratification of the self or the self-image (and not necessarily of one's instincts) becomes the main motivational factor at a conceptual level of development.* Concepts like inner worth, personal significance, mental outlook, appraisals reflected from others, attitudes toward ideals, aspirations, capacity to receive and give acceptance, affection, and love are integral parts of the self and of the self-image, together with the emotions which accompany these concepts. To think that these emotional factors, which are sustained by complicated cognitive processes, are only displacements or rationalizations which cover more primitive instinctual drives is a reductionist point of view.

d. Neglect of Nonmotivational Factors

As Thomas (40) and others have emphasized, not all factors which have a dynamic or psychological effect are to be subsumed under the heading of motivation. Physical factors also may have dynamic effect. For instance, a child may, on account of physical or biological deviance, present a type of behavior which will have an adverse effect on the mother. The mother's negative reaction may in its turn have an adverse effect on the child. The circular chain of events will have psychogenetic effects which are not motivated.

Another important characteristic, which deserves to be stressed more than it is generally done in psychoanalytic circles, is that the consequence of behavior is different from the intention or motive of such behavior. Thus an aloof, detached person, who is so because of shyness or difficulty in interpersonal relations, may be experienced by others as having a superior, disdainful attitude. This interpretation leads to a negative attitude on the part of the others, which in its turn leads to a reinforcement of the aloofness or detached behavior in the patient. Paranoid behavior too leads to hostile reactions, which in their turn reinforce the paranoid attitude of the patient. That the effect of behavior goes far beyond the intention of the person who manifests such behavior is common knowledge to the students of other sciences of man, such as sociologists and historians, but some of us, psychiatrists and psychoanalysts, have forgotten this truism.

Psychopathology may originate from false interpretations or distortions which are not necessarily motivated. The lingering of primary process cognition in children who are exposed to adverse environmental conditions may impart some abnormal conceptions of the world and behavior habits which will continue to affect the individual as symptoms, even in the adult life (8). Also conceptions, habits, and emotional responses, automatically acquired from the family or society at large and taken for granted as correct, may lead to distortions and pathological developments, not motivated as such.

e. Confusion Between Motivation and Volition

Most psychoanalytic authors seem to deny will altogether and accept only the existence of motivation as the psychological determinant of action. According to this point of view, every act is motivated (or caused by a wish or drive), not freely chosen. Thus the will does not determine the choice, but the motivation (conscious or unconscious) does, or the strongest of the possible contrasting motivations. If motivation removes the possibility of free choice, then the only act of free will would be the one which is not motivated. But an act which is not motivated at all is not performed voluntarily by any human being—it is automatic.

Some psychoanalysts believe that everything follows conscious or, most of the time, unconscious determinism and that we fool ourselves into believing what we choose. For instance, acting against wish A is an effect of wish B. But even wish B, which on the surface looks like a willful determination, rests on another unconscious wish C. At this stage of knowledge it is impossible to dismiss altogether the psychological importance of will and choice as different from wish-directed motivation (7). Yet will and free choice do not play an important role in the mainstream of psychoanalytic thought.

*f. Therapeutic Effect as Resulting Only from Making
Conscious What Is Unconscious*

Psychoanalytic therapy in its classical conception is viewed more or less as an act of liberation. The suffering individual is liberated from unconscious burdens, fixations, repressions, defenses, etc., and once this act of liberation has been accomplished the personality is supposed to make its own adjustment. In order to be cured, the patient is supposed not just to acquire insight, that is, knowledge that his symptoms are manifestations of illness, but also to undo the repressions and restore to consciousness the full conflict which was eliminated from awareness because it was unbearable. The patient thus must understand the origin, development, and dynamic meaning of his symptoms.

Classic psychoanalytic theory adds that the energy used for the repression of so much psychological material is now free and can be used for constructive purposes toward achieving normality. Very few psychiatrists today would deny the great importance of insight and of the restoration to consciousness of the unconscious. What is debatable is whether these techniques are the only effective ones in therapy and whether they are enough. A frequent complaint is that the patient has acquired insight or has obtained awareness of what used to be repressed, and yet the symptoms do not disappear. This situation is often explained with the expression that the patient has acquired intellectual but not emotional insight. The meaning of this expression is obscure. Perhaps it is meant that although the patient has acquired some understanding about the origin, development, and meaning of some aspects of his inner or external behavior, this new understanding does not confer to him the power to change his attitude about certain aspects of his life and consequently his behavior.

Probably improvement requires that the patient rearrange many constellations of thoughts and emotions which affect much larger areas of life than those directly involved in the specific symptomatology. Improvement and cure presuppose also corrections of those factors mentioned under headings *c* and *d*.

NON-FREUDIAN AND NEO-FREUDIAN PSYCHOANALYTIC SCHOOLS

In a brief review of the status of psychiatric theory, only a passing remark needs to be made about the two major non-Freudian psychoanalytic schools. The Jungian school is continuously losing ground, especially in the United States. On the other hand, some of Adler's important concepts, like that of the feeling of inferiority, have been so widely accepted that we forget that Adler introduced them.

Concerning the neo-Freudian schools of psychoanalysis, we can state that they have avoided some of the errors made by the classic school. All of them have rejected the notions of the libido theory and the id. We can also add that they have fallen into the genetic fallacy to a much lesser degree than the classic school. For most of them, however, we could repeat the criticisms made under headings *d, e,* and *f.*

Because of space limitations it is not possible to review the important contributions by Fromm, Horney, and others, and we shall take into consideration only Sullivan's theoretical position. Sullivan's contributions have greatly enriched the field of psychoanalysis and general psychiatry (36-38). We shall focus on two major aspects.

a. The Interpersonal Theory

More than any other author Sullivan has the merit of having shown that one becomes a person by virtue of relations with other human beings and not by virtue of inborn instinctual drives (30). To add to the field of psychiatry the gigantic dimension of the interpersonal is a gigantic contribution. However, it is impossible to encompass the whole field of psychology and psychiatry in an exclusively interpersonal framework. This framework deals with what goes on between A and B, but not with what goes on inside A and inside B. Yet every psychological phenomenon starts and ends intrapsychically; every interpersonal phenomenon is coupled with an intrapsychic one. The intrapsychic counterpart is at least as important as the interpersonal, especially in such phenomena as cognition, symbolism, and emotion.

Obviously Sullivan did not integrate the inner and outer reality in a superior synthesis. Nobody has been able to do so at the present stage of our knowledge. By concentrating on interpersonal relations the Sullivanian school minimizes the relevance of the inner self or of the total psyche of man: it focuses on an extremely important, but nevertheless partial, interpretation. In the same vein, by visualizing the self as made of reflected appraisals or other external influences, it overlooks the self's autonomous characteristics.

People influenced by Sullivan have continued his pioneer work within the interpersonal frame of reference. They have opened new areas of psychiatric inquiry by studying the person in the social context in which most psychological phenomena originate, develop, and deviate. However, in what seems to be the deeper vision of the large context, we must carefully avoid the danger of not respecting the person in his own separateness, individuality, and autonomy. These characteristics are as important as those which derive from the person's belonging to a social structure. For instance, under the indirect influence of the Sullivanian school, some authors see schizophrenia exclusively as a social or intra-familial drama. They do not take into consideration the fact that the drama has to be internalized in specific abnormal ways in order to lead to the psychosis (8).

b. Psychological Dynamisms as Modes of Fulfilling Needs for Satisfaction and Security

Sullivan's dynamic conceptions (or theory of motivation) are subsumed under his theory of need fulfillment. Satisfaction of basic needs (food, shelter, sleep, rest, lust) replaces the instinctual gratification of the Freudian system, but does not play such an important role as instinctual motivation does in the Freudian system. In my opinion this is a useful corrective to the biological emphasis of the Freudian system. The need for security (or need to remove anxiety) is the focus of Sullivan's dynamic theory. For Sullivan, security depends on good interpersonal relations and on an adequate amount of self-esteem. I agree fully with Sullivan: no longer is the human being seen exclusively as being at the mercy of animal instincts or of a restrictive society. However, interpersonal relations, self-esteem, and security are based on cognitive and symbolic processes, whose origin, development, and functioning have not been clarified by Sullivan. Moreover, Sullivan's dynamics do not include motivation which transcends the need for satisfaction and security (for instance, ethics and creativity).

SOME ADDITIONAL ISSUES

Perhaps because of my own biases, I feel that one of the areas more urgently in need of consideration is that of cognition. As I wrote elsewhere, cognition is the Cinderella of the field of psychiatry (5). This by no means implies that proper attention should not be paid to noncognitive physiological-behavioral factors. They too are extremely important. However, man cannot be studied like subhuman animals. Whereas his biological nature makes him part of the biological world, his cognitive functions make him enter a universe of symbols which transcends prehuman biology. Human psychology and psychopathology deal more with this universe of symbols, and with high-level emotions related to these symbols, than with instincts and primitive physiological mechanisms. That is the reason why studies in subhuman animals can elucidate only a few elementary psychological and psychopathological mechanisms but leave us completely in the dark about many others.

I distinguish three types of cognition—primary, secondary, and tertiary.

Primary cognition, or immature types of cognition as they occur in the mechanisms included by Freud in the primary process (1, 2, 4, 5), is exemplified by schizophrenic thinking and dream cognition.

Secondary cognition consists chiefly of conceptual thinking (7, 9).

In contrast to primary cognition, the content is here much more important than the form. A great deal of human life has to do with conceptual constructs. It is impossible to understand the human being without such important cognitive constructs as the self-image, self-esteem, self-identity, identification, hope, projection of the self into the future, etc. All these cognitive constructs are connected with or give origin to high-level emotions and consequently become an integral part of human motivation.

Tertiary cognition, or the creative process, must also receive psychiatric consideration (6, 7).

Incidentally, the study of cognition may help avoid an error commonly made by psychiatrists: that of confusing the form with the content, that is, structural psychopathology with psychodynamics. The origin and meaning of the conflict do not explain the psychological form or the specific symptomatology in which the conflict is mediated or represented. For instance, if a schizophrenic hears a voice calling her a prostitute, it is not enough to know that the hallucination is a symbolic reproduction of the threatening voice of the patient's mother. It is also important to study how and why such a voice of the past is transformed into an hallucination and not, let us say, into simple guilt feeling, compulsion, obsession, phobia, etc.

Another field which requires attention is that of psychiatric nosology and/or nomenclature. We are still following a classification of mental diseases which is more or less based on the original one by Kraepelin. The truth is that at the present stage of our knowledge we cannot do much better. Perhaps this is the only field in which further work should be postponed until greater knowledge of mental disorders is achieved. For the time being, we must do the best we can with the unsatisfactory classifications that are at our disposal.

The relations between psychoanalysis and psychotherapy require close attention. It is my feeling that the two fields will converge and possibly fuse, mainly because psychotherapy will incorporate the most valid aspects of psychoanalytic practice and theory. If such is the case, it will be necessary for psychotherapists to receive training similar or comparable in length and depth to that received by candidates in psychoanalysis. In this case, as in others, sponsors of present training methods must adopt more flexible positions. To a large extent changes will depend again on the theoreticians who prepare the ground not only for therapeutic practice but also for the training of new generations of psychiatrists.

Rather than to try desperately to make consistent what is inconsistent and to explain the fallacy of a theory in terms abstracted from the good points of the theory to which they feel committed, theoreticians should be open to all vistas and should work toward constructing bridges between equally plausible orientations. No reductionism of any kind but a pluralistic approach must prevail in psychiatry. Those of us who are more humanistically oriented may even conclude that there is no sharp demarcation between the study of psychiatric illness and the concern with the meaning of life.

REFERENCES

1. ARIETI, S.: Special logic of schizophrenic and other types of autistic thought. *Psychiatry,* 11:325-338, 1948.
2. ARIETI, S.: *Interpretation of Schizophrenia.* New York: Brunner, 1955.
3. ARIETI, S.: Manic-depressive psychosis. In *American Handbook of Psychiatry,* Vol. 1. Edited by S. Arieti. New York: Basic Books, 1959, pp. 419-454.
4. ARIETI, S.: The microgeny of thought and perception. *Arch. Gen. Psychiat.,* 6: 454-468, 1962.
5. ARIETI, S.: Contributions to cognition from psychoanalytic theory. In *Science and Psychoanalysis,* Vol. 8. Edited by J. Masserman. New York: Grune & Stratton, 1965.
6. ARIETI, S.: Creativity and its cultivation: Relation to psychopathology and mental health. In *American Handbook of Psychiatry,* Vol. 3. Edited by S. Arieti. New York: Basic Books, 1966, pp. 722-741.
7. ARIETI, S.: *The Intrapsychic Self: Feeling, Cognition and Creativity in Health and Mental Illness.* New York: Basic Books, 1967.
8. ARIETI, S.: New views on the psychodynamics of schizophrenia. *Amer. J. Psychiat.,* 124:453-458, 1967.

9. ARIETI, S.: Some elements of cognitive psychiatry. *Amer. J. Psychother.*, 21:723-736, 1967.

10. ARLOW, J. A.: Report on panel: The psychoanalytic theory of thinking. *J. Amer. Psychoanal. Assn.*, 6:143-153, 1958.

11. ARLOW, J. and BRENNER, C.: *Psychoanalytic Concepts and the Structural Theory.* New York: International Universities Press, 1964.

12. BERTALANFFY, L. VON: General systems theory. In *General Systems Yearbook of the Society for the Advancement of General Systems Theory.* Edited by L. von Bertalanffy and D. Rappaport. Ann Arbor: University of Michigan Press, 1956.

13. BERTALANFFY, L. VON: The mind-body problem: A new view. *Psychosom. Med.*, 24:29-45, 1964.

14. COBB, S.: *Borderlands of Psychiatry.* Cambridge: Harvard University Press, 1943.

15. DEUTSCH, F. (Ed.): *On the Mysterious Leap from the Mind to the Body.* New York: International Universities Press, 1959.

16. ECCLES, J.: *The Physiology of Nerve Cells.* Baltimore: Johns Hopkins Press, 1957.

17. ECCLES, J.: Quoted in *Recent Advances in Biological Psychiatry.* Edited by J. Wortis. New York: Plenum Press, 1966.

18. FREUD, S.: Project for a scientific psychology (1895). In *The Origins of Psychoanalysis.* New York: Basic Books, 1960.

19. FREUD, S.: *The Interpretation of Dreams* (1900). New York: Basic Books, 1954.

20. FREUD, S.: Three essays on the theory of sexuality (1905). In *Standard Edition of the Complete Psychological Works of Sigmund Freud.* London: Hogarth Press, 1953.

21. FREUD, S.: New introductory lectures on psycho-analysis (1932). In *Standard Edition of the Complete Psychological Works of Sigmund Freud.* London: Hogarth Press, 1964.

22. FREUD, S.: *An Outline of Psychoanalysis.* New York: W. W. Norton & Co., 1937.

23. GOLDSTEIN, K.: *The Organism.* New York: American Book Co., 1939.

24. HEBB, D. O.: *The Organization of Behavior.* New York: John Wiley & Sons, 1949.

25. HOLT, R. R.: The development of the primary process: A structural view. In *Motives and Thought: Psychoanalytic Essays in Honor of David Rappaport.* Edited by R. R. Holt. *Psychol. Issues 5:* Monogr. 18, 19, 1967.

26. JACKSON, J. H.: *Selected Writings of John Hughlings Jackson.* London: Hodder & Stoughton, 1932.

27. LASHLEY, K. S. and COLBY, K. M.: An exchange of views on psychic energy and psychoanalysis. *Behav. Sci.*, 2:230-240, 1957.

28. MACLEAN, P. D.: Psychosomatic disease and the "visceral brain": Recent developments bearing on the Papez Theory of Emotion. *Psychosom. Med.*, 11:338-353, 1949.

29. MORUZZI, G. and MAGOUN, H. W.: Brain stem reticular formation and activation of the E.E.G. *Electroenceph. Clin. Neurophysiol.*, 1:455-473, 1949.

30. MUNROE, R.: *Schools of Psychoanalytic Thought.* New York: Dryden Press, 1955.

31. PAPEZ, J. W.: A proposed mechanism of emotion. *Arch. Neurol. Psychiat.*, 38:725-743, 1937.

32. PENFIELD, W. and RASMUSSEN, T.: *The Central Cortex of Man.* New York: Macmillan Co., 1952.

33. PIAGET, J.: *The Child's Conception of the World.* New York: Harcourt, Brace & World, 1929.

34. RAPAPORT, D.: The structure of psychoanalytic theory—A systematizing attempt. *Psychol. Issues*, 2:1-158, 1960.

35. SCHUR, M.: *The Id and the Regulatory Principles of Mental Functioning.* New York: International Universities Press, 1966.

36. SULLIVAN, H. S.: *Conceptions of Modern Psychiatry*. Washington, D. C.: William Alanson White Foundation, 1947.
37. SULLIVAN, H. S.: *Interpersonal Theory of Psychiatry*. New York: W. W. Norton & Co., 1953.
38. SULLIVAN, H. S.: *Clinical Studies in Psychiatry*. New York: W. W. Norton & Co., 1956.
39. SZASZ, T. S.: *The Myth of Mental Illness*. New York: Hoeber Medical Division (Harper & Row), 1961.
40. THOMAS, A.: Purpose Versus Consequence in the Analysis of Behavior, read at a meeting of the Society of Medical Psychoanalysts, New York, N. Y., November 8, 1967.
41. WERNER, H.: *Comparative Psychology of Mental Development*. New York: International Universities Press, 1957.
42. ZILBOORG, G.: *A History of Medical Psychology*. New York: W. W. Norton & Co., 1941.

13

A Re-examination of the Phobic Symptom and of Symbolism in Psychopathology

---

The study of phobias has been one of my major interests since the beginning of my psychiatric career and continues to be for me an area of study and research. This paper, published in 1961, is my first writing on phobia, and reexamines the phobic symptom and symbolism in general in psychopathological conditions.

In spite of some important exceptions (9, 10, 14, 15), the study of phobias has been neglected recently. And yet if a symptom should be the representative of psychiatric disorders no other one could be better selected. In fact phobia or fear may appropriately represent one of the most common states of man, who in spite of, or rather, because of, his advancement and understanding, has become so aware of the precariousness of his condition as to transform danger from something to be prevented to something to be always concerned with.

The reasons why phobias have been relatively neglected in the literature are two: first, whereas phobias were seen as constituting a syndrome in themselves (called phobic state or anxiety hysteria), recently they are more frequently recognized just as symptoms of a total psychoneurotic clinical picture (and much less frequently psychotic). For the last two decades the emphasis has been on studying total syndromes rather than isolated symptoms. The second reason is the fact that after Freud's classic interpretation of phobias (8), no important diverging or supplementary hypotheses have been advanced.

Although the present writer agrees that the study of the total syndrome is more important than the study of the individual symptoms, he feels that a re-examination or reassessment of established conceptions is from time to time warranted.

THE PSYCHOLOGICAL STRUCTURE OF PHOBIAS

Freud's interpretation of phobia consists in seeing this symptom as a displacement (8). For instance, little Hans is actually afraid of his father, but in his neurosis the fear is displaced to horses. According to Freud the displacement hides a sexual threat and thus becomes symbolic of what it replaces. For instance, fear of being bitten by a horse replaces fear of castration by the hands of father.

According to the present writer, the displacement is not necessarily from one object (father) to another (horse). More than a displacement a concretization takes place. The patient may be in fearful expectancy of vague, intangible threats, which may be difficult to define or recognize: hostility from father, possibility of abandonment by mother, atmosphere of hate and resentment in the household, etc.

In several phobic patients the psychiatrist may easily recognize the concretization of a more general anxiety situation: fear of sexual relations hides a bigger fear in sustaining loving relationships; fear to travel hides a bigger fear of making excursions into life; fear of many little things generally hides a general state of insecurity. Odier (15), in a certain way understood this phenomenon when he wrote that "Behind the phobogenic object hides a concept, an idea, a vague intuition."

In the writer's opinion what happens in phobias is the expression of a general principle of psychopathology, viz.: that which cannot be sustained at an abstract level because it is too anxiety provoking, or for other reasons, is concretized. This concretization of concepts and idea-feelings is not merely the expression of a reduction to a concrete level, as Goldstein (11, 12) has described especially in organic cases, but an active process of concretization, that is, an active changing of the abstract into the concrete. For instance, before the onset of a psychosis a patient has the vague impression or feeling that the whole world is hostile toward him. After the onset of the psychosis the vague feeling becomes transformed into a concrete delusion: "They are against him" (3). Concretization reaches the point of perceptualization in hallucinations (1). For example, before the psychotic outbreak the patient had a self-effacing attitude, a pervading feeling of inadequacy and unworthiness. After the onset of the psychosis he hears voices accusing him of being a failure, a homosexual, a spy, etc.; that is, at a perceptual level he hears expressions of his own undesirability.

Phobias share with many other psychiatric symptoms the phenomenon of concretization. However, they have characteristics of their own, which have to be re-examined and reinterpreted for a more complete understanding of the phenomenon. These characteristics appear more evident if contrasted with those of delusions:

1. Whereas in delusions the threatening objects are other human beings (the persecutors), in phobias there is a dehumanization of the source of fear. For instance, bridges, cars, high buildings are frequently the phobogenic "objects." Characteristic enough is the fact that animals (horses, dogs, cats, insects) are often the phobogenic objects, but not human animals. Some human beings such as dentists, policemen, monks, may become phobogenic not because they are human but because of their role or the uniform they wear. In other words, the phobogenic object is either their role or their uniform.

2. Although the phobic patient attributes great power to the phobogenic object, he concentrates his attention on himself, that is, on the effect of the fear on himself. Whereas the deluded patient is mostly concerned with the bad qualities of the persecutor, the phobic is mostly concerned with the disturbance he will undergo if he is exposed to the danger.

3. The phobic patient retains some possibility of action within the framework of his symptomatology: he may escape the danger by avoiding the phobogenic object. In other words, it is up to him to avoid the fear-provoking situation. He is not a passive or helpless agent of persecutors, as is the deluded patient.

4. Contrary to the deluded patient the phobic retains the capacity to test reality. He understands that his fear is absurd and not syntonic with the rest of his psychological functions. As a matter of fact a great part of his conflict consists in his being obligated to react in a way that he himself considers absurd.

Can these characteristics of phobias be interrelated and explained? An attempt will be made toward a pathogenetic interrelation of the various aspects of the symptom, but an etiological interpretation is beyond the purposes of this paper.

The fundamental mechanism in phobias is introjection, not projection. In other words, the phobogenic object is not perceived as an entity in itself but as a disturber of the organism. As I have described more extensively in other works (5), a primitive form of perception consists in experiencing the external object only as a disturber of the organism. The perception does not mirror reality. It is an inner status of disequilibrium that the external stimulus produces. What counts is the alteration of the inner status of the organism more than the mirroring of the external object (4). In phobias this primitive type of perception occurs. The phobogenic object is introjected as a disturber of the organism, not *per se*. Obviously an unrealistic quality is *projected* to the phobogenic object, but the introjection of the alleged emotional disturbance is the main characteristic and reaches exaggerated proportions.

In all forms of altered introjections or of increased emotional disturbance (for instance in depressions) appreciation of external reality is not distorted or only to a minimal degree: only the inner status is. The phobic patient retains a grasp on external reality: on the other hand the deluded patient does not. The latter does not introject pathologically; he projects pathologically. Pathologic projection requires a transformation in cognition; the focus is on the cognitive functions not only of the patient, but also of the external world. But the only cognitive powers in the external world are other human beings. In phobias no cognition of other people is taken into account. The phobogenic object is not considered as a malevolent being who plots the destruction of the patient; it is seen only as a disturbing agent, not as a willed object.

It may be useful at this point to use Buber's terminology (6). In the phobic patient there is an I-It relationship between the patient and the phobogenic source; an I-Thou relationship in the paranoid. In both cases the relationship is distorted, and seen by the patient as a one-way relationship, that is from the external object to the patient and not from the patient to the external object. As I had occasion to discuss elsewhere (2), the pathological I-Thou relationship of the deluded is a more primitive one than the I-It pathologic relationship.

Human beings do not have merely an I-Thou relationship, but also an I-It relationship; that is, a relationship between the person and the non-human world. Many neurotic persons who have difficulties in interpersonal relations try to change the I-Thou relationship into an I-It relationship. They try to treat people as things; they depersonalize them. For instance, people become machines, sexual relations only a biological function, human relations become scientific experiments, and so on. Even the therapist becomes a therapeutic machine which renders a service. In the phobic patient the I-It relationship becomes accentuated. As I have described elsewhere (2), in the deluded patient this neurotic mechanism is absent. The patient cannot translate the personal into the impersonal. As a matter of fact one sees the opposite process: the impersonal tends to be personalized. Whatever of significance happens is never attributed to chance or to physical events (or to that particular chance which is bad luck). Almost everything is anthropomorphized and seen as a consequence of a personal will. One could object that in phobias too there is a certain kind of animism inasmuch as a special power is attributed to special situations and to inanimate things. Furthermore, animals, that is animated entities, are ofter phobogenic objects. This is true, but to a much more limited extent than in the psychotic patient. In phobias the phobogenic object acquires a special power only as a disturber of the organism, not as a plotting agent. Only human beings can be plotting agents.

The fact that the phobogenic object is an "It" permits the patient to retain a certain active role, that of mobilizing his defenses. In this respect the phobic differs from the psychotic and is similar to other psychoneurotic patients. The phobic defends himself with avoidance (of the danger); the hysteric with bodily impairment (so that he will not be able to face danger), the compulsive with a ritual (which, like magic, will protect him from danger).

SYMBOLIZATION

The study of phobias may help us to re-examine the general problem of symbolism in psychopathology, as phobias stand out among the most typical examples.

Since the beginning of the psychoanalytic era psychopathological symbolism has been intensely studied, but has not yet been correlated with the general symbolic process of the human mind, with which neurologists as well as philosophers and semanticists have been concerned. In this paper only the salient features of the general symbolic process will be reviewed in order to show later how they differ in pathological symbolism.

As Cassirer (7), Langer (13), and others have mentioned, a symbol is something which stands for something else. A most primitive type of symbol is the signal, which is a clue for something else which, however, is implied or present, although not obviously so. For instance, a certain rash is, for the physician, the signal of measles in the child, a certain odor is for the cat the signal that a mouse is around.

A real symbol, however, is something that stands or may stand for something which is absent. For instance, the name John may stand for John when John is absent. Language is a community of symbols. At first a symbol may stand for an external object: for example, the word "mother" stands for the child's mother, in the child's mind, but eventually for every mother. That is, the word will not denote only one object, one mother, but will refer to the whole category of females who beget children. Furthermore the symbol mother is not only communicated to others, but shared with others. That is, all who hear it know the denoting or conceptual meaning of the word "mother."

With the evolution of culture, symbols are created which stand for higher and higher categories. For instance, numbers are symbols which may stand for anything (the symbol 3 may stand for three apples, three books, three men, etc.). Algebraic symbols may stand for every number. Higher symbols are obtained by abstracting parts from lower classes. The new symbol will represent the new class formed by all the members possessing that abstracted part. For instance, from the symbol "animal" we may abstract the symbol "animal with vertebral column," constituting thus the class of vertebrates. From "vertebrate" we may abstract "mammals" which are those vertebrates which nourish their young with maternal milk, and so on. The members of the higher class acquire some qualities without losing the qualities of the lower class.

The above remarks are insufficient to encompass the complex phenomenon of symbolism but perhaps sufficient to throw some light on the differences between normal and pathological symbolization.

Let us take again as a paradigm the case of Freud's patient, little Hans:

1. The horse as a phobogenic object, at a conscious level is not a symbol, but a signal. In other words, it must be present in order to evoke fear. It is true that the memory of the horse may be frightening to Hans, but this case is already a complication of the situation: the memory is a symbol of the signal "horse."

2. The phobogenic situation is a very concrete situation, and cannot be abstracted from its actuality.

3. The horse as a phobogenic agent is not a symbol which can be shared with others. Hans can communicate his fear to others, but the fear will not be shared by others.

4. Fear of the horse replaces at a conscious level many other fears, which are still present, although not acknowledged. Fear of interpersonal relations may coexist with the fear of the horse, although the patient concentrates on the horse and not on the interpersonal relations.

5. With the development of the illness, a phobia, like the fear of horses, may stand for an increasing number of events and interpersonal situations which evoke fear or anxiety. Larger classes of anxiety or fear-

provoking situations or objects can be constructed, but these classes cannot as abstracted from lower ones, as the class of mammals was abstracted from the class of vertebrates. The larger classes do not retain the properties of the smaller classes. Finally we can see that only one element is common to these phobogenic classes: the phobogenic quality. They are thus very arbitrary classes, non-Aristotelian and abnormal classes.

6. This common phobogenic quality, on which the abnormal class is built, at the level of consciousness is not shared by the members of the class. As a matter of fact the patient represses more or less the phobogenic qualities of all the members of the class, except the one which appears in the symptom. In other words, the patient becomes unaware of his anxiety about interpersonal relations, and becomes aware only of the fear of horses. Thus the abnormal class exists only in a state of unconsciousness.

It is important to distinguish these two categories of symbols, which the human mind is capable of conceiving. To confuse them is not only poor semantics; it means to remain oblivious to the two arrows of human symbolism: the arrow directed toward higher constructs and that directed toward lower constructs. Whereas the normal symbol acquires the property of entities which are not only absent but in some cases even impossible to see or confirm, like the infinite decimal and the imaginary numbers, the pathological symbol (called by me paleosymbol) (1) tends to *reduce to one property* the many characteristics of arbitrary classes. It is not leading to higher constructs and is not interpersonal. Its only constructive use consists in being a pathological defense for the patient, who without his symptom would be even more incapable of coping with more general anxiety-provoking situations.

SUMMARY

Phobias are seen as expression of the general psychopathologic phenomenon of concretization. The fears are concrete representations of more abstract anxiety-provoking situations and relationships.

Phobias have certain characteristics, like dehumanization of the phobogenic object, alteration of the emotional status, retention of active role and of reality test, which can be correlated.

Symbolism in psychopathology presents some characteristics, like concentration on signals and formation of arbitrary classes, which differ from those of normal symbolism.

REFERENCES

1. ARIETI, S.: *Interpretation of Schizophrenia.* New York: Brunner, 1955.
2. ARIETI, S.: *Psychiatric Quart.*, 31:403, 1957.
3. ARIETI, S.: Schizophrenia: The manifest symptomatology, the psychodynamic and formal mechanisms. In *American Handbook of Psychiatry.* Edited by S. Arieti. New York: Basic Books, 1959, Vol. 1, p. 455.
4. ARIETI, S.: The experiences of inner status. In *Perspectives in Psychological Theory.* Edited by B. Kaplan and S. Wepner. New York: International Universities Press, 1960.
5. ARIETI, S.: *The Intrapsychic Self. Feeling, Cognition and Creativity in Health and Mental Illness.* New York: Basic Books, 1967.
6. BUBER, M.: *I and Thou.* Edinburgh: Clark, 1953.
7. CASSIRER, E.: *The Philosophy of Symbolic Forms.* New Haven: Yale University Press, 1953.
8. FREUD, S. (1909): Analysis of a phobia in a five-year-old boy. In *Collected Papers,* Vol. 3, 149. New York: Basic Books, 1959.
9. FRIEDMAN, P.: *Psychoanal. Quart.*, 21:49, 1952.
10. FRIEDMAN, P.: The phobias. In *American Handbook of Psychiatry.* Edited by S. Arieti. New York: Basic Books, 1959.
11. GOLDSTEIN, K.: *The Organism.* New York: American Book, 1939.
12. GOLDSTEIN, K.: Functional disturbances in brain damage. In *American Handbook of Psychiatry,* Vol. I, 770. Edited by S. Arieti. New York: Basic Books, 1959.
13. LANGER, S.: *Philosophy in a New Key.* Cambridge: Harvard University Press, 1942.
14. LEWIN, B. D.: *Psychoanalyt. Quart.*, 21:295, 1952.
15. ODIER, C.: *Anxiety and Magic Thinking.* New York: International Universities Press, 1956.

14

New Views on the Psychodynamics of Phobias

Written 16 years after the previous paper, the present article summarizes many years of additional experiences with phobias. Although the approach remains related to the Freudian, the psychodynamic interpretation acquires new perspectives. The possibility is discussed of enlarging to completely different areas the field of unconscious motivation in phobias and in other psychiatric conditions. A case report is included.

PHOBIAS AND PSEUDOPHOBIAS

SOME OF YOU who are acquainted with my works on schizophrenia and depression may be surprised to find me talking in a symposium devoted to phobias. If I am permitted to begin this presentation with a personal note, I will be able to reassure the audience that I am not venturing into a new field. In my youth I knew a leader whom I greatly respected and admired and who suffered from phobias. The whole town knew that he was afraid of animals, especially of dogs. It was actually the interest I had in him, the striking contrast between his unusually endowed personality and the ridiculous predicament in which his condition would at times put him that disclosed to me the mystery of mental illness and inspired me to study psychiatry. I plan to write about the life of this man elsewhere. I wish to add also that because of my interest in this leader, the first studies I pursued in psychiatry were on phobias, and my very first patient—whom I treated when I was still a student in the department of psychiatry, where I was preparing the thesis required by

Presented at the Eighteenth Emil A. Gutheil Memorial Conference of the Association for the Advancement of Psychotherapy, New York City, October 23, 1977.

European medical schools to graduate—was a person suffering from agoraphobia.

Although the subsequent course of my life led me to focus my research on other areas of psychiatry, the study of the phobic condition has remained always among my most vivid interests, and in the course of over thirty-five years I have accumulated quite a number of unusual cases.

I have seen many patients purely on a consultation basis, for the purpose of making a differential diagnosis between phobias and other conditions similar to phobias, which I shall call pseudophobias. I shall devote the first and shorter part of my presentation to these pseudophobias, which are interesting not merely from the point of diagnosis, but because they will help us to understand better what are the essential characteristics of real phobias and what is behind their manifest symptomatology.

First of all, we must clarify a point which is not as evident as it seems. Not every fear or even abnormal fear is a phobia. I have seen, for instance, a large number of women who, from a few days to a few years after they had given birth to a baby, had developed the fear of hurting the child, maybe of killing him with a knife, or of throwing him out of the window. These women were generally brought to me to determine whether they were suffering from post-partum schizophrenic psychosis, or from phobias. The family also wanted to be informed as to whether the patient really constituted a danger for the child. These women are neither phobic, nor schizophrenic, unless, of course, they have other symptoms which are schizophrenic in nature. There is no definite avoidance of the child in these women or state of panic at the sight of the child, as it exists in phobic patients in the presence of the phobogenic object or situation. The fear is not acute, but remains in them almost constantly, as an obsession. As as matter of fact, these patients have an obsessive-compulsive psychoneurosis either precipitated or re-exacerbated by childbirth. Hidden behind the manifest symptomatology is the anxiety about the role of mother and motherhood, and an identification with the patient's mother, the child's grandmother. In these cases there is no danger to the child. I have not seen one case in which the child was hurt. Schizophrenic post-partum psychoses are very common, and may constitute some danger to the child, but they have a different symptomatology. A definite danger for the baby exists in post-partum depressions. The suicidal mother may include the baby or all her children in what she considers the suicidal resolution.

Pseudophobias occur frequently in schizophrenia, especially in relatively mild cases. I am not referring to definite fears which stem from paranoid delusions, like the fear of being poisoned, kidnapped, or ridiculed by a persecutor. I am referring to symptoms intermediary between phobias and delusions. For instance, a patient is reluctant to go to bed because she is afraid that during the night a man may come out of the closet and strangle her. The fear persists although she has checked and seen that nobody is in the closet. The hostility of the world, or the hostility of the persecutors, assumes the symbolic aspect of the man who comes out of the closet and will take advantage of her and kill her and abuse her sexually while she is sleeping. The irrationality of the fear is often recognized, but not completely. A doubt remains that the fear may be justified. When the patient improves, the symptom loses the characteristic of the delusion and is replaced by a more typical phobia. Pseudophobias which occur in schizophrenic patients are as a rule less resistant, more fleeting in character than in typical psychoneurotic phobic patients, and generally have a more favorable prognosis as far as the symptom is concerned.

Even children who seem to be afraid to go to school are suffering from pseudophobias. I am happy that the term school phobia is much less used today. As Bowlby (1) has described, these children are not afraid of school, but of leaving mother, for whom they have a strong attachment, connected with undue anxiety. The fear of leaving mother is there, conscious, and is not replaced by symbolic symptoms.

In these pseudophobias that I have mentioned, and in many more which I could describe if time would permit, the manifest symptomatology is a concrete representation of the anxiety which rules the life of the patient, or of the drama which the patient is living consciously or unconsciously. However, even in the manifest symptomatology we can see the interpersonal character of the drama, for instance, the drama between the mother and the newborn child, between the woman and the male world of which she is afraid to the point of not being able to make romantic liaisons with any man. The child who does not want to go to school has an interpersonal problem with his relation with his mother, based on strong feelings of dependency and of uncertainty about such dependency.

The interpersonal drama is not so evident in the manifest symptomatology of real or typical phobias. First of all, what is the definition of phobia? A phobia is the perception of a specific and definite danger and the emotional reaction to danger, in situations where there is no objective danger. The patient experiences fear, for instance, when he crosses a bridge, when he sees a dog or a horse, and so forth. The patient realizes the irrationality of his feelings. Nevertheless, he cannot control his apprehensions and must avoid the phobogenic objects and situations.

THE PSYCHODYNAMICS OF PHOBIAS

The typical phobic condition is one of the few psychiatric syndromes which have been known since ancient times. The earliest description of a case is found in one of the books attributed to Hippocrates (2) and probably written around 400 B.C. Although Stanley Hall (3) and Pierre Janet (4) did accurate studies of this condition, a new era of deeper understanding started with Freud's work "Analysis of a Phobia in a Five-Year-Old Boy" (5). Freud described hom little Hans saw a horse fall and after that incident he developed the fear that a horse would fall down and would bite him.

Freud explained how horses had really nothing to do with the little boy's fears. Hans was experiencing sexual desire for his mother and had developed death wishes for his father, who was his rival. At the same time Hans developed fear of punishment for entertaining such wishes. According to Freud the phobia was implemented by displacement: the horse replaced the father, and the dreaded bite from the horse replaced the dreaded castration by the hands of the father.

Other psychodynamic schools have stressed that phobias are not necessarily based on repressed infantile sexual strivings and fear of punishment. The neo-Freudian schools of psychoanalysis connect the origin of phobias and other neurotic manifestations with disturbed relations during childhood and adolescence between the patient and the other members of the family, especially the parents. These disturbed relations would cause a state of anxiety, which later would manifest itself in a definite psychoneurotic symptomatology, and at times specifically in the form of phobias. Odier (6) wrote that behind a phobogenic object hides a concept, an idea, a vague intuition. In a previous contribution (7) I tried to investigate Odier's concept, and I described how often the phobia is not just a displacement, as described by Freud, but also a concretization, that is, a concrete representation of a vague or intangible threat. I also pointed out that the phobic person retains a certain freedom of action in the context of his symptomatology. He believes he can escape the threat by avoiding the phobogenic objects. In other words, it will be up to him to avoid the situation which arouses fear. I also pointed out that one of the most important characteristics of phobias, contrary to what happens in the majority of delusions, is a dishumanization of the source of fear. Frequently the phobogenic objects are bridges, cars, high buildings, etc. Animals (like horses, dogs, cats, insects) are often phobogenic objects, but humans are not. If some humans, like policemen or nuns, are experienced as phobogenic, it is by the virtue of special role they play or of the uniforms they wear. In other cases the phobogenic object is an infective disease, and human beings are phobogenic not in themselves but insofar as they are innocent vehicles of the infection. Using Martin Buber's terminology (8), I pointed out that the phobic person who used to experience difficulty in interpersonal relations makes an attempt through his phobias to change the anxiety-provoking I-Thou relation into an I-It. I shall return to this point later.

Since I wrote the mentioned article, I have made additional observations which led me to reconsider and to reevaluate all the phobic patients whom I have seen in over three decades of psychiatric practice.

An observation that I have made in many (but not all) cases which I studied psychodynamically is that these patients had been very sensitive and gifted in childhood. A rather large number of them had a happy early childhood, characterized by a basic optimistic attitude toward people in general, life, and the promise of the future. These patients, however, became badly disappointed later, at times as early as in late childhood, often in adolescence, and in rare instances in young adulthood. From a "state of innocence" they brusquely passed to a second stage during which they considered themselves exposed to the mysterious unpredictability of life, to the sneak attack of danger, or to the errors and malevolence of others. At times it is an episode like the death of a parent which brings about the stage of general insecurity and dangerousness. At other times it is the discovery of a previously unsuspected horrendous or dishonorable aspect of life, or the realization that people whom the patient trusted very much are untrustworthy and even dangerous in a physical and moral sense. In only a few cases could I trace back the onset of this second stage of insecurity to the occurrence of typical Oedipal situations and fears of castration, as described by Freud.

In this second stage most patients are not phobic yet, but live in a state of not fully conscious anxiety. In my experience, they may become phobic much later, even from 5 to 20 years after the beginning of this second stage.

The patient is not phobic in this second stage, but lives in a state of controlled anxiety.

The earlier "state of innocence" which I have referred to may coexist with the state of instinctive dominance of the child described by Freud.

Its loss, when the second stage starts, may be even more powerful in its effect than the primitive instinctual drives. This interpretation is not an application of Jean-Jacques Rousseau's idea that man is born innocent and society makes him bad. The "state of innocence" may also come from the external world; it may be an unverbalized assumption that the child makes in his early interchanges with his mother and with the acceptance of her great unconditional love. Having shaped the world according to the early image of love, derived from Mother or from both parents, he is badly disappointed later for a series of reasons which have to do with other persons but vary in every case. We cannot exclude that a particular biological predisposition may make the patient particularly sensitive to this type of anxiety, experienced as a pervasive feeling that life is not safe but suffused with dangerousness. The danger is vague, diffused, invisible, intangible, and yet it seems immense and omnipresent because at a certain point in life it may become manifest as something unexpected and unpredictable.

The future patient now has to confront a dangerous universe. In a way which he cannot clearly verbalize, he experiences this danger as being of vast proportions, maybe connected with the whole of life or a large part of it. The life of everybody is always in a precarious state and uncertain equilibrium, threatened by diseases, earthquakes, motor accidents, fires, hurricanes, and so forth. But the patient who eventually becomes phobic is particularly vulnerable to what other human beings can do to his life. They may scold him, neglect him, ignore him, ridicule him, belittle him, disregard his rights, offend his human dignity, consider him not up to par, cheat him, rob him, enslave him, injure him, kill him, and so forth. They may do worse things to him. They may transmit their evil, corrupt him, make him become dishonest, a cheater, and so forth.

With similar feelings the patient could become a very detached person, overtly hostile, unable to love, but he does not become this way. He could become a paranoid schizophrenic, but he does not. Whether it is a cosntitutional predisposition or the love that he experienced in his early childhood which saved him from this fate, we do not know. He becomes phobic instead. He will become afraid of some specific objects and situations (bridges, squares, germs, dogs, horses, etc.), and he will continue to accept the rest of the world and to make overtures of friendship and love.

Generally it is either an important episode related in meaning to the dramatic child episode or an accumulation of life anxieties which brings about the third stage, characterized by typical phobias. In some cases the phobic condition starts or is exacerbated when new interpersonal situations develop which are threatening, for instance, when the patient gets married, has to go to live with the parents-in-law or in proximity of the parents-in-law or with a step-parent, or has given birth to a baby. In these cases and many others, the human agents, like spouses, parents-in-law, babies, etc., are not consciously experienced as threats or only to a mild degree.

By becoming phobic the patient puts into effect several defensive maneuvers:

1) He reduces a diffuse or global anxiety to a definite concrete fear; for instance, he is now afraid only of crossing bridges.

2) Although it is true that the specific fear is always potentially present in him, he has now found a method to deal with it; for instance, he will avoid crossing bridges.

3) He has been able to change the source of fear from human beings to non-human phobogenic objects or to special environmental situations. The danger is also limited to his physical integrity, does not include the moral or psychological. For instance, the patient is not afraid of being corrupted, but of being infected with a contagious disease. As I said earlier in this presentation, the patient is able to change threatening I-Thou relations into an I-It situation.

It is on this third aspect of phobias that I wish to focus. First of all, we can say that contrary to what happens in pseudophobias, even in the manifest symptomatology of real phobias, the human relation which constitutes a threat or is threatened, is no longer visible.

Martin Buber is critical of the human being who relates to his fellow man as if he were a thing, an *It*, and not a person, a *Thou*. Buber is right, of course, when he refers to relations among normal persons. However, when the phobic displaces the source of danger from a person (or persons) to a thing, to a germ, or to an animal, not only does he do that to diminish his anxiety, but also to protect his fellow human beings, whom otherwise he would see in a way unfitting the human image. It would be horrendous for a human being to be so threatening; only an *It* could be in that way. The phobic is the opposite of the slave-owner who reduces a human being to a tool. By resorting to his neurotic mechanism he is able to maintain a dialogic relationship with other persons, even those who caused his original anxiety.

The fact that quite often animals are selected as phobogenic objects is also of paramount significance. The phobic patient rejects the ancient dictum *Homo homini lupus* (Man is a wolf to man) and changes it into another: *Lupus homini lupus* ([only] a wolf is a wolf to man). The wolf here stands for any animal, or a non-human entity, which is inhuman to fellow men. Human beings are exonerated and the patient can continue to live in harmony with the human community. The animal becomes a real scapegoat. Freud actually hinted at this process when he wrote that by becoming afraid of horses little Hans could continue to love his father. He changed *Pater Johanni equus* (Father is a horse to Hans) into *Equus Johanni equus* ([only] a horse is a horse to Hans).

I believe that what I have so far illustrated will permit us to reconsider and possibly enlarge the motivational aspect of the psychiatric symptom. Although I am referring now exclusively to phobias, in works now in preparation I make an attempt to explain that, with some important modifications, this particular enlargement of the motivational aspect of the symptom has to be found also in schizophrenia and in depression.

Imitating what Claude Bernard had done for general medicine, Freud showed that the psychiatric symptom has not only a regressive aspect, resulting from the damage or dysfunction caused by the illness, but also a restitutional aspect. Freud stressed that the symptom is also an attempt to repair, an effort to repress the unacceptable, a compensation, a way to achieve disguised or displaced goals. All this is true, but I think we can go even further in understanding the purposeful activity of the human psyche in health and in mental disease. The motivation goes beyond the protection of the patient himself. Often it includes an effort to maintain respect for fellow human beings and to retain a sense of their human dignity. By attributing the cause of his trouble to non-human sources, the patient protects the human image. Since he is human, he defends himself, too, but also the whole of humankind. This motivation, which transcends the interest of the patient himself, could even be called a spiritual motivation, or the spirituality of the human being as emerging even in mental illness. However, it is with a certain hesitation that in this environment I use these words, which are difficult to define, lead easily to misinterpretation, and seem more appropriate in philosophical and theological circles.

CASE REPORT

I shall speak now about a case which I intend to report in much greater detail in a future presentation. What I shall present here is only an excerpt of a long clinical history, but enough in my opinion to show

how Freud's original discoveries and the observations and interpretations reported in this paper can blend in some cases.

The patient, a 53-year-old Italian-born patient whom I shall call Guido, came to see me for an illness which had plagued him for over 20 years. He had resided in the United States for many years and had consulted many psychiatrists both in the United States and in Europe, but nobody succeeded in helping him. The illness started when, in his late twenties, he was about to leave Italy and come to the United States. He then became afraid to touch anything or to be touched by any thing or human being, for fear of becoming infected. Guido told me that life had been torture, a living death to him for many years.

In the course of treatment he said that he could trace back the onset of the illness, the actual initial moment. He was in Sicily, in the village where he was born, and he went to a barber to have a haircut. He noticed that the person who was sitting in the chair where he was supposed to sit next was an elderly and sickly man who appeared to Guido to be suffering from tuberculosis. The time came for Guido to sit on that chair, and he did, but soon developed the idea that he had been infected. From that day on he became afraid of touching any person living in the village, lest he become infected.

Later Guido told me that although the episode at the barber shop was the definite beginning of the illness, premonitory symptoms or quasi-symptoms had occurred a few days previously. He had left Milan, where he worked, and had gone to his native village in Sicily to say goodbye to his mother before coming to America, and also to make there final preparations for the emigration. While he was in his village, he heard that Bruno, a good friend of his, who also worked in Milan in the same firm where he did, was seriously and possibly critically ill. Guido heard the news from the wife of Bruno, who asked him please to accompany her to Milan to see her sick husband. Bruno and his wife were much older than Guido and had been friends of Guido's parents for many years. The patient interrupted his preparations for the trip to America, went to Milan with Bruno's wife, and indeed when they arrived, they found Bruno seriously ill. What type of illness Bruno had, the patient has never been able to ascertain, and I doubt that it was an infective disease. Guido remembered that he was somehow hesitant and afraid to go to visit Bruno in the hospital. As a matter of fact, he remembered that the first time he left the hospital after visiting Bruno, he opened the revolving door with his foot. He did not want to touch it with his hand for fear of becoming infected. A few days later Bruno died, and after the funeral the patient returned to his village in Sicily.

A few days after the episode at the barber shop Guido's fear of becoming infected was no longer confined to people or things in his village, but spread to any person who would come from Milan or to any object manufactured in Milan. He could absolutely not touch any people or object coming from that city. When he came to the United States, he managed at first to do fairly well, and even got married and had three children; but the fear of touching any person or object coming from his village or from Milan persisted. Eventually he started to think that any person living in the United States could have touched somebody coming from Milan or from Sicily. Therefore he should avoid touching anybody.

I shall omit the detailed description of the symptomatology, which spread rapidly, paralyzed the activities of the patient, and caused anguish to an agonizing degree. Nevertheless, Guido was able to manage an Italian-style café and to make a moderately comfortable living. In spite of his illness he has remained a friendly and warm person, very much loved by his three children. The wife, however, could not tolerate his illness and left him. The children remained with him.

During the course of treatment he told me that the first seven or ten years of his life were wonderful. He also said that the family atmosphere underwent a drastic change for the worse when his father died. The father was much older than the mother, and had been a very successful man, as a matter of fact, one of the most successful and respected persons in the village. Before his death, in old age, he had been blind for several years. After his death the economic condition changed completely. The mother, whom the patient described as a very loving and maternal person, did not know how to support the family. The patient himself at the age of 13 left the village to go to work in Milan, as many people used to do in his village, and would go to see his mother at Christmas time.

Later in the treatment the patient told me that another very unusual thing had occurred before the father died. He was hesitant to tell me what it was all about; he had not revealed this information to any previous doctor. He remembers that one day, while his old and blind father was sick in bed, he, his mother, and Bruno, the friend whom I already mentioned, were in the bedroom visiting the father. At a certain moment Guido turned his head from the direction of the father's bed to the place where mother was sitting and saw Bruno putting his hand over mother's thigh, over the high part of the thigh as to caress it or grab it. The mother allowed Bruno to do so, in front of the moribund and blind husband. Guido understood; that gesture was indicative that much more was going on between Bruno and his mother. He said nothing, did nothing, showed no emotional display. As soon as possible, that is, when he was 13 and felt no longer like a child, he left his village to go to work in Milan; and in Milan again, in the circle of people who were coming from his Sicilian village—friends and relatives—was Bruno, who also had gone to Milan to work. Guido saw Bruno regularly in Milan. Bruno was well liked by the circle of friends and relatives, and Guido tried to like him, too, although he was conscious of a certain reluctance to accept him entirely. Several years late, when Guido was in his late teens, Guido confronted Bruno. He told him, "Bruno, I saw what you did that day in front of my sick father. You did have an affair with my mother." Bruno became confused; he did not deny the allegation, but became very anxious and told Guido, "Please, don't tell my wife. Promise that you will not tell my wife." Guido made that promise and kept it. As a matter of fact, when Bruno was very sick and Guido accompanied Bruno's wife to Milan to see her dying husband, he had many opportunities to be alone with her, but he did not reveal anything.

Thus everything seemed normal until Bruno's sickness, Bruno's funeral, and Guido's return to his village. Then the illness exploded in a furious manner, and even years later gained in tragic intensity.

I must admit that I have not yet understood completely this interesting case, and that I am open to suggestions. Nevertheless, even what we know from this fragment of the clinical history that I have reported seems to me sufficient to permit the formulations of probable hypotheses.

Before I attempt an interpretation, I must state that as to the timing of the reported events Guido could give only approximate but not definite dates. We are in a position, however, to recognize in Guido's history the three stages of psychodynamic development that I described earlier in the paper.

We have a first period or stage of Guido's life, free of anxiety or of suffering, the first seven to ten years. Whether this period was really so serene as Guido described it, or has been idealized later by the patient, is hard to say. In this period the figures emerge of the respected and honored father, and of a loving mother. The picture changes and the second stage begins when the father becomes blind, moribund, and a cuckold. The crucial moment took place when Guido saw a sign of the last thing he expected to see, the proof of his mother's infidelity.

If we visualize the cultural milieu of a very conservative and somewhat primitive Sicilian village, where matters of sex and honor are of paramount importance, we can understand how Guido reacted to the sight of Bruno's caressing mother's thigh. That gesture was more than a revelation; it was a cataclysm. It is fair to say that no child, no matter in what culture he was raised, would have liked to see such a compromising gesture in front of the dying and blind father; but in a Sicilian environment the episode acquired even more importance. That honest and trustworthy interpersonal world which Guido had envisioned in his mind all of a sudden threatened to collapse. But he did not permit it to collapse. Either because of psychological denial or for other reasons, Guido maintained his composure and silence, and, according to what he told us, continued to love dearly his mother and to maintain a certain restrained friendship for Bruno, too. It is very possible that the harmonious or relatively harmonious and loving environment of the first ten years helped him to build defenses. It is also important to note, however, that as soon as he could, he left his mother and went to live in Milan. There he met Bruno again.

Guido made an apparently successful attempt to maintain normal relationships with the interpersonal world. At a conscious level he never blamed his mother, who was married to an old man; nor Bruno, to whom he also felt bound by friendship and loyalty. During this second psychodynamic stage, however, Guido is not completely well. He is a very insecure and fearful individual. Nevertheless he is able to live and work adequately.

With the illness and subsequent death of Bruno, the third stage starts and the phobic condition manifests itself with a violence which seems to equate the force of repression which must have been needed for many years. How is all this to be explained?

After Bruno's death there is no need any more for Guido to repress totally the pathogenic antecedents. Milan and the Sicilian village represent Bruno and Mother and become the focuses of an infection which may potentially spread to the whole world. Bruno and Mother remain innocent; the trouble is with the infection, which has allegedly originated in the two places where live the culprits of what must have seemed to Guido's once immature mind the greatest crime. Guido continues to exonerate or condone the two guilty ones, but, similar to what happens in the Greek tragedy of Oedipus Rex, a plague or potential plague is threatening. However, it can infect only him, because he is the only one who knows the crime and does nothing about it.

Of course, we can also consider to what extent Guido's Oedipal feelings are involved. Guido's rival was not his father, but Bruno; and whatever Oedipal hate Guido had must have been directed toward Bruno. It could be that he wished Bruno's death, and that when Bruno actually died, he felt guilty, or in an imaginary danger of being punished by the deceased Bruno through an infection which Bruno originated. I believe, however, that it would be a reductive approach to attempt to explain the whole picture from the point of view of sexual desire for the mother and fear of punishment from a parental figure. I believe that other important factors to be taken into consideration in this case are the contrast between Guido's early childhood and his late childhood; the impact of the psychological cataclysm he underwent when he discovered mother's adultery, a discovery which could have engendered the collapse of his trusting attitude toward the world. The role he assumed was the opposite of vengeful Hamlet's. He made instead gigantic efforts to exonerate everybody, to continue to love everybody, and to attribute whatever disturbed him to a non-human source, a potential infection, incidentally transmitted by people. In my opinion, what is of crucial importance in this case is not a sexual drama, but a moral drama, not the fear of castration, but the fear of what appears evil to the patient. The phobia gets hold of Guido and removes all the conflicts. Unfortunately it becomes so ingrained in his life to the point that his life is paralyzed. What must have been to him the gigantic shadow of evil was transformed into the shadow of a gigantic neurosis. The world is saved from a potentially spreading evil, but he, Guido, must contend with the potential spreading of an infection.

PSYCHOTHERAPY

I shall discuss briefly now psychotherapy, not in reference to the case I have described, but in general. The therapy of typical cases of phobic psychoneurosis constitutes a real challenge. In my experience any type of drug therapy is ineffectual.

I have found psychodynamic therapy useful, but only to a moderate degree. Since I started to understand the psychodynamics of phobias in the vaster framework that I have outlined, and I have succeeded in helping the patient to become conscious first of his transition from the stage of innocence and happy childhood to the stage of generalized danger; second, of the unconscious effort made on his part to exonerate the human environment and to retain the capacity to love; and third, of the symbolic significance of certain late events in life, I have obtained considerable ameliorations of the disorder. However, even this larger psycho-dynamic understanding is not by itself sufficient to achieve a complete cure in a considerable number of cases.

This state of affairs is not difficult to understand. As I have explained in my discussion of the psychodynamics, the phobic symptom offers definite secondary gains, which are not really secondary but of paramount importance. It is difficult for a patient to relinquish a symptom which represses early pathogenetic traumas, eliminates a global climate of anxiety, and reduces it to a specific dangerous situation that in most cases he can avoid. In some cases, like Guido's case, there seems to be no reduction of anxiety because the phobogenic object is generalized. In these cases, too, however, the symptom permits the patient to retain warm interpersonal relations and the capacity to love.

In my experience, to be really effective, psychodynamic therapy has to be supplemented by two auxiliary treatments. The first consists of the gradual exposure of the patient to the dreaded situation, in the beginning while he is accompanied by the therapist. It will be much easier for the patient to overcome the fear if the anxiety is diminished by the presence of the therapist, especially when the interpretations given have decreased the phobogenic power of the stimulus. Eventually the patient will be able to face the alleged dangerous situation by himself.

The second and in my experience very useful auxiliary treatment consists of altering or rearranging the whole life, family environment, and routine of the patient, so that the unconscious climate of anxiety or suspicion toward the interpersonal world decreases in intensity and there is less need to transform it into the specific fears.

I have found that the adoption of these three methods brings about recovery or at least amelioration in a large number of cases.

SUMMARY

It is important to differentiate phobias from pseudophobias. They differ not only in their manifest symptomatology but also in their underlying psychodynamics. According to the author's observations, in many cases of phobias a stage of relatively happy childhood is followed by a stage in which a generalized, intangible fear, related to other human beings, is perceived. This stage is often precipitated by a traumatic event. When other events related to the original traumas occur, or when the climate of anxiety increases, a phobic symptomatology occurs, which attempts, through defensive maneuvers, to limit and concretize the dangers and to maintain warm relations with fellow human beings (third stage).

The modalities of a combined form of psychotherapy are outlined.

REFERENCES

1. BOWLBY, J.: Attachment theory, separation anxiety, and mourning. In S. Arieti (Ed.), *American Handbook of Psychiatry*, Second Edition, Vol. 6, pp. 292-309. New York: Basic Books, 1975.
2. HIPPOCRATES: *On Epidemics V.* Section 82, translated by S. Farrar. London: Cadel, 1780.
3. HALL, G. S.: A study of fears. *American Journal of Psychology*, 8:147-249, 1897.
5. FREUD, S.: Analysis of a phobia in a five-year-old boy (1909). *Collected Papers*, Vol. 3, pp. 149-289. New York: Basic Books, 1959.
6. ODIER, C.: *Anxiety and Magic Thinking.* New York: International Universities Press, 1956.
7. ARIETI, S.: A re-examination of the phobic symptoms and of symbolism in psychopathology. *American Journal of Psychiatry*, 118:106-110, 1961.
8. BUBER, M.: *I and Thou.* Edinburgh: Clark, 1953.

15

Psychopathic Personality: Some Views on
Its Psychopathology and Psychodynamics

*This paper is my only article on psychopathic personality.
Published in 1963, it was later incorporated into* The Intrapsychic Self.

MANY PSYCHIATRISTS are in agreement with Cleckley (4) in believing that
current classification of mental disorders, prepared under the auspices of
the American Psychiatric Association (6), is somewhat inadequate in
defining and in categorizing as personality disorders such disparate conditions as schizoid personality, sociopathic personality, sexual deviation,
antisocial reaction, enuresis, etc. The confusion is further increased when
we consider the fact that it is not often easy to distinguish personality
deviations which appear as secondary manifestations in practically all
psychiatric conditions, from the syndromes in which they constitute the
basic pathology.

With the term psychopath, there is generally designated a person of at
least average and often superior intelligence, who is given to recurring
acts of inadequately motivated antisocial behavior, who seems irrespon-
sible, lacking anxiety or guilt over his past or future actions, and who
seems unable to learn from experience about the unfeasibility of his antisocial behavior.

Thus, the antisocial character of his behavior appears as the most
salient feature. A Robinson Crusoe could not be a psychopath. In other
words, a psychopathic condition manifests itself only a societal environment. This statement does not imply that societal or interpersonal factors
are the only ones involved in these conditions. As we shall see later, the
interpersonal factors are very important in both originating the psychogenetic patterns of living and in the shaping or evolving of the overt symp-

tomatology; but they are not the only ones. Two other important aspects have also to be taken into consideration: the first concerns the specific formal mental mechanisms which are characteristic of the psychopath; the second refers to the particular way of experiencing of the psychopath. These three aspects will be taken into consideration in the following sections of this paper. Before doing so, however, I must mention that although I am aware that there are many mixed or transitional or unclassifiable cases, clinical experience and the study of literature have led me to adopt the following classification of psychopathic personalities.

First, the patients are divided into two groups: 1) the pseudopsychopathic personality (or symptomatic psychopath) and 2) the true psychopathic personality (or idiopathic psychopath). A similar grouping has been made by other authors (15), although with different views in mind.

The main part of the classification, however, concerns the true or idiopathic psychopath, of which the following types have been differentiated: a) the simple; b) the complex; c) the dyssocial; d) the paranoiac.

I. THE PSEUDOPSYCHOPATH (OR SYMPTOMATIC PSYCHOPATH)

The topic of pseudopsychopathy will receive only cursory treatment in this paper, the main aim of which is to offer new points of view on the true or idiopathic psychopathic condition.

The pseudopsychopath is an individual who only symptomatically manifests psychopathic traits or tendencies, but whose main psychiatric difficulties have to be interpreted as parts of other clinical entities. Many of these patients, when accurately examined, will be recognized as suffering from psychoneuroses or character neuroses. A large number of these patients have manifested psychopathic behavior in childhood, or adolescence. In the majority of them it is possible to recognize that what goes on is still a rebellion against the parents or symbolic parents. A pattern of behavior perpetuates itself, presenting antisocial features which at times seem impulsive, at other times compulsive in nature. The patient seems to have a hostile character structure which impels him to defy or to hurt others, especially when these others stand for parental authority.

To this group of pseudopsychopaths, in my opinion, belong also more complicated cases which occur in children and whose dynamism has been lucidly illustrated by Adelaide Johnson (14) and by Szurek (18). These two authors, however, consider such patients real psychopaths and not pseudopsychopathic neurotics.

According to Johnson and Szurek the delinquent child is an individual whose delinquency has been unconsciously sanctioned by the parents, generally the mother. The child's acting out would offer the parents a vicarious gratification of their poorly integrated forbidden impulses. Szurek and Johnson seem to believe that in all psychopathic children who do not belong to the "sociological group" this mechanism is always involved. For Szurek the psychopathic person is a delinquent child grown older.

The present writer recognizes that the contributions of Szurek and Johnson have been very important and believes that in many cases of juvenile delinquency the mechanism they have illustrated is certainly involved. However, he cannot agree that all delinquents or psychopaths, with the exception of the "sociological," belong to this group.

To the group of the pseudopsychopaths have to be added postpsychotic patients, who recover from their psychotic, generally schizophrenic episodes, but reintegrate only at what seems to be a psychopathic level. The patient has lost the overt psychotic symptomatology, but now indulges in antisocial or socially nonacceptable behavior. Generally these patients are persons who before becoming ill had strong wishes which they did not dare to satisfy or act upon. After the psychotic episode they cannot control the wishes.

II. THE IDIOPATHIC PSYCHOPATH

Idiopathic psychopaths are easily recognized as such by every psychiatrist. In the official nomenclature of the American Psychiatric Association they are designated as suffering from "antisocial reaction." The basic mechanisms underlying their symptomatology are difficult to interpret. We are dealing here with something beyond a fight against the superego or an acting out in accordance with the unconscious sanction of the patients. It is well known that psychoanalytic or dynamically oriented therapies are seldom successful with idiopathic psychopaths.

In the following section we shall examine in detail, first the formal and then the psychodynamic mechanisms of the simple psychopath. In the subsequent sections we shall examine the other types only in the characteristics which differ from those of the simple psychopath.

a) The Simple Psychopath

Formal Mechanisms. The simple psychopath is an individual in whom periodically a strong need arises which urges him toward immediate gratification, even when this gratification is not sanctioned by other people. The non-gratification of the need is experienced by the patient as an unbearable frustration or discomfort. Whereas the psychotic realizes his wish by changing his thinking processes or his symbolic world, the psychopath realizes his wishes by putting into effect actions which lead to a quick gratification, no matter how primitive or how much in contrast with the norms of society. He resorts to a short-circuited mechanism which promptly leads to a feeling of satisfaction. Theoretically the psychopath could satisfy his wishes in a more or less distant future, if he would resort to long-circuited processes which are necessary for a mature and socially acceptable attainment of goals. But he cannot wait. Future satisfaction of needs is something that he cannot understand and which makes no sense to him. He lives emotionally in the present and he completely disregards tomorrow. This point needs clarification. Intellectually the patient knows that the future exists and that he could obtain his aims in ways which are acceptable to society. But all this has for him, essentially a theoretical reality, is experienced only in a vague, faint way. At times he is able to visualize all the steps which he would have to go through were he to satisfy his needs in socially acceptable ways. He becomes terrified or feels helpless at such prospect and tries to suppress the ideas of all those steps. On the other hand, he continues to experience his present needs which urge him toward immediate gratification.

As I have written elsewhere (1, 2), psychoneurotic anxiety is predominantly long-circuited. It is not a fear of an immediate danger, but is connected with the expectation of danger, that is with something dangerous which may or may not occur in a near or distant future. The psychopath does not experience this type of anxiety. He experiences a short-circuited anxiety, which may be called tension or discomfort. Consequently he cannot even be too anxious about future punishment. He knows theoretically that he may be caught in the antisocial act and be punished, but again this punishment is a possibility concerning the future and therefore the idea of it is not experienced as something having emotional strength or the power to make him change the course of his present actions.

Normal people during the process of maturation have learned to postpone gratification of needs. This is the result of phylogenetic evolution which has enabled man to use more and more complicated neuronal cortical patterns, which permit him to visualize the future and to react with an increasing complexity of responses. Ontogenetically this is a process of development and socialization which Freud has described as the passage from the pleasure to the reality principle. The true psychopath acts in accordance with the pleasure principle. It is easier and quicker to steal or forge checks than to work, to rape than to find a willing sexual partner, to falsify a diploma than to complete long studies in a professional school.

In some psychopaths the need seems to consist of a primitive urge to discharge hostility through actions, without any apparent gain other than the pleasure of inflicting injury upon others. In these cases we have a complicated picture: not only is the patient more hostile than the average person, but, contrary to the average neurotic, is unable to change, repress, postpone or neutralize his need for hostility.

True psychopaths are said to have no loyalties for any person, group or code. They are also said to be unable to identify with others. These statements are correct but refer only to the by-products of the basic formal short-circuited mechanism. The urge to gratify the need is so compelling that the patient cannot respect any loyalty or identify with other people; that is, he cannot visualize the bad effects that his actions will have on other people. As we have already mentioned, the patient may intellectually visualize these future bad effects, but such visualizations are not accompanied by deterring emotions.

The short-circuited mechanism by which the psychopath operates is self-defeating and leads inevitably to complication, in spite of aiming at the avoidance of all complications. For instance, a psychopath may just want to rape a girl and he carries out his wish; but then the sudden fear comes to him that the girl may report him to the police. So the quickest way to avoid this complication is to kill the girl; but, sooner or later the killing of the girl will produce more serious complications.

In attempting to avoid complications or ramifications which have to do with future happenings, the psychopath repeatedly places himself in a web of new dangers.

Before concluding these remarks on the formal mechanisms and the experential modes of the simple psychopath, we must add that in the majority of these patients, new plans for actions leading to gratification or to release from the state of stress, occur as sudden insights. The patient thinks of ways to solve his problem as quickly as possible when he suddenly experiences some kind of "enlightenment" on "how to do it." This sudden "psychopathic insight" may appear as an act of creativity. In a certain way it is. Actually it consists chiefly of techniques by which it is possible to disregard some factors which to a normal person would have an inhibiting influence. Furthermore the patient tends to resort to the same "solution" all over again, so that after the initial act, we can no longer talk of psychopathic creativity. Eventually we can even talk of stereotyped responses.

Etiologic Considerations and Psychodynamics. Before going into the psychodynamics of the simple psychopath we must consider the possibility of organic factors as etiologic determinants. Why is the patient using a short-circuited mechanism? Does he have at his disposal all the neurons which permit the much more complicated patterns of thinking and behavior which are compatible with civilized life? Since Lombroso's (16) attempt in 1876, many authors have tried to find correlations between physical constitutions and psychopathic behavior. The results have been inconclusive. Glueck and Glueck (8) found that approximately 60 per cent of persistent delinquents were predominantly mesomorphic. Electroencephalographic studies seemed promising (7, 11, 12), but have led to no definite findings. We know, however, that the prefrontal lobe syndrome at times reproduces a picture which has many similarities to that of the simple psychopath. Since the famous case of Phineas Gage, reported by Harlow (9, 10), we know that prefrontal patients are tactless, impulsive, deprived of anxiety and given to antisocial behavior. More recently, similar pictures have been seen in some patients submitted to frontal leucotomy. However, as far as can be detected by present methods of investigation, there seems to be no evidence of frontal or cortical lesions in by far the majority of psychopaths.

It is thus appropriate to search for psychodynamic mechanisms which may determine or at least enhance the establishment of the short-circuited mechanism, or makes it so overpowering as not to permit the use of more complicated patterns. We can only offer hypotheses, which at the present time are supported by a relatively small number of cases. We know that the young child at first behaves in accordance with the short-circuited mechanism, but that at a certain phase of his development he learns to postpone gratification. He learns to do so, if he is consistently trained to expect substitute gratification at progressively increasing intervals. For instance, little George wants a second ice cream. He wants it at all costs; he says that he "needs it." But if mother keeps the child on her lap, caresses him and says, "No, George, you cannot have it now," little George will be able to accept this deprivation, because it is immediately compensated for by the tenderness of mother. Later in similar cases, as a compensation for the deprivation, instead of direct tenderness he will get the approval of mother. Still later he will get only a promise, that is the hope that something good will happen to him as a reward for not responding immediately to impulsive urges. Promises and hopes, although abstract visualizations of things which have not materialized, retain a flavor or an echo of mother's approval and tenderness. Now it could be that the future short-circuited psychopath did not go through these normal stages. What appeared to the child as deprivation held no compensations. The postponement was enforced in a crude way. No benevolent mother was there to help the child to make the transition from immediate gratification to postponement. He did not learn to expect approval and tenderness, to experience hope and to anticipate the fulfillment of a promise. Frustration remains a very unpleasant, even unbearable experience. Thus he continued to exercise his neuronal patterns in circuits which referred to the present and led to quick responses.

What we have so far illustrated in this infantile situation can explain why the patient becomes more adept with short-circuited mechanisms than with long-circuited ones. If, however, the whole psychopathology of the psychopath would be included in this mechanism, the patient would reveal himself to be quick-tempered, childish, immature, but not necessarily antisocial. To be specific, wanting two ice creams may be immature, but not necessarily psychopathic. To reveal psychopathic tendencies, the child must steal the second ice cream.

Thus, the psychopathic mechanism is more complicated. The process may be understood if we remember what has already been mentioned in passing: that the psychopath does not experience, at least in sufficient quantity, anxiety or worry with regard to future happenings. A person may be immature and desirous of quick gratification, but if he has the ability to experience a sufficient quantity of anxiety he will not become a psychopath. A person who has no anxiety can mentally scan all possible ways by which he can obtain quick gratification. For a person who experiences adequate amounts of anxiety, such scanning, in so complete and prompt-to-action way, is not possible. The antisocial possibilities are automatically inhibited or suppressed by the anxiety and in many cases may remain totally unconscious or repressed. The psychopath does not find himself in this situation.

Again, in a hypothetical manner we can state that the mother-child relationship has a great deal to do with this lack of anxiety. If at a certain stage of development the parents have impressed the child with the possibility of bad future consequences as a result of his behavior, if they have threatened the child with future punishment, and have carried out the punishment at a certain interval after the misbehavior, the child is not likely to become a psychopath. These words may sound strange. In fact for many years opposite points of view have repeatedly been expressed in psychiatry: For instance, with regard to how harmful it is to provoke anxiety in children, and how excessive anxiety originated in the relationships with the parents may lead to severe psychoneuroses and to schizophrenia. These points of view are substantially correct. However, it may be equally correct that the great permissiveness and nonanxiety provoking attitude that parents have recently assumed, partially because of "psychological sophistication," are contributing factors in the recent increase in juvenile delinquency all over the world, and incidentally, for the decrease in obsessive-compulsive psychoneuroses.

We must once more conclude that the patient is in a difficult situation, between psychological Scylla and Charybdis. If he or she evokes too much anxiety in the child, one sort of mental disorder may be facilitated; if too little anxiety is elicited, the likelihood of occurrence of another sort of mental disorder may be greater. Let us not be too discouraged! Most parents seem capable of veering away from these two excesses and of maintaining a normal route. At times we find psychopathic children in very strict and severely punishing families. This is not necessarily a contradiction of the foregoing. In these cases the punishment, generally physical in nature, was imparted by the parents immediately after the misbehavior. Thus the child could experience immediate fear and pain, but not anxiety about the future.

At times we find complicating features in the picture of the simple psychopath. In some cases, the short-circuited mechanism is adopted only in very limited areas of life. Perhaps the parents were able to elicit a normal amount of anxiety in most aspects of living but none in others. Numerous gradations are possible, which deserve accurate pyschodynamic studies.

In a considerable number of simple psychopaths we find also, a basically inadequate personality. We have, for instance, the following picture: The patient harbors relatively big aims and wishes although he is psychologically inadequate to realize them. He tries several times, but every time he tries, he gets into a predicament. Eventually, the relatively quick mental processes which led him to ill-planned adventures lead him to find quick antisocial solutions to his predicaments, for instance to request money from relatives or to actually steal. Here a basically inadequate personality operates together with the short-circuited mechanism.

In some cases of simple psychopathy sociocultural factors seem to have played a facilitating role. The patient at times acknowledges these environmental factors, but simplifies their mode of operation by saying that he follows his impulses only when the environment allows him to do so.

b) The Complex Psychopath

I have mentioned how the simple psychopath has occasionally an illumination or insight on "how to do it." The insight of the complex psychopath is more complicated. It can be summarized in the formula, "how to do it and get away with it." To this group of psychopaths belong the professional bank robbers and some unscrupulous political leaders.

At first it may seem difficult to explain the mechanisms of the complex psychopath, as they seem to contradict the mechanisms which have so far been explained. Finding ways to rob a modern bank and, even more so, ways of reaching and retaining political power, seem to require long-circuited mental processes. We must add at this point that every mental mechanism has to be considered in relation to the general mental set. Complex psychopaths are very intelligent people and relative to their intellectual potential or to what normal ways of making goals would entail, the methods they use, like eliminating political adversaries by murder, are quick methods. Moral considerations are not allowed to delay the urge for gratification, although relatively long-circuited mechanisms have to be adopted and endured, to avoid further delays or in order to make the gratification possible. Here the ego, which retains considerable strength, is used in the service of the relatively quick gratification. Long-circuited mechanisms are in the service of short-circuited ones.

My limited clinical experience has so far not permitted me to distinguish psychodynamic factors, or early environmental factors, which differ from those of the simple psychopath. I must add, however, that the whole philosophy of life of the complex psychopath seems different from that of the simple psychopath. The simple psychopath seems to eliminate the conflict between the pleasure principle and the reality principle by completely acceding to the pleasure principle. The complex psychopath operates at a much higher level. He solves the conflict that the normal man may have at times between what he considers self-realization and social morality by following without hesitation what seems to him self-realization. The complex psychopath believes that he deserves, or is entitled to, or that it is congruent with his personal endowment, to seek that particular gratification. He does not care how he is going to get it. The norms of society are not going to stop him and should not apply to him. Whereas the simple psychopath can be seen as following a style of life based on the philosophy of Epicurus, or, more correctly, on the philosophy popularly attributed to Epicurus, the complex psychopath follows a style of life consonant with some tenets of Nietzsche and some teachings of Machiavelli.

c) The Dyssocial Psychopath

To this group belong individuals who are occasionally called "sociological psychopaths." The word "dyssocial," proposed by the Committee on Nomenclature and Statistics of the American Psychiatric Association (6), seems to this author more appropriate. In fact these patients are not socialized in a usual sense. They substitute for everybody's society a smaller and special society, which permits and enables them to be antisocial toward the members of the large society. They may be capable of strong loyalties for their group.

These patients are people who in their young age were often members of juvenile or delinquent gangs. As adults they become members of groups of professional criminals. Some authors consider these patients not as psychopathic personalities but as members of special occupational groups (Jenkins) (13).

Jenkins (13) also believes that "the professional criminal is a cultural product." Others authors, like Cohen (5), and Shaw and McKay (17), have given great importance to sociological-cultural factors in the etiology and psychogenesis of the dyssocial psychopath. I agree that sociological-cultural factors are very important, but I do not share Jenkins' point of view that the dyssocial psychopath is completely separated from the other types. In fact there are many mixed cases; for instance of people who at times have individually given vent to their antisocial behavior and at other times only when they had the support of a special group to which they belonged.

This type of psychopath does not belong only to gangs of juvenile delinquents or to association of thieves, but at times to groups which in particular environments are socially acceptable. Undoubtedly one of the most famous and, I can add, infamous of the dyssocial psychopaths was Adolph Eichmann. His group was the Nazi gang, to which he gave his loyalty to the very end. Even while he was about to be executed he invoked his loyalty, as a justification of his deeds. He said: "I followed my flag and the law of war." Implicitly, he meant that he followed the laws of that criminal gang which was the Nazi party and the then German government, which permitted him to kill millions of innocent human beings.

How can we interpret the formal and the dynamic mechanisms of the dyssocial psychopath? Obviously his phenomenology is more complicated than that of the simple psychopath. In the dyssocial psychopath too there is a strong urge to gratify a primitive need for greed, or for discharge of hostility by resorting to relatively short-circuited mechanisms (gas chambers, armed robbery, multiple murders, etc.). However, the short-circuited mechanism must *be released* or sanctioned by the authority of a special group. The patient is not simply disregardful of his conscience or superego, like the simple psychopath. He substitutes the normal conscience with the ideology or the laws of the special group of which he has become a part. Adoption of the short-circuited mechanism is thus as important in the dyssocial psychopath as in the simple and complex. Here, however, its use has to be accompanied or preceded by an abnormal displacement of conscience (or superego, or parental identifications, in accordance with the various terminologies). This displacement was probably facilitated by several factors: 1) the patient did not receive in childhood or early in life that parental approval, recognition, etc. that he needed to build up his self-esteem; 2) availability for sociological-cultural-historical reasons, of a group which can give the patient this approval and recognition, at the same time that it permits him to use short-circuited mechanisms for the gratification of primitive needs. At times unusual features complicate the picture of the dyssocial psychopath. In some rare cases the group to which he is loyal and whose support he needs is replaced by a single person, for instance a friend, a father-in-law, a fellow prisoner, etc.

Are these mechanisms that we have so far described in the simple, complex and dyssocial psychopaths related to psychotic mechanisms? Psychopaths are generally not considered psychotic either in psychiatric classifications or by the law. Cleckley, however, by suggesting that they have only a "mask of sanity" perhaps implies that they should be considered insane (3). If Cleckley means that these people should be considered psychiatrically very ill, that they cannot in some circumstances control their actions and that the law and our attitude in relation to them should be revised, then I fully go along with Cleckley. However, I am reluctant to use the words "psychotic" or "insane" in reference to them. With the words "psychotic" we do not mean simply a person who is seriously mentally ill. We mean a person who has undergone a basic symbolic transformation (like the schizophrenic) or a basic emotional transformation (like the manic-depressive) or has sustained a severe cognitive defect (like some organic patients), and who also accepts his transformation as a normal way of living. The psychopath has an intellectual awareness that some of his actions are not acceptable to society. His insight, however, is not accompanied by an appropriate emotional tone and remains superficial. Furthermore, his need to carry out the psychopathic act by means of a short-circuited mechanism prevails over this insight.

That the psychopath has some insight is also manifested by the fact that he makes promises concerning the future. He makes repeated resolutions for good future behavior. He goes to the extent of showing to the therapist that he is fully aware of the troubles he will encounter if he repeats the same patterns of behavior. Nevertheless when the future becomes the present, the impelling need to repeat the short-circuited mechanism overcomes any consideration.

d) The Paranoiac Psychopath

To this last group belong rare individuals who present a peculiar mixture of paranoiac and psychopathic features. After accurate examination of them we can state that in addition to being psychopaths they are psychotics in the usual sense of the word.

Paranoid features are seen in many psychopaths who belong to the simple, complex and dyssocial types. They are, however, rather superficial, inconsistent, and often obvious defenses or patched-up rationalizations used to justify the abnormal behavior. In the paranoiac psychopath the paranoiac mechanisms are well systematized and accompanied by apparently logical cognitive processes. There is preservation of the personality and the general picture is closer to Kraepelin's classical paranoia than to the other paranoid syndromes or conditions. For this reason the term paranoiac rather than paranoid is used.* No hallucinations or obviously regressive features of the paranoid type of schizophrenia are encountered in these patients. Instead we find in some cases, periods of drug or alcoholic addictions.

These patients differ from the usual paranoiac inasmuch as their acting out in accordance with their delusions becomes the most salient feature of the syndrome. Undoubtedly many regular paranoiacs and paranoids act out in accordance with their delusions; but in the paranoiac psychopath the acting out is more extensive and the psychopathic traits generally *anteceded* a definite paranoiac symptomatology, or in some cases, periods of acting out with no freely expressed delusions *alternate* with obvious delusional periods. These paranoiac psychopaths are in many cases similar to the other cases of paranoia and perhaps they constitute only a variety of this syndrome. In fact, like the regular paranoiacs, they are generally

---

* In the psychiatric literature a confusion is often made between "paranoiac" and "paranoid." Paranoiac is the adjective related to the noun "paranoia," whereas "para-state, paranoid type of schizophrenia, etc.

single men, of superior intelligence, incapable of sustaining heterosexual relations, and present latent homosexual trends, hidden by sadistic features.

Whereas the dyssocial psychopath needs a group, which releases his tendencies to act out, the paranoiac psychopath needs a system of delusions which allows him to act out. He creates a delusional system which justifies his actions. Whereas in order to justify his use of the short-circuited mechanism the dyssocial psychopath needs a long-circuited mechanism based on his allegiance to a group or to a special code, the paranoiac psychopath finds his justifications by creating a long-circuited mechanism consisting of delusions. When the paranoiac psychopath is prevented from acting out, for instance, by imprisonment or hospitalization, he becomes more paranoiac. On the other hand, if he is discharged and especially if external situations permit him to act out, he becomes slightly less paranoiac and more psychopathic.

Some of these paranoiac psychopaths remain unrecognized for many years. Moreover the brilliancy of their intellect may hide their pathology and the peculiarity of their mental processes may assume demogogic persuasion and find resonant echo and wild acclaim in particular historico-cultural circumstances.

The classic example of a paranoiac psychopath is Adolph Hitler, if future historical and psychiatric research will confirm what already appears from an incomplete and preliminary evaluation of his personality. His grandiose plans which were well calculated, were often actualized at first by resorting to "the big lie" which, as he boasted, is easily believed, and later to crimes, at a scale never before seen on the surface of the earth.

In order to act out, Hitler needed a paranoiac system. Prominent in this system were the Jews, who were behind all evils and had to be exterminated. With the waning of his grandiose plans in consequence of his military defeats, his delusions became more pronounced and his need to act out more impelling. A vicious circle thus was repeating itself. Even in the last few months of his life he continued to blame the machinations of the Jews for his defeats. But even then, the end of his power was still in the future and not experienced emotionally by him as a real possibility. The enemy had to be at the doors of Berlin, in its physical actuality, before Hitler could feel the full import of the disaster. The last sentence of his will, which he dictated shortly before committing suicide, reiterated his delusions about the Jews.

Not all acting out of the paranoiac psychopath is antisocial. Some patients become alcoholic, drug addicts, or addicts to surgery, requesting operations which are unnecessary. Whereas psychotherapy of the symptomatic psychopath or pseudopsychopath may yield good results, the results with idiopathic or true psychopaths have seldom been satisfactory. Specific techniques, aiming for instance at establishing a normal experiencing of anxiety, have not yet been devised. In particular, psychotherapy of the paranoiac psychopath seems beyond the realm of present possibilities. If we, psychiatrists, must accept today's limitations of the therapy of the idiopath, we must alert ourselves to their prompt diagnosis and alert others to the danger which these patients may constitute when their condition is unrecognized.

REFERENCES

1. ARIETI, S.: The processes of expectation and anticipation. Their genetic development, neural basis and role in psychopathology. *J. Nerv. & Ment. Dis.*, 100:471, 1947.
2. ARIETI, S.: Writings in preparation.
3. CLECKLEY, H. M.: *The Mask of Sanity*. St. Louis: C. L. Mosby Co., 1955.
4. CLECKLEY, H. M.: Psychopathic states. In *American Handbook of Psychiatry*. Edited by S. Arieti. New York: Basic Books, 1959.
5. COHEN, A. K.: *Delinquent Boys: The Culture of the Gang*. Glencoe, Ill.: Free Press, 1955.
6. COMMITTEE ON NOMENCLATURE AND STATISTICS: *Diagnostic and Statistical Manual of Mental Disorders*. Washington, D. C.: American Psychiatric Assoc., 1952.
7. EHRLICH, S. K. and KEOGH, R. P.: The psychopath in a mental institution. *A.M.A. Arch. of Neurol. & Psychiat.*, 76:286-295, 1956.
8. GLUECK, S. and GLUECK, E. T.: *Physique and Delinquency*. New York: Harper, 1956.
9. HARLOW, J. M.: Passage of an iron rod through the head. *Boston Med. Surg., J.*, 39:389-393, 1848.
10. HARLOW, J. M.: Recovery from the passage of an iron bar through the head. *Mass. Med. Soc. Publ.*, 2:327-46, 1868.
11. HILL, D.: EEG in episodic psychotic and psychopathic behavior. *Electroencephal. & Clin. Neurophysiol.*, 4:439, 1952.
12. HILL, D.: Electroencephalography. In *Recent Advances in Neuropsychiatry*. Edited by W. R. Brain and E. B. Strauss. London: G. A. Churchill, Ltd., 1955.
13. JENKINS, R. L.: The psychopathic or antisocial personality. *J. Nerv. & Ment. Dis.*, 131:318-334, 1960.
14. JOHNSON, A.: Juvenile delinquency. In *American Handbook of Psychiatry*, Vol. 1. Edited by S. Arieti. New York: Basic Books, 1959, pp. 840-856.
15. KARPMAN, B.: On the need for separating psychopathy into two distinct clinical types: Symptomatic and idiopathic. *J. Crim. Psychopath.*, 3:112-137, 1941.
16. LOMBROSO, C.: L'uomo delinquente in rapporto alla antropologia, alla giurisprudenza ed alle discipline sociali. Milan, 1876.
17. SHAW, C. R. and McKAY, H. D.: *Social Factors in Juvenile Delinquency*. Washington, D. C.: National Commission on Law Observance and Enforcement, Report on the Causes of Crimes CPO, 1931.
18. SZUREK, S. A.: Notes on the genesis of psychopathic personality trends. *Psychiat.*, 5:1, 1942.

16

The Psychotherapeutic Approach
to Depression

This short paper, published in 1962, advances two new ideas which came to play a predominant role in my subsequent studies of depression: the differentiation of two types of depression (the "claiming" and "self-blaming" type), and the concept of the dominant other. The first elements of a dynamic-cognitive psychotherapeutic approach to depression are presented.

MY PAPER has several limitations. It will not deal with full-fledged depressions of the manic-depressive or involutional types, or with the treatment of patients, who, on account of the severity of their symptoms, are not suitable for psychotherapy and must be treated with physical methods. It will also not deal with the treatment of patients who have already overcome the acute attack of depression. Since Abraham's work (1), many reports have dealt with the psychoanalytic treatment of the patient during the symptom-free intervals. My paper, on the other hand, will pertain to those cases where depression is present and active, although not so pronounced as to prevent meaningful communications or to necessitate immediate relief with physical therapies.

Before discussing psychotherapy, however, I want to examine the formal mechanisms, the psychodynamics and some new nosological concepts of depression. These concepts apply to patients who are treated with psychotherapy as well as to patients treated with physical methods.

Formal Mechanisms of Depression

What is the biologic meaning of depression? Depression, or anguish, is mental pain, an experience to which the name pain is often given, because of the similarity to physical pain. Physical pain is a sensation which in-

216

forms the conscious organism that a loss to the continuity of the proper functioning of the body has taken place. By being unpleasant, pain is a warning that something is wrong. In lower species an attempt at removal of pain is made by withdrawal from the source of pain. In higher species, especially in man, a voluntary action generally attempts to remove the source of pain, so that the regenerative forces of the organism will permit healing. I do not think we shall be in error if we see something similar in that form of mental pain, depression. Something has happened which has brought about this unpleasant emotional state. A loved person, or the love of this person, a symbolic situation, a status, a concept of ourselves, an ideal have been lost. The depression is the reaction to the loss of what we consider a normal ingredient of our psychologic life. Like physical pain, mental has one purpose: it wants to be removed.

Let us assume that a person dear to us has died. For some time after the death all thoughts connected with the departed person will bring about a painful, almost unbearable feeling. Any cluster or constellation of thoughts even remotely connected with the dead person will evoke a feeling of sadness. We cannot accept the idea that the dear one is not with us anymore; we cannot adjust to his absence. But if that person was so dear, so important to us, a great number of our thoughts or actions are directly or indirectly connected with him and therefore will bring back sadness.

Nevertheless, after a certain period of time, we get adjusted to the idea that the person is dead. By the very fact of being unpleasant the sadness has a purpose—it wants to be removed. It will be removed only by forcing the individual to reorganize his thinking, that is, to untie the clusters of thoughts concerning the departed, to reorganize thoughts into different constellations which do not bring about sadness. By doing so the individual is compelled to rearrange his life to a certain extent, and the departed one is not considered any longer indispensable either psychologically or at the level of practical reality.

At times, however, this process fails and another mcehanism occurs which manifests several degrees of pathology. The depression, rather than forcing a reorganization of ideas, slows down the thought processes. In this case the psychologic mechanism seems to have the goal of decreasing the quantity of thoughts in order to decrease the quantity of suffering. At times the slowing down of thought processes is so pronounced (as in the state of stupor) that only a few thoughts of a general or atmospheric quality are left; these are accompanied by an overpowering feeling of melancholy. Thus the slowing-down of thought processes is a self-defeating mechanism. The decrease in motility, found in these patients, is secondary to the slowing down of thought processes, so that even the ideomotor activity preceding movements and actions is decreased (Arieti, 2).

Recently Ostow (3), has reached similar conclusions. He writes that one of the functions of depression is to impel the sufferer to retrieve the lost object. He also writes that "Depression is a form of psychic pain, and it motivates the individual to perform whatever act will relieve the pain most quickly." Ostow, however, sees depression also as an egoenervation, or of loss of psychic energy in the ego, which would explain the reduced activity—activity which would be wasted, as the lost object is irretrievable.

Psychodynamic Mechanisms

Very early in the life of people who are prone to become depressed there was a period of intense gratification of needs. The mother or mother-substitute was compelled by a sense of duty to be as lavish as possible in her care and manifestations of affection. This attitude predisposed the child to be very receptive to others, to introject the others, and later to be an extrovert and a conformist.

At a later period but still in early childhood, generally during the second or third year of life, but in some cases even much earlier, the family situation undergoes a drastic change. The mother now takes care of the child considerably less than before and makes many demands on him. This change in the mother's attitude may be due to the fact that in the meantime another sibling was born and the mother is now lavishing her care on the newborn with the same duty-bound generosity that she previously had for the patient. At other times the mother dies, is ill, or has to disappear for different reasons. More often, however, the reason for the change is to be found in the personality of the mother, who believes that when a child is a small baby, he has to be fully taken care of, but as soon as he shows the first signs of an independent personality, he should start to be given increasing responsibilities, a sense of duty, of obligation, and the like. No transitional stages are allowed.

For some not fully understood reasons, this process occurs in more pronounced aspects between mothers and daughters, and this fact may at least partially explain the greater prevalence of depression in women.* The child finds himself changed from an environment which predisposes him to great receptivity to one of great expectations. These dissimilar

---

* Perhaps mothers expect their daughters especially to assume heavy responsibilities and relieve them of their obligations.

environments, which are predisposed by cultural factors that I have outlined elsewhere (2, 4), are often actually determined by a common factor: the strong sense of duty that compelled the mother to do so much for the baby is now forcibly transmitted to the child. If no compensatory mechanisms occur, the child undergoes the trauma of the paradise lost. The child, however, tries to find solutions or pseudosolutions. Generally he adopts one of the two following mechanisms, which he will repeat also throughout his adult life. The first is an attempt to make himself even more babyish, more dependent, aggressively dependent, so that the mother or the important adult who later on will symbolically take her place, will be forced to reestablish an atmosphere of babyhood and of early bliss.

Another mechanism consists in trying to live up to the expectations of mother, no matter how high the price, how heavy the burden. Only by complying and working hard love or the lost paradise will be recaptured. If love is not obtained it is because the patient is at fault. He must atone or work harder.

Implied in these defenses is the belief that love is still available, but not as a steady flow. The patient has to find it with these mechanisms, but they too do not seem to work. No matter how aggressively dependent the individual becomes, he does not recapture paradise. No matter how compliant and hard working he is, he does not obtain what he wants. This realization brings about the depressed feeling. The actual manifest symptomatology of depression occurs when a symbolic reproduction of the early trauma takes place later in life. A loss has been sustained and the patient feels that his way of living has caused such a loss. Other mechanisms, like the manic defense, are not mentioned here because they are beyond the purpose of this paper.

Clinical Types of Depression

My clinical experience has led me to divide the cases of depression which are not part of a typical circular manic-depressive psychosis or of a typical involutional psychosis into two types which I call "claiming depression" and "self-blaming depression." Some people may find some similarities between these two types which I am going to describe and the so-called reactive and endogenous depressions. Actually the two classifications do not coincide. In fact I do not know what the endogenous factors consist of, and if they do exist I am not in a position to exclude their role even in the so-called reactive type. On the other hand, I am sure that even in those cases which some psychiatrists would call endogenous, psychogenetic and precipitating psychologic factors operate.

Although the self-blaming type of depression reaches psychotic proportions more often than the claiming type, my classification is not particularly concerned with the psychotic or neurotic status of the depression. As I have described elsewhere (2), a depression is to be considered psychotic not necessarily when it is severe, but when the emotional transformation is accepted by the patient as a way of living. In neurotic types the depression is instead unaccepted and fought by the patient. Although a considerable number of cases exist in which the claiming and self-blaming types are mixed, I believe it is important to distinguish these two main kinds, for at least two reasons: 1) in order to reach a better psychodynamic understanding of them; 2) because when occurring in pure culture they require a different psychotherapeutic approach, at least during the acute depressive attack.

I want to say, however, that the cases which have come under my observation irrespective of which of the two types of depression they belonged to, had an important characteristic in common. Contrary to what happens in schizophrenia, where the psychosis is a reaction to a failure of cosmic magnitude involving the relation with the whole interpersonal world, the failure of the depressed patient, even if apparently the result of a nonpersonal event, was sustained mainly or exclusively in relation to one person in his immediate environment. I shall call this person the *dominant other.*

The dominant other is represented most often by the spouse. Far less often in order of frequency, follow the mother, a person to whom the patient was romantically attached, an adult child, a sister, the father.* Also frequently the dominant other is represented, through anthropomorphization, by the firm where the patient works, or a social institution to which he belongs, like the Church, the political party, the army, the club, and so forth. All these dominant others are symbolic of the depriving mother, or to be more accurate, of the once giving and later depriving mother. If the mother is the dominant other she will act in two ways, as her present role is symbolic of her old one. If the dominant other dies he becomes even more powerful through the meanings attached to his death.

In the following discussion I shall refer to the patient as to a male; but actually from 65 to 70 per cent of the patients are women.

---

* This sequence is the result of bona fide clinical observations, not of statistically controlled data.

Claiming Depression

Contrary to what occurred until approximately 15 years ago, claiming depression is the most common type in psychiatric practice. For this type of depression I agree with Rado (5) that the patient's symptomatology is a cry for help. The patient is anguished, but makes you very aware of it. All the symptoms seem to have a message: "Help me; pity me. It is in your power to relieve me. If I suffer it is because you don't relieve me of this suffering. If I sustained a loss, it is because you don't give me what I need." Even the suicidal attempt or prospect is an appeal: "Do not abandon me," or "You have the power to prevent my death. I want you to know it." In other words, the symptomatology, although colored by an atmosphere of depression, is a gigantic claim. Now it is the gestalt of depression which looms in the foreground with the claim lurking behind; now it is the claim which looms with the depression apparently receding. Badly hidden are also feelings of hostility for the dominant other who does not give as much as the patient expects. If anger is expressed, feelings of guilt and depression follow. Some authors, for instance Bonime (6), have stressed the importance of this hostility.

If we remember the psychodynamic mechanisms that I have described, it will be easy to recognize that in claiming depression the patient is still claiming the lost paradise or the state of bliss of the early life, when he was completely dependent on the duty-bound mother. The patient makes himself dependent on the dominant other and becomes more and more demanding—the more deprived he feels. Any unfulfilled demand is experienced as a wound, a loss, and brings about depression. Moreover, the depression in these cases does not lead to the breaking of the old patterns or to new ways of thinking, but tends to perpetuate itself, to increase, and to slow down all activities.

I shall now outline briefly the main points of the treatment of this type of depression while the depression is active. In those cases where relatedness is easily established, we soon recognize that the patient wants to find in the therapist a substitute for the dominant other who has failed; or, in other words, he wants to find a substitute for the lost love object. To the extent that the patient's demands are realistic, the therapist should try to go along with these requests and satisfy some of the needs for affection, consideration, companionship. Even clinging and nagging have to be accepted. Occasionally, we even have to prolong the session for a few minutes, as at the last minute the patient feels the urge to make new demands or to ask "one more question." This attitude may seem a too indulgent one.

The fact is that at the beginning of the treatment we cannot expect the patient to give up mechanisms which he has used throughout his life. Many patients, especially at the beginning of the session, are not able to verbalize freely, and should not be requested to explain their feelings in detail or to go into long series of associations. On the contrary, the therapist should take the initiative and speak freely to them, even about unrelated subjects. As a patient of Clara Thompson (7), requoted by Rose Spiegel (8), said, the words of the analyst are often experienced as gifts of love by the depressed person. Following the suggestions made in Rose Spiegel's papers (8, 9), the therapist will soon learn to communicate with the depressed, in spite of his lack of imagery and the poverty of his verbalizations. It is in the feeling itself, rather than in verbal symbols, that he often expresses himself.

When this immediate craving for being given acceptance is somewhat satisfied, the depression will considerably diminish, but will not disappear. However, now the depression will no longer be in the form of a sustained mood, but will appear in isolated, discrete fits. At this stage it will be relatively easy to guide the patient to recognize that the fit of depression comes as a result of the following conscious or unconscious sequence of thoughts or of their symbolic equivalents: "I am not getting what I should—I am deprived—I am in a miserable state."

The patient is guided to stop at the first stage of this sequence: "I am not getting what I should." Can he substitute this recurring idea with another one, for instance, "What ways, other than aggressive expectation and dependency, are at my disposal in order to get what I want?" In other words, the patient is guided to reorganize his ways of thinking, so that the usual clusters of thoughts will not recur and will not reproduce the old sequence. The psychologic horizon will enlarge and new patterns of living will be sought. However, the patient will be able to do so only if the new relationship with the therapist has decreased his feeling of deprivation and his suffering, so that the old pathogenic sequence will not reproduce itself automatically and with such tenacity. Excursions into paths of self-reliance will be made more and more frequently by the patient. At the same time gradual limitations are imposed on the demands made on the therapst. Once the fits of depression have disappeared, the treatment will continue along traditional lines. The patient will learn to recognize his basic patterns of living which had led him to the depression, and the special characteristics of his early interpersonal relationships which led to the organizations of such patterns. Such characteristics as superficiality, insensitivity, marked extraversion covered by depression, recurrence of clichés, infantile attitudes, such as "love me like a baby," will be recognized as defense mechanisms and will disappear.

Self-Blaming Depression

This type of depression, which is much closer to the classic type described in circular manic-depressive psychosis, is declining in frequency.

The pictures of stupor or of overpowering melancholia which used to be seen, for instance in women who stated that they had consumed all their tears, who would pull their hair, would say that they had lost all their internal organs, are a rarity today. Nevertheless, cases characterized by a milder symptomatology of self-accusation do occur and have to be promptly recognized because they require a psychotherapeutic treatment which differs from the one just described.

These patients do not appear shallow or superficial as do the patients suffering from claiming depression. It is true that they are also very conventional but their conventionality finds sources in the traditions of the culture to which the patient belongs. It is true that they are poor in verbal symbols or in imagery, but their symbols often retain an augustinian or medieval flavor, with duty, sin, guilt, punishment, as the recurring themes. God often becomes the dominant other. In these cases the message the patient conveys is not, "Help me," but "I do not deserve any help, any pity." When suicidal ideas exist the message is not, "You should prevent my death," but, "I deserve to die; I should do to myself what you should do to me, but you are too good to do it." The classic Freudian interpretation of the suicide is that the patient in killing himself wants to kill the love object, but I could not confirm this point of view in the numerous patients that I have treated.

In a considerable number of patients we find a strange combination of depressive and obsessive-compulsive symptoms, resulting in an apparently serious syndrome, easily confused with the schizophrenic. Some of these patients are by some psychiatrists treated with electric shock: the depression will then subside, at least temporarily, but the obsessive symptomatology will flourish.

It is easy to recognize that in self-blaming depression the basic mechanism consists of an attempt to retrieve the loss, or to recapture the bliss of the first years of life by expiating, often by living up to impossible expectations. The second psychodynamic mechanism that I have described in the foregoing is here at work. Guilt feeling→atoning→attempted redemption is the pattern. The patient wants peace at any cost but peace cannot be found. The symptoms are often ways of changing anxiety into guilt feeling. For instance, the patient does not go to church on Sunday. Now he has something to feel guilty about. As painful as the guilt feeling is, the patient is aware that the possibility of suffering and thus of redeeming himself is in his power, whereas with anxiety he is at a loss; he does not know what to do about it.

The obsessive-compulsive symptoms occurring in many cases, are attempts to channel guilt feelings and to find measures to relieve them, so that the lost love will be recaptured. Actually they do not solve but aggravate the situation. For instance, the patient may have the obsession of thinking about something profane or sacrilegious, or about the oncoming death of a relative, and then he feels guilty about having such thoughts. Similarly, compulsions may obligate the patient to perform actions condemned by the ritual of his religion, and again he feels guilty.

There are relatively few recent reports on the psychotherapy of this type of depression, as almost all recent works concern the claiming type. The reason for the scarcity of reports is to be found not so much in the declining number of self-blaming patients as in the difficulty inherent in their treatment, so that most of them are given physical types of therapy. It is my feeling, however, that cases of relatively moderate intensity do respond to psychotherapy even better than to other treatments.

With this type of patient the therapist cannot assume the role of the benevolent giver, as in the claiming type. The patient would feel even more guilty and meaningful communication would not be established.

One of the first things we have to take care of instead is to affect the environment. Several sessions with the dominant other will reveal hidden mechanisms operating in the relationship. The dominant other quite often, because of repressed hostility or of obsessive-compulsive attitudes, unwittingly increases the patient's feeling of duty and guilt. Such sentences as, "You are too sick to do the housework now," or "For many years you took care of me, now I take care of you," increase the guilt feeling of the patient. Several changes have to be discussed with the dominant other or a substitute to relieve as much as possible the patient's feeling of guilt, responsibility, unaccomplishment, loss.

This technique helps, just as the relationship with the therapist helped in the claiming type, and will change a lasting mood of depression into one characterized by isolated, discrete fits of depression. At this point it will be possible to show to the patient how he translates any feeling of loss or disappointment into one of self-accusation and guilt. The sequence has to be interrupted. One of the fundamental things is not to allow depressive thoughts to expand into a general mood of depression, that is, to lose their discrete quality. The clusters of thought which lead to depression must be untied and new ones formed.

This approach has no lasting effect, of course, unless followed later on by deeper technique. Its value, however, at the beginning of the treatment, lies in breaking as many clusters of thought as possible which lead to depressive fits. A little later it will be possible to show the patient that the little disappointments or losses which lead him to self-accusation, guilt, depression, are actually symbolic of earlier, greater disappointments or losses.

Still later it will be possible to show the patient how he tends to transform anxiety into guilt. Finally, he will learn to face anxiety rather than to reproduce the sequence which will lead to depression. Eventually in these cases too the early interpersonal relationships and the basic patterns of living must be analyzed and interpreted. The treatment is more difficult than it would seem because vicious circles are formed or stumbling blocks are encountered which tend to perpetuate the depression. For instance, the patient may become depressed over the fact that he may so easily become depressed; any little disappointment triggers off the state of sadness or guilt. Again he has to be reminded that the little disappointment is symbolic of a bigger one. Another difficulty consists in the fact that some clusters of thought seem harmless to the therapist and are allowed to recur; actually they lead to depression because of the particular connections that they have only in the patient's mind. Eventually, however, the emotional pitch of the therapist will become more and more attuned to that of the patient.

I want to stress that alertness on the part of the therapist is always necessary in the treatment of depression. At times, when the depression has improved very much, a dangerous relapse may occur if the patient is allowed to feel guilty for the allegedly undeserved improvement or because a not yet used depressing cluster of thoughts is allowed to expand. The patient may become so discouraged over his relapse as to want to discontinue psychotherapy and actively seek shock treatment. This, I think, we may be able to prevent in most cases, if we maintain our vigilance and keep our feelings attuned to those of the patient.

REFERENCES

1. ABRAHAM, K.: Notes on the psycho-analytical investigation and treatment of manic-depressive insanity and allied conditions. In *Selected Papers on Psychoanalysis*. New York: Basic Books, 1953.

2. ARIETI, S.: Manic-depressive psychosis. In *American Handbook of Psychiatry*, Vol. 1. Edited by S. Arieti. New York: Basic Books, 1959, pp. 419-454.
3. OSTOW, M.: The psychic function of depression: A study of energetics. *Psychoanal. Quart.*, 29:355, 1960.
4. ARIETI, S.: Some socio-cultural aspects of manic-depressive psychosis and schizophrenia. In *Progress in Psychotherapy*, Vol. IV. Edited by J. H. Masserman and J. C. Moreno. New York: Grune & Stratton, 1959.
5. RADO, S.: Psychosomatics of depression from the etiologic point of view. *Psychosom. Med.*, 13:51, 1951.
6. BONIME, W.: Depression as a practice: Dynamic and psychotherapeutic considerations. *Compreh. Psychiat.*, 1:194, 1960.
7. THOMPSON, C. M.: Analytic observations during the course of a manic-depressive psychosis. *Psychoanal. Rev.*, 17:240, 1930. (Quoted by R. Spiegel, 8.)
8. SPIEGEL, R.: Communication in the psychoanalysis of depression. In *Psychoanalysis and Human Values*. Edited by J. Masserman. New York: Grune & Stratton, 1960, pp. 209-222.
9. SPIEGEL, R.: Specific problems of communication in psychiatric conditions. In *American Handbook of Psychiatry*. Vol. 1. Edited by S. Arienti. New York: Basic Books, 1959, pp. 909-949.

17

Psychoanalysis of Severe Depression:
Theory and Therapy

This paper (1976) summarizes some ideas already expressed in my chapter on Affective Psychoses, published in the second edition of the American Handbook of Psychiatry, and advances a number of new ideas. The psychoanalytic treatment of a case of post-partum depression is described.

INTRODUCTION

SINCE THE CLASSIC WORKS of Abraham and Freud (13), psychoanalysis has made considerable steps forward in the interpretation of depression. For example, Rado's (19, 20) conception that melancholia is a despairing cry for love, an attempt of the ego to punish itself in order to prevent the parental punishment, by enacting guilt, atonement, and forgiveness; Klein's (16, 17) interpretation of this condition as a pathological outcome of the depressive position; Bibring's (10) concept of depression as a conflict of the ego, a state of helplessness consequent to loss of self-esteem, are important contributions from either the Freudian or the Kleinian schools. A noteworthy contribution in the cultural school, is Bonime's (11, 12), who sees depression as a practice. According to Bonime, "The depressive is an extremely manipulative individual who, by helplessness, sadness, seductiveness, and other means, maneuvers people toward the fulfillment of demands for various forms of emotionally comforting response" (12).

In spite of these significant advances, one can repeat for depression what can be said for practically every area of psychiatry: no conclusive or decisive statement has been made, and no major breakthrough leading to a definitive position has occurred. As a matter of fact, some authors have reached pessimistic conclusions about this state of affairs. Grinker and his associates (15), considered the dynamic formulations of depression stereotyped and inadequate. Mendelson (18), in concluding his book on psychoanalytic concepts of depression, wrote: "It would have been pleasing to be able to report that this body of literature represented, in essence, a progress through the years of a Great Investigation. It does so in part. But perhaps even more does it represent a Great Debate with the rhetorical rather than scientific implications of this world."

Mendelson adds that his book on depression represents the summary of an era. "The era was chiefly characterized by boldly speculative theoretical formulations and by insightful clinical studies. . . . This era is drawing to a close."

Is Mendelson right? Is this era drawing to a close? Must we stop groping? Why have the contributions mentioned above remained involved only with some aspects of the large human phenomenon of depression?

Depression, as a pathological variety of sadness, penetrates and involves the whole person, from his core to his highest and spiritual manifestations. We cannot limit our vision of it in order to fit it in the procrustean bed of a theory based on instincts. When Freud (14) added to his theoretical framework the death instinct, or Thanatos theory, this concept, as far as depression was concerned, did nothing to clarify further his previous, and very useful concepts, of incorporation and introjection.

The cultural point of view that sees depression as a practice, that is as a system of manipulating techniques, is a very useful concept, especially in cases of mild depression. Even in more severe cases, in patients whom I have called suffering from the claiming type of depression, I (3, 7) have independently differentiated symptoms identical or similar to those described by Bonime. This claiming, demanding, clinging, appealing attitude, covered by the cloak of depression, is easily recognized in a special group of patients. But these maneuvers, which might explain the use of depression in some cases, do not clarify the nature of depression itself, as a specific subjective experience, nor its psychotic manifestations, nor its invasion of every aspect of human existence, to the point of endangering that existence. New ways of understanding both the feeling of sadness, which belongs to the repertory of normal emotions, and depression, an abnormal type of sadness that occurs in some psychiatric conditions, are needed. In this work I shall discuss some major points of my cognitive approach to depression, and report a successfully treated case of severe depression. Lack of space does not permit me to describe other cognitive approaches, such as the one by Beck (8).

A COGNITIVE APPROACH TO DEPRESSION

In the emotional repertory of every human being, sadness plays an important role; usually as a reaction to something unpleasant, generally a loss—physical, psychological, or moral. Eventually the individual puts into effect special mechanisms, like a reorganization of his thinking or determinate actions in order to hasten the coming of better days (Arieti 2, 4, 5). But it is not so in depression, an emotion related to sadness, which occurs in psychiatric conditions. Pathological depression, especially in its severe forms, seems excessive relative to the events that have elicited it, or inappropriate in relation to its known cause or precipitating factors, or a substitute for a more appropriate emotion when it takes the place of anxiety, anger, or hostility. In many cases depression does not seem to have been caused by any antecedent factor of which the person is conscious.

According to my studies of patients treated psychoanalytically, there is always a preceding ideology, or a way of seeing oneself in life in general, or in relation with another particular person, that prepares the ground for the depression. Although it is true that a depressive affect searches for and finds pessimistic ideas that justify the affect, initially the opposite takes place. The patient's ideology preexisted and was kept alive for a long time, in conscious or unconscious forms. Although the patient might have been aware of the importance of these systems of cognitive constructs, he was unconscious of their origin, of how much they involved, or of all the ramifications, assumptions, presuppositions, and feelings connected with them. These cognitive domains in most cases originated in childhood but continued to accrue throughout life.

At a certain time in the life of the individual, either an external event or an inner reappraisal of one's life brings about the twilight, disintegration, or loss of one or more of these fundamental constructs. Depression is the reaction to this inner loss, as well as to the inability to repair the loss. Although an external event of great importance, like the loss of a loved person, or of a position, or of a great hope, may have precipitated the episode, the significance of such loss by far exceeds the involved reality. The external event brings about the collapse of conscious or unconscious assumptions. The loss is the loss of a part of the psychological self. The sorrow at times acts as a representative of what was lost, because as long as at least the sorrow remains, the loss is not complete. The sorrow is the shadow of the absent, the echo of a voice that was heard repeatedly, perhaps with ambiguous resonance but also with love, respect, and hope.

The impact of these psychological changes produces an exaggeration or distortion of reality, or may include reality and unreality in a surrealistic transformation of affects.

These cognitive constructs that suddenly or gradually undergo disintegration generally have a double entity; they consist of what seems a psychological bifurcation. One branch of this bifurcation deals with the self-image. Thus the destruction of the construct implies a new evaluation of one's self and of one's life, with all the hidden meanings, implications, and ramifications, causing a tremor to the whole psychological fabric of the individual, a profound intrapsychic process.

On the other hand, the construct has an interpersonal branch which has to do with another person, very important to the patient. I have called this person the *dominant other* (3, 7). The dominant other has until now provided the patient with the evidence, real or illusory, or at least the hope that acceptance, love, respect, and recognition of his human worth were acknowledged by at least another person. Thus the interpersonal branch of the bifurcation is intimately connected with the intrapsychic, with the self-image, the way the patient experiences himself. The dominant other is represented most often by the spouse. Far less often, in order of frequency, follow the mother, a person to whom the patient is romantically attached, an adult child, a sister, the father. Also, the dominant other is represented frequently through anthropomorphization, by the firm where the patient works, or a social institution to which he belongs, like the church, the political party, the army, the club, a group or class of people, and so forth. As I have previously illustrated (2, 7) all these dominant others are often symbolic of the depriving mother, the mother unwilling to give the promised love. If the real mother is still living and is the dominant other, she will act in two ways—as her present role actually is, and also symbolically of her old one.

Often the precipitating factor of the psychotic depression is directly connected to the dominant other: The dominant other left or died, and the patient feels without sustenance, believes that he has finally been deprived of his love, as he was once deprived of the love of his mother. Or the dominant other has died before the relation with the patient was clarified. As Bemporad has illustrated (9), the patient finds that now he cannot depend any more on the dominant other for his self-esteem, approval, narcissistic supplies. It becomes obvious that he is incapable of autonomous gratification.

The second important situation which brings about this discontinuity is the realization, often only subliminally perceived or admitted, of the failure of the relationship with the dominant other. This symbolic parent, generally the marital partner, is recognized, or half-consciously recognized, as a tyrant who took advantage of the compliant, submissive attitude of the patient, rather than as a person to be loved and cherished. The patient has tolerated everything, wanting peace at any cost, but it becomes impossible for him to continue to do so. He feels that he has wasted his life in devoting himself to the spouse, in loving her or forcing himself to love her at any cost, just as he did with his mother in childhood. The realization that the spouse deserves not devotion but hate, is something the patient could not easily accept because it would have undermined the foundation of his whole life, would have proved the futility of all his efforts. In some cases the dominant other at a reality level has been active only in the past, but, by having been introjected, remains alive even if he happens to be dead. The dominant other might have been a parent who imposed an impossible goal or ideal on the patient. The patient must become a great man, win the Nobel Prize, become a great writer, a big financier, a doctor, an actress, a dancer, a devoted, self-sacrificing mother of six children, etc. When the patient senses, suddenly or gradually, that he is not going to attain this life goal, the cognitive construct is imperiled, both in the interpersonal branch of the bifurcation, with implied loss of love from the dominant other, and the intrapsychic branch, with loss of the cherished self-image. If the patient identified with the parent, the situation is even more complicated: there is a total destruction of the self-image and of the positive aspect of the relation with the dominant other. When these appraisals threaten to emerge, or actually do emerge to consciousness, a rupture to the psychological equilibrium occurs. Metaphorically, the patient bleeds profusely. Although he is alive, the hopes, ideals, and meanings for which he lived are dying or dead already. Thus he must die too, put an end to this meaningless life where only sorrow is meaningful. In these pathological cases the process of cognitive reorganization, that occurs in cases of normal sadness, is doomed to fail. The patient cannot replace the collapsing constructs with new ones, cannot renew his life or emerge again to a different mode of existence. Instead, another process occurs which brings about several degrees of pathology. The depression, rather than forcing a reorganization of ideas, slows down the thought processes. In this case, the psychological mechanism seems to have the purpose of decreasing the quantity of thoughts in order to decrease the quantity of suffering. At times the slowing down of thought processes is so pronounced (as in the state of stupor) that only a few thoughts of a general or atmospheric quality are left; these are accompanied by an overpowering feeling of melancholy.

But this is a self-defeating mechanism. When the depression becomes overwhelming, it takes possession of practically the whole psyche. Thinking is reduced to a minimum and the patient is aware only of the overpowering feeling of depression. If the patient is asked why he is depressed, he may even say that he does not know. Often the ideas or thoughts that have triggered off the depression become almost immediately submerged by the depression; they become unconscious. In these cases, the depression serves the same function that repression does in other psychiatric conditions. The cognitive components are repressed, but the painful feeling is very intensely experienced at the level of consciousness. I must add that in a considerable number of patients, although a smaller number than used to be, the depression is accompanied by a profound guilt feeling. The patient feels responsible for whatever has happened that brought about his psychological collapse. If some energy is left, it must be used for self-punishment. Vaguely it is felt that enough punishment will restore the acceptable self-image. In this group of patients the idea-feeling of guilt is often the last thought to remain conscious before it is also submerged by the oceanic feeling of depression.

In previous contributions (3, 7) I have described in detail the role of the psychotherapist in the treatment of severe depression. Contrary to what happens in schizophrenia, where the psychosis is a consequence of a failure of cosmic magnitude, involving as a rule the relation with the whole world, the failure of the depressed patient is experienced mainly or exclusively in relation to what I have called basic cognitive constructs and in relation to the dominant other. The task of the therapist is to study these basic constructs and the relationship with the dominant other, and the injuries that they have undergone.

When the therapist enters the life of the very depressed patient, and proves his genuine desire to help, to reach, to nourish, to offer hope, he will often be accepted, but only as a *dominant third* (7). Immediate relief may be obtained, because the patient sees in the analyst a new and reliable love-object. Although the establishment of this type of relatedness may be helpful to the subsequent therapy, it cannot be considered a real cure; as a matter of fact, it may be followed by another attack of depression when the patient realizes the limitation of this type of therapeutic intervention. The analyst must be not a dominant third, but a *significant third*, a third person with a straightforward, sincere, and unambiguous type of personality, who wants to help the patient without making threatening demands. He will help the patient to give up the old constructs and build new ones. He will show to him that if he had remained fixated to the old ideology or to the past ways of life, they would have fossilized his existence. Renewal and self-emergence are possible, and with them the potential for a more meaningful life.

The following case will illustrate in a paradigmatic fashion the theoretical premises that I have mentioned, as well as some therapeutic modalities. This report deals with one of the most severe cases of depression that I have ever seen; a case where the threat to previously established basic constructs and the change in relation with the dominant other were brought about by a significant event in the life of the patient: the birth of her child. Although I believe that I have clarified and brought to solution the main aspects of this case, by no means do I claim that I have understood it in its entirety. The reader will certainly discover several still untapped possibilities and issues which are in need of further discussion.

CASE REPORT

Lisette was 24-years-old when I first saw her. She was a white woman from Australia, and was in this country with her husband, who had won a scholarship to do postgraduate research in New York City. Here is a brief account of the events that brought her to me. Several months previously she had given birth to a girl. Immediately after the birth she became depressed; however, she and her family did not give too much importance to her condition, and she received no treatment. Her condition became much worse, and eventually she had to be hospitalized for a few months. She was treated with drug therapy; she improved and was discharged. A few weeks later, however, she started again to be seriously depressed. She started treatment with a psychoanalyst of classic orientation, but there was no improvement. On the contrary, the situation was deteriorating rapidly. The patient became unable to take care of the baby and was completely incapacitated. Her mother-in-law, who lived in Australia, was summoned to New York to help the patient. When she arrived, the patient resented her very much, so she returned to Australia. Then the patient's mother came and remained with her for several months. Suicidal ideas were freely expressed by the patient and suicide was an impending threat. She could not be left alone. When I first saw her entering the waiting room of my office, she was accompanied by her mother and husband, who were sustaining her on each side, almost to prevent her from falling. When I looked at her face for the first time, I saw a picture of intense sadness and abandon, so picturesque as to give me a fleeting impression that perhaps it was not genuine, but histrionic and theatrical. I had never seen such scenes before except in Italian movies. But when Lisette was alone with me in my office, her real suffering revealed itself; it was a genuine, uncontrollable, overpowering, all evolving, all absorbing, all devastating depression. The feeling of hopelessness and despair, as well as the motor retardation prevented her from talking freely. Nevertheless she managed to tell me briefly that her therapist was not doing her any good; she was sick and wanted to die. When I spoke to her mother and husband later (she was being closely watched in the waiting room by another person), they told me that I was supposed to be only a consultant. They wanted to know whether the patient should receive electric shock treatment; it was no longer possible to manage her at home. They were consulting me to find out whether I was firmly opposed to electric shock treatment in this case. In view of the failure of drug therapy, of psychoanalytic treatment, and the seriousness and urgency of the situation, I told the husband that shock treatment should be tried, and that they should consult me again afterward. The patient received 15 shocks. This is a large number for depressed patients, who generally receive an average of five. The treatment was eventually stopped, however, because there was no improvement. I remembered, from my early experiences at Pilgrim State Hospital, that depressed patients who do not improve even after such a large number of treatment have poor prognosis. When Lisette returned to see me, she was still very depressed, very suicidal, still hopeless. In spite of 15 grand mals there was practically no memory impairment. She told me that she strongly resented going back to her analyst or for more electric shock treatment, and begged me to accept her in therapy.

I wish to describe my feelings when she made this request, partially because of narcissism on my part, but also because I believe that it is important to evaluate the feelings of the analyst at the beginning of the treatment of every seriously ill patient. I told myself, "This is another one of those hard cases that end up in my office. Will I ever get to see an easy-to-treat neurotic?" At the same time, however, I experienced a desire to face the challenge. I was touched by that profound, seemingly infinite pain. I was also perplexed. I already understood that all this had to do with the birth of the child, but how a birth could produce such devastating depression was still a mystery to me. What basic construct or what relation was undergoing a disintegration capable of producing such a violent and seemingly unhealing process in that young, promising, intelligent, and sensitive young woman?

When I discussed the matter with her previous therapist, he did not object to terminating his treatment, so Lisette came to me. Here is a brief history of the patient, as it was collected during the first few months of treatment.

The patient was born in a small town, contiguous to a big city in Australia. The parents belonged to the upper middle class. The father was a successful divorce lawyer, blessed with a cheerful character that made him see the world with rose-colored glasses, and helped him to make a brilliant career. His refined form of shallowness, with such effervescent optimism, made him navigate surely and fast, but without leaving a wake. The patient felt much closer to her mother, who actually was a much more demanding person. Her mother had a humanistic education, would speak about art, literature, poetry in particular, and seemed to have much more in common with the patient. She helped her with her homework while the patient was in high school and college. Her mother also made many demands and, according to Lisette, in her face there was almost a constant expression of disapproval.

Mother had been engaged to a man who died during the engagement. She often referred to this man with enthusiastic terms never used in relation to father. Although father adored mother, mother had for father only a lukewarm, amicable relation. The marriage of the parents was defined by Lisette as fairly good, but not marvelous. The patient knew that sexual life between the parents was not a thrilling one. Mother had told her that she merely obliged.

Earlier in life mother had suffered from epilepsy and also depression. Mother's epilepsy and depression had both started with the birth of the patient's brother. Mother became depressed to such a point that four-year-old Lisette had to be sent to live with her grandmother for a while. Incidentally, this grandmother, mother's mother, is the only person throughout Lisette's childhood who shines as a giver of affection, love, warmth, and care. Lisette always loved her dearly. In spite of grandmother's affection, separation from mother was experienced as a trauma by Lisette. Mother recovered quickly from her depression, but as already mentioned, she had also developed epilepsy. There was an atmosphere of secrecy in the family about mother's epilepsy. In fact, Lisette had never seen mother having an attack until she, Lisette, was 20. On that occasion, Lisette called God to help mother, but in mother's face was God's denial of her request. The truth could no longer be concealed, and she experienced a sense of horror, moral horror because of the denial by God.

Although the patient was always very good in school, during adolescence she felt inferior and unattractive. She had a negative attitude toward life. Everything that appeared good or likable, also appeared superficial, like father. Everything that was deep and worthwhile appeared inaccessible, like mother's approval. There was no doubt in her mind that mother had always preferred her brother, for whom she had strong rivalry and jealousy. She went through a period of rebellion, during which she felt people were empty, superficial, made of plastic. She did not care how she looked and was neglectful of her appearance. Because she was not well dressed and because of her bohemian ways, she felt she was disapproved of, not only by her mother but also by the upper middle class of the small town where she lived. And yet as much as Lisette was critical of these people, she seemed to need their approval and acceptance.

When Jack, a young man of the lower middle class, started to pay attention to her, she was grateful that somebody had noticed her presence. Soon she felt very much in love with him, admired his idealism, intelligence, interest in research; and when Jack graduated from school, they got married. The patient stated that her marriage was a happy one from the very beginning. The only thing that she resented in her marriage was her husband's family, and especially her husband's mother. Jack's mother was different from her son, cheap, vulgar, materialistic. Very coarse, she would eat with her fingers, and sniff tobacco. She was also narrow-minded. To the degree that Jack was desirable, his mother was undesirable. Jack won a research fellowship in the United States, and everybody was very happy. In the meantime, however, Lisette had become pregnant. The pregnancy was accidental, and came at a very inopportune time. The patient was angry about it and experienced nausea. Although the pregnancy was a complication, Lisette and her husband came to the United States in May, during her fifth month of pregnancy. The baby was expected in September.

Lisette told me that during her pregnancy she had had a peculiar idea. I must make it clear that when I first heard about it, the idea did indeed appear so peculiar as to make me think of a schizophrenic disorder. Lisette told me that during her pregnancy she had the feeling that her mother-in-law had entered her. "What do you mean?" I asked, and apparently I unwittingly approached her with an obvious feeling of perplexity or even consternation. Lisette told me with a reassuring voice,

"Don't worry. I did not mean it literally. My husband's sperm that had impregnated me contained genes inherited from his mother. I was displeased that inside of me a baby was growing that was partially a derivation of my mother-in-law."

In spite of this reassurance the idea seemed bizarre to me, and, in a different context, I still would have considered the possibility of schizophrenia. In fact, we know that in preschizophrenics and schizophrenics certain expressions used metaphorically are forerunners of delusions. In these cases the delusion eventually denotes literally what was previously meant in a metaphorical sense. However, in this case nothing else was schizophrenic or schizophrenic-like. I had to rely on my clinical experience with schizophrenics to evaluate the clinical picture in its totality and exclude such possibility. The future development of the case supported my clinical evaluation that there was no schizophrenia.

The patient gave birth in the month of September, and the symptomatology of a depression started to be manifested first in mild and later in very pronounced form. The childbirth represented a focal or central point from which the whole manifest symptomatology originated and irradiated in various directions. For a long time Lisette could not even talk about the birth of Clare in more than fleeting, passing remarks. The episode of the birth itself, as experienced by Lisette, was painful to such a tragic degree as to prevent discussion of it until the ground had been prepared by the treatment. At this point it may be useful to evaluate, however, what we already know about Lisette's case and to delineate some basic constructs.

In the life of this patient there was a dominant other, and this person was not the husband but the mother, the mother so much needed for approval, and from whom the approval was so uncertain; the mother with whom she would like to identify, but can no longer. This dominant mother as a basic construct has a satellite, the mother-in-law. The patient did not have to be as careful in her conceptions about the mother-in-law as she had to be in reference to her mother. Without guilt or compunction of any sort, and strengthened by some realistic facts, Lisette displaced to the mother-in-law some of the bad characteristics of her mother, and the feeling that she had for her mother. The mother-in-law was not only vulgar and disapproving, but she herself had made Lisette become a mother. The mother-in-law becomes, although at a quasimetaphorical level, the phallic mother who entered Lisette and made her pregnant. The husband is totally dismissed; the mother-in-law, who had made her become a mother, was a monstrous distortion of Lisette's mother. If Lisette accepted her pregnancy, she had to accept her mother and her mother-in-law, and what they stood for. If they stood for motherhood, that was a motherhood she wanted to reject. Accepting their type of motherhood meant being as they were and giving up the self-image, a cognitive construct about herself which was cherished and gratifying. The fact remains, however, that during the pregnancy Lisette was apparently all right. It was the childbirth itself that precipitated the condition; but Lisette did not want to talk about the birth for a long time.

From the beginning of treatment I got the impression that Lisette could open up to me. I was immediately accepted by her as a dominant third, and when she trusted me fully and saw me as an undemanding, accepting, and not disapproving person, I became a significant third. I had the feeling that although she did not consider me a source of love, she saw me as a source of strength, clarity, and hope.

For several months the sessions were devoted to studying her relations with her mother; how Lisette lived for mother's approval. A look, a gesture of disapproval would make her sink into a deep state of depression. To be disapproved of by her mother meant utter rejection, unworthiness. She required to be taken care of, fussed over by mother, as grandmother did. Grandmother was really the person to whom the patient was close. Her affection was a profuse, steady flow, and Lisette had no fear of interruption because of sudden disapproval. In contrast, mother's approval could always end abruptly whenever she decided Lisette had made an infraction, no matter how little. There is no doubt that the patient put into operation manipulations and other characteristics as Bonime has described. There was, however, in addition, the constant need for mother's approval, as Bemporad has illustrated. Not only did she want to be mothered by mother, but she wanted mother to have a good opinion of her. Mother seemed to be the only person who counted in her family constellation. And yet many of mother's actions or words were interpreted in a negative way by Lisette; not with the suspicious distortion of the paranoid, but with the adverse appraisal of the depressed. For instance, when mother said that the patient had been lucky in comparison to her, she implied that the patient was spoiled, and had an easy life. When mother said how wonderful Jack was, she meant that Lisette did not measure up to her husband. If mother was making a fuss about Clare and was calling her darling, Lisette would become very depressed, wishing mother would call her in that way. She resented mother terribly and yet could not contemplate the idea of being left alone with

Clare if mother went back to Australia. Then she would be overwhelmed by her duties and she would feel completely lost.

Using the insightful formulation of Bemporad (1970), I repeatedly pointed out to Lisette that at present she was incapable of autonomous gratification. Any supply of self-esteem and feeling of personal significance had to come from mother. Mother was not just a dispenser of love, but was put in a position of being almost a dispenser of oxygen and blood. By withdrawing approval, the supply would end and Lisette would become depressed. At the least sign of forthcoming disapproval the supply would be interrupted. Disapproval would bring about in her not only depression, but guilt feelings as well, because she felt she deserved to be disapproved of. And yet a part of her wanted to be like her mother, although her mother was not like her grandmother.

I explained to Lisette that she sustained a first important trauma after the birth of her brother, when she was sent away from the depressed mother and experienced a feeling of deprivation. Moreover, she associated deprivation, loss of love, and depression with childbirth. I have found that in postpartum psychoses, of both schizophrenic and depressed types, the patient makes a double identification, with her mother and with her child. Inasmuch as Lisette identified with her mother, she was a mother incapable of giving love, a mother who would become depressed, a mother who would only love an intruder like Clare. Little Clare became the equivalent of Lisette's brother, who once deprived her of mother's love. If Lisette identified with the child, she felt depressed as a child deprived of love feels. These feelings were confusing and, of course, self-contradictory.

Lisette came to experience treatment as a liberation from mother. Mother's disapproval gradually ceased to mean loss of love and loss of meaning of life. And indeed treatment was a liberation; not so much from mother as a physical reality, but from mother as the mental construct of the dominant other. The relation with the analyst, the significant third, permitted her to stop identifying with mother without losing the sense of herself as a worthwhile human being. Moreover, anticipation of maternal disapproval did not bring about depression or guilt feeling. At the same time that mother lost importance, the satellite constructs of the mother-in-law, as well as of the upper middle class of the little town, lost power. During the early periods of the treatment, in fact, when Lisette could talk about the people in her home town, she was still worried about what they would think of her, in spite of the distance of more than ten thousand miles. At the same time that mother, as an inner object, and the related constructs, were losing value, the husband was acquiring importance. The patient had always admired and respected the husband, but the husband had never been put in a position where his withdrawal of approval would be of vital importance. Now the husband could be enjoyed as a source of love. Lisette's desire for sexual relations returned. The patient became also more capable of sharing interest in Jack's professional and scientific activity. Before, she was interested only in humanistic subjects, as mother was.

Up to this point, treatment had consisted of changing the value of some basic constructs so that their loss would not be experienced as a psychological catastrophe, and so that new, more healthy constructs could replace the disrupted and displaced ones. In other words, the patient was searching for and finding a meaning of life which was not dependent on the old constructs, not connected with pathological ideas.

After several months of treatment it was felt that the patient could manage her life alone and mother returned to Australia. The patient had a mild fit of depression, caused by their separation, but no catastrophe occurred. After a while Lisette was asking herself how she could have tolerated her mother in her home for so long.

It took some time after mother left for the patient to bring herself to talk about a most important issue: the experience of childbirth. Lisette explained that when she discovered that she was pregnant, she decided to take a course for expectant mothers on natural childbirth. According to the basic principle of natural birth, the woman in labor does not succumb to the pain, she maintains her grip on herself. The woman in labor should not scream; the scream is ineffectual despair, is being no longer in control of oneself. In spite of the preparation, however, Lisette, while in labor, could not bear the pain and screamed. It was a prolonged, repeated, animal-like scream. While she was screaming, she wanted to kill herself because to scream meant to give up as a human being, to disintegrate. But she screamed; she screamed, she screamed! What a horror to hear herself screaming, what a loss of one's human dignity.

During many sessions the patient discussed her cognitive constructs about childbirth. She resented being a biological entity, more an animal than a woman. Biology was cruel. Women were victims of nature. They became slaves of the reproductive system. You started with the sublimity of romantic love and you ended with the ridiculous and degrading position of giving birth. While giving birth, you were in a passive, immobile position, which was dehumanizing. Nurses and doctors who meant nothing to you, saw you in an animal-like, degrading position. You revolted and screamed and lost your dignity. Lisette wanted her husband to be present in her moment of greatness, during her childbirth, but instead he was witness to her descending to her utmost degradation. Childbirth was the death of love, the death of womanhood. You were no longer you, but a female of an animal species. You became what these dominant adults made you, and, what is even worse, you needed them. You wanted to be liked and loved by them when actually you despised them. You were no longer yourself; already dead because the ideal of yourself, of what you were or what you wanted to become was no longer tenable. You gave up the promise of life. You went through dissolution of thoughts and beliefs. The pain increased, became insurmountable.

Eventually Lisette felt only pain, physical pain, but also moral pain. She could not think any more. She felt depressed, and the waves of depression submerged her more and more. But at the periphery of her consciousness, some confused thoughts faintly emerged: She did not want to be a mother; she did not want to take care of the child; she would not be able to take care of the child; she could not take care of her home; she should die. It was impossible for her to accept what she had become—a mother—and the concept of motherhood did not hold for her the sublimity which culture attributes to it: rather it held negative, animal-like characteristics. She felt she had probably become an animal-like mother, like her mother-in-law.

At an advanced stage of the treatment Lisette was able to recapture all these thoughts that had occurred to her after the birth of Clare, thoughts which had become more indistinct, almost unconscious, as the depression occupied more and more her consciousness. Treatment permitted the ideas that precipitated the depression, and that the depression had made unconscious, to emerge.

Although they were revealed to me in an intricate confused network, it was not difficult for me to help Lisette disentangle and get rid of them because we had already done the preliminary work. Once we dismantled mother as the inner object of dominant other and as an object of identification, it was easier to bring the associated ideas back to consciousness. When Lisette gave birth, she rejected motherhood, together with her own mother; and yet she was identified with her mother, who had become depressed after giving birth to Lisette's brother. Thus, by rejecting her mother, she was rejecting herself. In the beginning of treatment she became aware gradually that her suffering was partially due to her not receiving approval and gratification from her mother, but later on she became aware of her greater suffering due to the loss of her basic constructs, which were not replaced by others. Lisette realized that the depression had been so strong as to prevent her from searching for other visions of life. She understood that the physical pain that she sustained during childbirth was symbolic of the greater and more overpowering pain caused by the incoming twilight of the basic constructs without experiencing depression. Even her attitude about being a member of an animal species changed greatly. She came to accept that we are animals and procreate like animals but we can transcend our animal status. And there is beauty in our animal status, too, provided we are able to fuse it with our spiritual part. The patient was able to reassess old meanings in a nonpathological frame of reference and came to accept new meanings. Treatment made rapid progress. My fear that it would be difficult to change the husband's role in Lisette's life proved unfounded. Contrary to the other males, the father and brother, who were not significant figures, the husband rapidly acquired importance and was fully experienced as a source of love, communion, and intimacy.

Treatment lasted a little over two years. The family has returned to the native country. In a span of seven years there have been no relapses.

Some general thoughts about psychotic depression occur to me when I compare this condition to schizophrenia. Both the schizophrenic and the psychotic depressed lament what they have come to know and feel about life. However, whereas the schizophrenic rejects and symbolically destroys the cruel world, and attempts through projection and special cognition to rebuild his own private universe, the person who is depressed to a psychotic degree does not reject the world, as a mother does not reject a bad child. The psychotic depressed does not even reject his suffering, but accepts it, all of it, and the suffering expands more and more, relentlessly and endlessly into a psyche that seems endless in its capacity to experience sorrow. This sorrow is not completely unfounded. There is always a resonance in our heart for the sorrow of the depressed, which is similar to ours, and a partial truth which is connected with the human predicament. When we successfully treat a patient who is depressed, we do not ask him, of course, to give up his identity, but, rather, whatever lie or impossible value had become connected with that identity. We do not help a human being to lose a sense of commitment, but only the commitment that seduces and saps the self. When we successfully treat a patient who was depressed to a psychotic degree we experience a burst of joy because we have helped a suffering person who is happy to have known us. But we also feel a secret joy, because we have come to know him, and in knowing him we know more of ourselves.

Lisette reminded us that we are barely out of the jungle and we can easily resume a purely animal status, not because we are animals—which we are—but because we are humans with ideas. Lisette showed us that no matter how unusual, drastic, or unpleasant the external circumstances happen to be, we ourselves are the great contributors to our own sorrow because of the strange ways in which we mix and give meaning to our ideas and feelings. The study of the circumstances of life is important; but even more important is the study of our ideas about these circumstances, of our ideals and what we do with them, and of how we use them to create feelings. This study may enlighten not just our pathology, but our so-called normality, not just our despair but our hope, not just our loneliness, but our ways of helping each other and reinforcing the human bond.

REFERENCES

1. ABRAHAM, K. (1911): Notes on the psycho-analytical investigation and treatment of manic-depressive insanity and allied conditions. In *Selected Papers on Psychoanalysis*. New York: Basic Books, 1953.
2. ARIETI, S.: Manic-depressive psychosis. *American Handbook of Psychiatry*, 1st ed., Vol. 1. Edited by S. Arieti. New York: Basic Books, 1959.
3. ARIETI, S.: The psychotherapeutic approach to depression. *Amer. J. Psychother.*, 16:397-406, 1962.
4. ARIETI, S.: *The Intrapsychic Self: Feeling, Cognition and Creativity in Health and Mental Illness*. New York: Basic Books, 1967.
5. ARIETI, S.: Depressive disorders. In *International Encyclopedia of the Social Sciences*. New York: Macmillan Co. and The Free Press, 1968.
6. ARIETI, S.: The intrapsychic and the interpersonal in severe psychopathology. In *Interpersonal Explorations in Psychoanalysis*. Edited by E. Witenberg. New York: Basic Books, 1973.
7. ARIETI, S.: Affective disorders: Manic-depressive psychosis and psychotic depression: Manifest symptomatology, psychodynamics, sociological factors, and psychotherapy. In *American Handbook of Psychiatry*, Vol. III. Edited by S. Arieti. New York: Basic Books, 1974.
8. BECK, A. T.: *Depression. Clinical, Experimental, and Theoretical Aspects*. New York: Hoeber, 1967.
9. BEMPORAD, J. R.: New Views on the psychodynamics of the depressive character. In *The World Biennial of Psychiatry and Psychotherapy*, Vol. 1. Edited by S. Arieti. New York: Basic Books, 1970.
10. BIBRING, E.: The mechanism of depression. In *Affective Disorders*. Edited by P. Greenacre. New York: International Universities Press, 1953.
11. BONIME, W.: Depression as a practice: Dynamic and therapeutic conderations. *Comprehen. Psychiat.*, 1:194-198, 1960.
12. BONIME, W.: Psychodynamics of neurotic depression. In *American Handbook of Psychiatry*, Vol. 3. Edited by S. Arieti. New York: Basic Books, 1966. (Republished in this issue, p. 301.)
13. FREUD, S. (1917): Mourning and melancholia. In *Collected Papers*, Vol. 4. New York: Basic Books, 1959.

14. FREUD, S.: *Beyond the Pleasure Principle*. London: International Psychoanalytic, 1922.
15. GRINKER, R. R., MILLE, R. J., SABSHIN, M., NUNN, R., and NUNNALLY, J. C.: *The Phenomenon of Depressions*. New York: Hoeber, 1961.
16. KLEIN, M.: (1935): A contribution to the psychogenesis of manic-depressive states. In Melanie Klein, 1948, 282-310.
17. KLEIN, M.: *Contributions to Psychoanalysis*. London: Hogarth Press, 1948.
18. MENDELSON, M.: *Psychoanalytic Concepts of Depression*. Springfield, Illinois: Thomas, 1960.
19. RADO, S. The problem of melancholia. *Int. J. Psychoanal.*, 9:420-438, 1928.
20. RADO, S.: Psychodynamics of depression from the etiological point of view. *Psychosomatic Medicine*, 13:51-55, 1951.

18

Psychotherapy of Severe Depression

In this paper I discuss further my clinical experiences in treating severely depressed patients with psychotherapy. The depressive cognitive patterns of the patient must be recognized in their longitudinal and psychodynamic unfolding. I attempt to show the therapist how he can guide the patient to recognize these patterns and how to motivate him to try other ways of living.

PSYCHOTHERAPY of affective psychoses is still in the pioneer stage. Although depression has been treated with psychotherapy for a long time, generally the cases treated had not reached the psychotic level. It is true that, unlike schizophrenia, psychotic depression was treated psychoanalytically relatively early in the history of psychoanalysis (1, 2). However, these cases have been very few and as a rule the patients were treated in the intervals between the attacks of depression.

According to my clinical experiences, the intensity of the depression should not deter the therapist from making psychotherapeutic attempts (3). Psychotherapy becomes a necessity when drug therapy and shock therapy have been ineffective, when the syndrome recurs in spite of these treatments, or when the patient refuses to try physical therapies again. Contrary to common belief, most cases of psychotic depression do respond to psychotherapy if a proper therapeutic procedure is adopted.

The procedure I am going to describe was applied to 12 cases of extremely severe depression treated on an ambulatory basis. A much more extensive report of these cases will appear elsewhere (4). The patients were 9 women and 3 men; 10 of them had suicidal ideation. The patients were treated for at least 18 months with a minimum of 2 sessions a week. After at least 3 years from termination of treatment I can now report that full recovery with no relapses was obtained in 7 patients, marked improvement in 4, and failure in 1.

It may be useful before proceeding to compare the psychotherapist's tasks in treating a case of psychotic depression and a case of schizophrenia. Both the schizophrenic and the very depressed patient lament what they have come to know and feel about life. In both conditions there is a close interweaving of a drama of the present with a drama of the past. In both conditions the therapist must understand each of the two dramas. The schizophrenic rejects and symbolically destroys the world, which he perceives as hostile, and attempts through projection and special cognition to rebuild his own private universe. Thus his failure and his concern tend to become of cosmic magnitude. The person who is depressed to a psychotic degree does not reject the world, and acts to a certain extent like a mother who does not reject a bad child. The psychotically depressed patient does not even reject his suffering, but accepts it, all of it, and the suffering expands more and more, into a psyche that seems endless in its capacity to experience sorrow.

PSYCHODYNAMIC VIEW OF PSYCHOTIC DEPRESSION

Normal Sadness

The patient cannot put into operation the mechanisms adopted by a normal person who recuperates from a feeling of sadness, grief, or bereavement (5). For example, a normal individual hears the news of the unexpected death of a person he loves. After he has understood and almost instantaneously evaluated what that death means to him, he experiences shock, then sadness. For a few days all thoughts connected with the deceased person will bring about a painful, almost unbearable feeling. Any group of thoughts even remotely connected with the dead person will elicit sadness. The individual cannot adjust to the idea that the loved person does not live any more. And, since that person was so important to him, many of his thoughts or actions will be directly or indirectly connected with the dead person and will therefore elicit sad reactions.

Nevertheless, after a certain period of time, that individual adjusts to the idea that the person is dead. By being unpleasant, sadness seems to have a function—its own elimination. It will be removed only if the individual is forced to reorganize his thinking and to search for new ideas so that he can rearrange his life. He must rearrange especially those ideas that are connected with the departed, so that the departed will no longer be considered indispensable—indispensable, that is, to equilibrium of the psychological structure of the survivor. Like pain, sadness stimulates a change in order to be removed, but it is a psychological change, an ideational change, a rearrangement of thoughts and clusters of thoughts. Eventually actions will also be altered as a consequence of this cognitive rearrangement. Bowlby (6-8) has described the active search in children deprived of their mother, and Parkes (9) has reported the various ways in which widows search to repair their losses. In other words, in normal sadness, after a period of slowness, or inactivity that prevents quick responses there is a reorganization of functions, first cognitive and then motor, which aims at bringing about a return to a state of normality.

The person who is severely depressed cannot use these recuperative mechanisms. He finds himself in a psychological trap from which he cannot escape. The overpowering feeling of depression keeps him in a state of unconsciousness or dim consciousness cognitive structures and patterns of life that started at an early age. In other words, depression has, among other functions, that of repressing cognitive structures.

Ideology of Psychotically Depressed Patients

My studies of patients treated with psychotherapy indicate that there is always a preceding ideology, a way of seeing oneself in life in general, in relation with another particular person, or in relation to a goal to be achieved that prepares the ground for the depression. Although depressive affect prompts the person to search for and find pessimistic ideas that justify the affect, the opposite initially occurs. The patient's ideology preexisted and was kept alive for a long time in conscious or unconscious forms. Although the patient might have been aware of the importance of these systems of cognitive constructs, he was not conscious of their origin, of how much they involved, or of all the ramifications, assumptions, presuppositions, and feelings connected with them. These cognitive domains in most cases originated in childhood and continued to accrue throughout life.

In many cases these cognitive structures and patterns made the patient live not for himself but for another person, whom I have called the dominant other. The dominant other is represented most often by the spouse, less frequently by the mother, a lover, an adult child, a sister, the father. The dominant other may be represented through anthropomorphization by the firm where the patient works, a social institution, or class of people. Some other patients live for an inaccessible aim, which I have called the dominant goal.

When the patient realizes the failure of his pattern of living, he also recognizes that he is unable to change it. Thus he finds himself in a state of helplessness and hopelessness. A frequent example is that of a woman who used to consider her husband a dispenser of love and affection, a protector, a friend, a partner in every respect. She then starts to see him as an authoritarian person who imposed his rule, at times in a subtle, hardly visible way, at other times in a manifest manner. The patient's own life, at first believed devoted to love and affection, is seen now as not genuine. The patient has been excessively compliant, submissive, and accommodating. By doing always what the husband wanted and denying her wishes, she has not been true to herself; as a matter of fact, she feels she has betrayed herself. The patient may exaggerate and see the authoritarian husband as a real tyrant, somebody who deserves not love, but hate, somebody who enslaved her and changed her real nature. In most cases she does not realize that she also played a role in establishing this type of interpersonal relation. By following a pattern of submissiveness that started early in life she developed ingratiating attitudes and was willing to accept fully a patriarchal type of society and family and to keep the dominant other in the belief that she was perfectly contented or even happy in her way of living.

The emerging new ideas about the husband, however, cannot be accepted. A woman who had not followed the pattern of submission and dedication at any cost would now try new ways for what remains of her life (e.g., separation, divorce, new affection), but the patient cannot do this. She cannot conclude that she has wasted so much of her life. She still needs the same dominant other to praise her and to approve of her to make her feel worthwhile. How could he continue in that capacity if she expresses hate, rebellion, or in some cases, even self-assertion? The patient has reached a critical point at which a realignment of psychodynamic forces and a new pattern of interpersonal relationships are due, but she is not able to muster them. This is her predicament. She is helpless. She either cannot visualize alternative cognitive structures that lead to recuperative steps or, if she is able to visualize them, they appear insurmountable. At other times these alternatives do not seem unrealizable, but worthless, since she has learned to invest all her interest and desires only in the relationship that failed.

Depression following realization of failure to reach the dominant goal is more common among men. The patient realizes that he is not going to be a great doctor, lawyer, politician, writer, actor, industrialist, lover, or musician, but he cannot change the direction of his goal. If the goal is not achieved, life is worthless. If he wanted to be a great conductor, a

Toscanini, now he has to face the fact that he is not a Toscanini, that he is himself, John Doe. But he has no respect for John Doe, as he should. He believes John Doe is nothing. There is some tangential and partial justification in the patient's assessing himself in this negative way because he spent so much of his thoughts in being Toscanini, and his psychological life without this overpowering fantasy seems empty. The limitations of the patient, determined by his rigidity and adherence to an inflexible pattern of life, do not provide him with alternatives. As in the patient who experiences failure in the relation with the dominant other, the patient may visualize alternatives but they seem either insurmountable or worthless.

If space permitted, I would also touch on the inability to find alternative cognitive structures in patients who become depressed after loss of spouses, parents, positions, hopes, etc. The post-partum depression occurring in the woman who cannot accept the new pattern of life required by motherhood is another very complex situation (10).

In these cases sadness cannot be removed and is transformed into deep depression. When unpleasant ideas occur they are submerged by the wave of depression. The cognitive basis of the condition is repressed, but the painful feeling is very intensely experienced at the level of consciousness. This last remark may seem at variance with what we observe in many patients who express depressive ideas about the way they view themselves, the world, and the future. Beck (11-13) has carefully described the cognitive elements that keep the patient in a state of depression. In my experience with cases of severe depression, these depressive thoughts are used by the patient to justify his preexisting depression. They replace much more basic and more intense depressive trends, which have to be studied longitudinally, since they go back to the early life of the individual (5).

THERAPEUTIC PROCEDURE

Initial Tasks of the Therapist

The first task of the therapist is not that of interpreting to the patient the inappropriateness of his patterns of living or the maladaptive quality of his endless sorrow but that of entering into his life with a strong and significant impact.

The therapist assumes an active role. He is a firm person who makes clear and sure statements. He is compassionate, but not in a way that can be interpreted as acknowledgment of helplessness. He tells the patient that he knows how deep his anguish can be, but that he also knows that depression does not come from nothing. There is always a reason, which the patient, alone, cannot find. In other words, the patient is invited to lean on the therapist.

When the therapist succeeds in establishing rapport and proves his genuine desire to help, to reach, to nourish, to offer more clarity about certain issues and hope about others, he will often be accepted by the patient, but only as a dominant third, i.e., a third person in addition to the patient and the dominant other. Immediate relief may be obtained because the patient sees in the therapist a new and reliable love object. Although the establishment of this type of relatedness may be helpful to subsequent therapy, it does not constitute a real cure; as a matter of fact, it may be followed by another attack of depression if the patient realizes the quality and limitation of this relation. The therapeutic approach must proceed toward a more advanced stage, in which the therapist is no longer a dominant third, but a significant third—a third person who, with his firm, sincere, and unambiguous type of personality, wants to help the patient without making threatening demands or requesting a continuation of the patient's pathogenetic pattern of living. Whereas the dominant other is rigid and static, the significant third will change rapidly and will eventually appear as a person who shares life experiences without aiming at domination.

The point must be stressed, however, that in the initial stage of the psychotherapy of severe depression, like in the psychotherapy of schizophrenia, the therapy must somewhat conform to the patient's pathology and, often, in less pronounced forms, even repeat it. Otherwise treatment is immediately experienced by the patient as dangerous and is rejected before a meaningful therapeutic relatedness has been established.

Once the therapist has been able to gather enough information, the relation with the dominant other must be interpreted. The patient must come to the conscious realization that he did not know how to live for himself. He never listened to himself; in situations of great affective significance he was never able to assert himself. He cared only about obtaining the approval, affection, love, admiration, or care of the dominant other. As Bemporad (14) described, the patient was incapable of autonomous gratification; he had to obtain it from the dominant other.

Potential Problems

When the therapist succeeds in making some headway in understanding the patient's psyche, several developments that must be promptly coped with may occur. The patient may become less depressed but angry, either at the dominant other or the therapist, whom he would like to transform into a dominant third. The anger and hostility toward the dominant other (most frequently the spouse) is at times out of proportion. Once the ideations which were repressed or kept at the periphery of consciousness come to the surface, the dominant other may be seen as a tyrant, a domineering person who has subjugated the patient. The therapist may have a difficult task in clarifying the issues. At times the dominant other has really been overdemanding and authoritarian and has taken advantage of the placating, compliant qualities of the patient. Often, however, it is the patient himself who, by being unable to assert himself and by complying excessively, has allowed certain patterns of life to develop and persist. Now, when he wants to change these patterns, he attributes the responsibility for them to the dominant other. No real recovery is possible unless the patient understands the role that he himself has played in creating the climate and pattern of submissiveness. Similarly, if the major pathogenetic constellation of his psyche is his concern with the dominant goal, he must understand why he gave such supremacy to the achievement of that goal. Did he see in such a goal the only possible meaning of his life, and why?

The therapist must not only help the patient bring to full consciousness cognitive patterns and their effect on his life; he must also gradually guide the patient to visualize different patterns and to invest them with hope and desires. The patient who has understood the role he has played in the dynamics of his condition will lose a sense of passivity and will feel less helpless and less inclined to accept a feeling of hopelessness. He will learn to assert himself and to aim at what is really meaningful to him and gratifying.

Bemporad and I have elsewhere (4) described the varieties and details of the complicated psychotherapeutic approach to the severely depressed. However, even in a short presentation like the present one, a few more important issues cannot be omitted.

In a considerable number of patients, although a smaller number than used to be, the depression is accompanied by a profound guilt feeling. The patient feels responsible for whatever has happened that brought about his psychological collapse. If some energy is left, it must be used for self-punishment. He feels vaguely that enough punishment will restore a self-image acceptable to him. The guilt is often actually based on hate for the dominant other, in a way reminiscent of the sadistic trends of the depressed that Freud (2) described as directed against the incorporated love object. The guilt feeling has repeatedly helped the patient to choose a pattern of atonement and submission to the dominant other in order to placate him and to obtain his love and approval. If such approval is not obtained, the patient's guilt feeling increases because in his cognitive structure lack of approval means not having done enough to deserve it. Moreover, in accordance with his patterns of living he has learned to transform anxiety into guilt. As painful as the guilt feeling is, the patient is aware that the possibility of suffering, atoning, and placating is within his capabilities, whereas with anxiety he is at a loss; he does not know what to do about it. It is important to explain these mechanisms to the patient. However, the greatest relief from guilt feeling will occur when he has transformed his relation with the dominant other.

When the patient has somewhat improved and is able either by himself or with the help of the therapist to realize that alternative ways of living are available to him, he may state that he is afraid to embark upon them, even though the depression has lifted and the motor retardation is no longer present. The patient may be afraid of attempting new ways of living because they are unknown and unfamiliar. Other inhibiting factors stem from the fact that these new ways seem extremely remote and do not arouse in him motivation toward their achievement. The patient, who has been for so long entrenched in his complexes and enduring patterns of living, has never day-dreamed about or invested feelings in these alternatives. Again the therapist must help the patient gradually to develop the lacking motivation for different paths of living.

The patient who has partially recovered continues, nevertheless, to feel more at home with the feeling of depression than with other moods. He may exploit any negative event or thought to become depressed again. We must repeatedly show him how he uses every minor unpleasant event or thought to justify his depression, which initially stemmed from a deeper source.

At other times the patient entertains ideas half-way between these superficial depressive ideas that he exploits and ideas that are genuinely related to the deep problems of which he has now acquired awareness. He may brood over what he did not have or may have a feeling of self-betrayal. He has some realization that some aspirations have to be given up; he has the feeling that he cannot count on the recurrence of opportunities that he did not grasp, and so on. The therapist must guide the patient so that he can catch himself in the act of having these ideas or in an attitude in which he expects to be or to become depressed. If he becomes aware of these ideas and of expecting to be consequently depressed, he may be able to intercept the process and to avert the depression. He will become more and more receptive to alternative ways of living.

As a final point, I wish to mention that psychotherapy as described in this paper does not exclude concurrent drug treatment with antidepressants such as MAO inhibitors or tricyclics. I have resorted to such combined treatment with satisfactory results. I want to stress again, however, that psychotherapy alone can be an effective treatment in severe depression and that it may have to be used to the exclusion of other types of treatment in the conditions which I mentioned at the beginning of this paper.

REFERENCES

1. ABRAHAM, K.: Notes on the psycho-analytical investigation and treatment of manic-depressive insanity and allied conditions. In *Selected Papers*. New York: Basic Books, 1953, pp. 137-156.
2. FREUD, S.: Mourning and melancholia (1917). In *Collected Papers*, 6th ed., vol. 4. Edited by E. Jones. London: Hogarth Press, 1950, pp. 152-170.
3. ARIETI, S.: The psychotherapeutic approach to depression. *Amer. J. Psychother.*, 16:397-406. 1962.
4. ARIETI, S. & BEMPORAD, J.: *Severe and Mild Depression. The Psychotherapeutic Approach*. New York: Basic Books (in press).
5. ARIETI, S.: Affective disorders: Manic-depressive psychosis and psychotic depression: Manifest symptomatology, psychodynamics, sociological factors and psychotherapy. In *American Handbook of Psychiatry*, 2nd ed., vol. III. Edited by S. Arieti, E. B. Brody; S. Arieti, editor-in-chief. New York: Basic Books, 1974, pp. 449-490.
6. BOWLBY, J.: Mother-child separation. In *Mental Health and Infant Development*, vol. 1. Edited by K. Loddy. New York: Basic Books, 1956, pp. 117-122.
7. BOWLBY, J.: Grief and mourning in infancy and early childhood. In *The Psychoanalytic Study of the Child*, vol. 15. Edited by R. S. Eissler, A. Freud., H. Hartmann, et al. New York: International Universities Press, 1960, pp. 9-52.
8. BOWLBY, J.: *Attachment and Loss*. New York: Basic Books, 1969.
9. PARKES, C. M.: Bereavement and mental illness. *Brit. J. Med. Psychol.*, 38:1-26, 1965.
10. ARIETI, S.: Psychoanalysis of severe depression: Theory and therapy. *J. Amer. Acad. Psychoanal.*, 4:327-345, 1976.
11. BECK, A. T.: Thinking and depression. I. *Arch. Gen. Psychiatry*, 9:324-333, 1963.
12. BECK, A. T.: *Depression: Clinical, Experimental, and Theoretical Aspects*. New York: Hoeber, 1967.
13. BECK, A. T.: Depressive neurosis. In *American Handbook of Psychiatry*, 2nd ed., vol. III. Edited by S. Arieti, E. B. Brody; S. Arieti, editor-in-chief. New York: Basic Books, 1974, pp. 61-90.
14. BEMPORAD, J. R.: New views on the psychodynamics of the depressive character. In *The World Biennial of Psychiatry and Psychotherapy*, vol. I. Edited by S. Arieti. New York: Basic Books, 1970.

19

Psychiatric Controversy: Man's Ethical Dimension

Although determinism may permeate human existence, man's moral values raise him above the level of a subhuman animal and enable him to direct his own life. In this paper, read at the 127th Annual Meeting of the American Psychiatric Association in 1974, I suggest that psychiatrists should not encourage the patient to see himself as a passive agent molded by external circumstances, but should rather influence him to exert his will, make conscious choices, and, above, assume a sense of responsibility for his own actions. In order to free the patient from whatever conditions hinder his will and to help him make choices, psychiatric treatment must consider man's ethical dimension.

COMMITTED AS WE ARE to the scientific method, we psychiatrists divide, dissect, and examine the psyche of the human being piece by piece. This is a legitimate procedure, provided that after the analysis we reach a synthesis, give the proper consideration to those aspects of the personality that could not expand, and, more important, do not leave out any basic human dimension.

We do not always follow this procedure. In our double allegiance to science and to man, who in his totality is not reducible to the accepted canons of science, we tend to adhere to traditional science exclusively and to minimize man's ethical dimension. In what I call the "ethical dimension" I include such vast areas as moral values and the phenomena of will, conscious choice, and responsibility.

I do not mean to suggest that the therapist should impose his values on the patient; I simply wish to stress that values always accompany and give a special psychological significance to facts and that when we deprive facts of their value, we fabricate artifacts which have no reality in human psychology. An individual may suspend his value judgment when he wants to examine a fact from a specific point of view, but then the ethical content has to be reestablished if the fact is to have human significance. If we remove the ethical dimension, we reduce man to a subhuman animal, an animal that is not *beyond* freedom and dignity, but whose organization *precedes* the experience of freedom and dignity—a subhuman animal to whom Skinnerian psychology can be safely applied.

It is easy for many of us who practice psychodynamic psychiatry to understand how Skinner's approach has only limited application to our work. The functions of the psyche that we study in our daily work—feelings, emotions, attitudes, introjection, guilt, expectation, purpose, goal, inner self, personality, determination, choice, will, etc.—are miraculous or imaginary entities for Skinner (1). According to Skinner, ideas, dreams, images, insights, and conflicts cannot be seen or observed and, therefore, do not count, nor can the existence of an inner life be inferred from them. Skinner follows a procedure antithetical to the medical procedure, for a physician does not simply observe his patient's behavior but also makes inquiries about what goes on inside of the patient.

Although I have never gathered statistics on a large scale on this subject, I am inclined to believe that many psychiatrists are ready to reject Skinner's position. But unfortunately, many of us are willing to accept other positions that do not consider adequately the ethical dimension. In contrast to the position of Rollo May (2), Leon Salzman (3), Leslie Farber (4), myself (5), and many others, a large group of psychiatrists and psychologists do not believe that there is such a thing as human will. Certainly a normal voluntary action consists of many steps, some of which are not yet susceptible to scientific analysis. We do not know when neurology ends and psychology begins. We do not know the intimate neurological mechanism that initiates a voluntary movement. Perhaps what we call will is the synthesis or result of many neuropsychological mechanisms plus newly emerging elements that in a tentative way we call autonomy, individuality, originality, creativity, and indeterminacy.

PREEMINENCE OF DETERMINISM

Determinism reigned supreme in the era of hard-to-imagine proportions that extended from the appearance of the atom to the development of the human cortex. The simplest entities (the subatomic particles) and the highest (some parts of the human cortex), respectively, opened and closed this vast era that unfolded over billions and billions of years. The most complex entity in our universe, the human cortex, again permits a certain independence from causality as it existed at the subatomic level studied by Heisenberg. However, the freedom of man, made possible by his cortex, is different from the so-called freedom of the subatomic particles. It is integrated with the essence of man. Although this freedom produces an interruption in the deterministic chain of causes and effects, it immediately rejoins determinism, thereby reestablishing continuity, for the will of man becomes a *cause* of action. It is a causality compatible with free will. It is for future research to establish whether subatomic "freedom" becomes incorporated in some particles of neurons and changes ideas into free actions and thus reintegrates itself into the essence of man.

For many psychiatrists, including myself, what we call will, that ability by virtue of which we conform our behavior to our determination, is the culmination of the psychological functions of the human being. Certainly we can bypass our will. We may meekly obey others, or we may behave in conformity with our conditioned reflexes. If we have some psychiatric disorder, our will is hindered in various ways. If we are hysterical, we lose control of some functions of our body. If we are phobic, the avoidance of the dreaded event rather than our determination will guide our actions. If we are obsessive-compulsive, we feel obligated to obey internal injunctions even when they seem absurd. If we are psychopathic, we cannot say no to ourselves; we are under the impulse to satisfy our urges immediately. If we are catatonic, we go through a stage in which even our smallest movement may be endowed with cosmic responsibility and guilt; consequently, we do not move at all. Those of us who have intensely studied the catatonic type of schizophrenia consider the catatonic state to be the nadir of the human condition (6). Although the catatonic is not physiologically paralyzed, he cannot respond to people who touch him, bump into him, smile at him, or caress him. He appears to be a statue, but unlike a statue he hurts in a most atrocious way, having lost the most precious and human of his possessions—his will. By studying cases of catatonic schizophrenia of different degrees of severity, we can learn a great deal about the existence, unfolding, and impairment of the will (6).

Psychiatric treatment attempts to liberate the patient from whatever condition limits his will, whether it is a mild neurosis or a severe catatonia. It should be understood, however, that total freedom and total self-causation are not available to any man. Even partial freedom is not something a human being is born with; it is a striving, a purpose—something to be attained. Being born free is a legal concept that, although valid in daily life, has philosophical limitations. Striving for freedom is an unceasing attempt to overcome the conditions of physico-chemistry, biology, psychology, and society that affect human life. The psychiatric patient has the additional burden of overcoming the conditions of his psychopathology, and the purpose of psychiatric treatment is to help him do so. It would be unrealistic to forget, however, that this self-causation is only a thin margin of a totality in which the majority of facts and events are ruled deterministically. But I feel that this thin margin is sufficient to change the world, to make history, to cause the rise or fall of man (5).

Classical Freudian psychoanalysis has a controversial (and I would say ambivalent) attitude toward the concept of will. On one side, Freudian psychoanalysis adheres to a strict deterministic view of reality and life that leaves no room for human choice. According to Freud, most of our actions are caused by unconscious motivation, and as long as our actions are the result of unconscious motivations, we cannot call ourselves free or feel responsible for what we do.

Like many other great thinkers, Freud contradicted himself on many issues, including the question of will. More than any of his predecessors or contemporaries he revealed the role of the unconscious wish as a determinant of human behavior. But Freud's great discovery does not imply that will has no role. Let us consider Freud's famous statement, "Where id was, ego must be." Freud meant that as a result of psychoanalysis, unconscious wishes, generally relegated to the id, must become part of the ego; i.e., they must become conscious. But what is the purpose of this? To make the id part of the ego does not mean unleashing the unconscious wishes or giving them free reign or unrestricted access to conscious behavior, although this is the way some people interpret Freud's statement. I believe that Freud meant that once the unconscious wishes become conscious, they will be regulated by the functions of the ego. The individual will be in a better position to accept or reject them. In other words, Freud conceived psychoanalysis not as a liberation of the id but as a liberation of the ego from the unwanted, unconsciously determined oppression exerted by the id. Thus, psychoanalysis has the function not of restricting but of enlarging the sphere of influence of the will. Its aim is to return a sense of responsibility to the human being for many actions, that previously were beyond his control. In this respect, psychoanalysis enlarges the ethical dimension.

POSITION OF SOME PSYCHODYNAMIC SCHOOLS

In addition to Freudian psychoanalysis, some schools of psychodynamic psychiatry have also neglected the role of autonomy and individuality, which are prerequisites for free will. Whereas some geneticists believe that most or all of our life is predetermined by our genetic code, some psychodynamic psychiatrists believe that our present life is entirely determined by our past experiences—by what our parents, families, schools, and society have done to us. Thus, although the psychiatrists who focus only on the environment do not invoke heredity, their basic philosophy is similar to that of the geneticists: man's destiny is shaped by forces external to the self.

WE CREATE OUR OWN SELF-IMAGE

Obviously we are influenced by external forces. Genetic, familial, and social factors are important, but not to the extreme degree that many psychiatric studies imply. Conceptions that view the individual only as a passive agent or tabula rasa, as a receiver, or as a puppet pulled by strings of different kinds have prevailed in daily psychiatric practice. For instance, when we elicit a history from the patient's family or (in most cases) from the patient himself, our aim is to establish how this history has made the patient what he is now. Some psychiatrists ignore completely the fact that the patient has always recreated that history. What he tells us is seldom what happened but more frequently what he perceived and interpreted, what he assimilated, and what his memory has constantly changed and given different meaning to. The child does not just reflect or absorb from the environment; he also tries to select what to give prominence to. The image that the child has of himself does not consist of reflected appraisals from parents or family members but of what the child did with those appraisals. In the same way, the image that he has of his parents and siblings, although related to the actual essences of these people, is not a mirror reproduction but rather a subjective interpretation. There is a definite discrepancy between the way reality and the significant people in one's life were in the past and the way one has perceived them. This discrepancy is particularly pronounced in the schizophrenic and preschizophrenic individual but also exists (to a lesser degree) in the neurotic individual and in all of us. This discrepancy is one manifestation of individuality. The image that the individual has of himself is particularly important because it is a major constituent of inner life or what is at times called the self. And, our self-image is not created exclusively by others but also by ourselves. We are among our own creative forces.

I must stress again that I do not mean that we are completely free. The self in whose creation we have cooperated is also the result of our specific biological endowment and a random mixture of external factors. The psychiatric patient has less possibility of contributing to the creation of his own self than the normal person because he was handicapped by external contingencies. However, the patient who has successfully progressed to an advanced stage of treatment will stop blaming his mother or father, his childhood, his spouse, or the conditions at work for all his troubles. The more he becomes conscious of his secret life (the more he understands his thoughts and motivation), the more he increases the area of responsibility. He recognizes the role that other people played in his life, but he assumes some responsibility for what happened to him and especially for the way he will direct his life in the future. Of course, it would be absurd for him to think that his destiny will be entirely in his own hands, but he is aware that he too is a determining force in his own life.

Insofar as psychiatric treatment increases the ability to make choices, it is constantly involved with man's ethical dimension. Any choice that affects others reveals our sense of responsibility, our concern or lack thereof not only for ourselves but for others. What we are responsible for is typically a product of our own self. Of course, when responsibility becomes one's only concern, it is distorted and assumes a tyrannical role; however, its absence, or a great decrease in it; produces in us the psychopathic variety of human life.

SELF-REALIZATION AND THE ROLE OF PSYCHIATRIC TREATMENT

A misinterpretation and a misapplication of some psychiatric and psychoanalytic concepts stand out among the many causes of the permissiveness and hedonism of our days. I refer particularly to the concept of self-realization that has persuaded many to strive for self-fulfillment, even if this means disregarding the rights of others. This misunderstanding derives not only from the already mentioned concept of id liberation, misconstrued from Freudian theory, but also from a broad generalization of some concepts of the neo-Freudian schools of psychoanalysis and humanistic psychology. Maslow, Horney, and Fromm believe that the highest ethic, as well as the aim of psychotherapy, is the one that leads to self-realization.

This point of view is controversial on many grounds. First, there is no preordained, specifiable potential in man that has to be realized. Man is indefinite and capable of unpredictable growth because of the multitude of possible encounters with different systems of symbols and concepts (7). Man must aim at continuous growth or self-expansion, but not a mythical realization of an assumed potential. Man is not an acorn that may become an oak. For man, there is no question of potentiality but of infinite possibilities. Second, "self-realization" is very deceptive as a subjective experience. Reading the writings of Mussolini and Hitler, and even of some politicians of our own times, one is forced to conclude that these people were sure of realizing themselves and their "own destiny" by following a mission or mandate given them by the people. Third, and most important, self-realization ignores the actual problem of ethics, one's moral relation to others. Self-fulfillment is not necessarily an ethical aim; it may be a form of hedonism and narcissism, again easily recognized in the lives of some politicians. What some authors mean by self-fulfillment is a legitimate aspiration. However, when self-fulfillment is pursued, it is not on ethical grounds but for personal gratification. To remain ethically justifiable, it must not interfere with ethical principles. We certainly should aspire to our psychological growth and happiness, provided we do not infringe upon the rights of others.

Ultimately, we must ask the question of whether psychiatric treatment itself conditions the patient by making him choose accepted behavior and reject what is considered socially unacceptable behavior. To the extent that treatment has this effect, it is not psychodynamic; it does not enlarge the freedom of man. We must be able to make a fine distinction. Influencing the patient (as psychodynamic treatment does) does not mean conditioning the patient; it means increasing the patient's vistas and his range of choices. The patient then does the choosing. As a matter of fact, as Halleck (8) has recently stated, the patient should have a voice even in the choice of his own treatment.

CONCLUSIONS

Often a defeatist philosophy of life, in which everything is presumed to be fallacious or illusionary, permeates psychotherapy. According to this view there is no escape from the determinism that regulates human life (9); human life is a part of a deterministic cosmos in which everything is caused by something else. Obviously a large part of our existence is determined by outside forces. Certainly we must agree with Freud that the part of the iceberg which is submerged is much larger than that above the surface. But from that part which is above water we can see the polar star and a large part of the firmament. Even though the deterministic forces prevail and ultimately overcome us, we should not feel defeated if we have added our will, our choice, and our sense of responsibility to the conditions that give meaning and direction to our existence.

REFERENCES

1. SKINNER, B. F.: *Beyond Freedom and Dignity.* New York: Alfred A. Knopf, 1971.
2. MAY, R.: *Love and Will.* New York: W. W. Norton, 1969.
3. SALZMAN, L.: Personal communication, 1972.
4. FARBER, L.: *The Ways of the Will: Toward a Psychology and Psychopathology of the Will.* New York: Basic Books, 1966.
5. ARIETI, S.: *The Will to Be Human.* New York: Quadrangle/New York Times Book Co., 1972.
6. ARIETI, S.: *Interpretation of Schizophrenia,* 2nd ed. New York: Basic Books, 1974.
7. ARIETI, S.: *The Intrapsychic Self: Feeling, Cognition and Creativity in Health and Mental Illness.* New York: Basic Books, 1969.
8. HALLECK, S. L.: Legal and ethical aspects of behavior control. *Amer. J. Psychiat.,* 131:381-385, 1974.
9. KNIGHT, R. P.: Determinism, freedom and psychotherapy. *Psychiat.,* 9:251-262, 1946.

Part III
COGNITION AND ITS RELATION TO
PSYCHODYNAMICS

20

The Processes of Expectation
and Anticipation

This is my first paper on cognition, written in 1947, when few studies had been done in this area. The mental processes of expectation and anticipation are studied in relation to comparative psychology, clinical psychiatry, psychoanalysis, anthropology, and neurology.

THE DEVELOPMENT of symbolic processes is one of the most important evolutionary changes occurring in the upper levels of the phyletic scale. A mental process may be called symbolic if it can stand for previous experience and if it can determine behavior responses by virtue of these past experiences. Past and present find a psychologic continuity through the functioning of these processes, some of which may be represented with such words as memory, imagination, thought, language, abstraction, etc.

There are, however, other symbolic processes, by far less well known and studied, which determine our present behavior in virtue of future experiences. They are the processes related to the functions of expectancy and anticipation. These two functions are related to one another, the second being a development of the first. Whereas the first process may be traced back to species as low as the crayfish (11), the second appears only in human beings at a certain stage of development.

By (immediate) expectancy is meant the capacity of the subject to anticipate certain events while a certain external stimulus is present. For instance, the monkey expects to secure a banana as reward while solving a problem (24); and the baby expects sucking at the sight of the mother's breast. This process is not just a conditioning; it is a more elevated function implying, let us say, something like a visualization or mental

265

representation of an event which has not yet taken place. The presence of an external stimulus (experiment set for the monkey, maternal breast for the baby) is necessary.

By (distant) anticipation is meant, instead, the capacity to foresee or predict future events, even when there are no external stimuli which are directly or indirectly related to those events. With a few exceptions, among which is outstanding the contribution of Freeman and Watts (6), the importance of these two functions in psychopathology has not been fully considered. There cannot be, however, any doubt about their psychopathologic importance if we consider the phenomenon of anxiety.

In fact, there cannot be anxiety without the capacity to expect or anticipate. Freud himself states, "Anxiety is undeniably related to expectation; one feels anxiety lest something occur" (7). He also defines anxiety as "a reaction to the perception of an external danger, of an injury which is *expected* and *foreseen*" (7) (Italics mine). Claude and Lévy-Valensi (4) propose the following definition "un sentiment pénible d'attente." Whereas fright is the reaction to a present, immediate danger, anxiety is, as if it were, the reaction to a danger which is not yet an act, and may be defined as an emotional state connected with the expectancy of a danger. Without entering here the intricate problem of the mechanism of the emotions, we may say that whereas the bodily resonance of fright may be considered as a preparation for an *immediate* danger or emergency, the mental and bodily changes accompanying anxiety, and the perceptions of some of these changes, may be considered as favoring a prolonged, though painful vigilance for a future event. The temporal element, present versus future, is one of the distinguishing features of these two emotional statuses. Of course, there are many other differences between fright and anxiety, both in the pure emotional experience and in the physiologic resonance, but in the opinion of this writer, the temporal quality is one of the fundamental differential characteristics.

The relation between expectancy and anxiety can be studied in experimental neuroses in animals. In the opinion of this writer, not all experimental neuroses in animals are states of anxiety, but only those which imply in their mechanism the process of expectancy. Experimental neuroses have been determined by Pavlov (20), by the application of a strong conditioned stimulus when the animal is accustomed to a weak one; by protracted inhibition, but especially by a clash of excitation and inhibition as in a too difficult discrimination (13). Similar results have been obtained by Gantt (10), Liddell and several others. When the animal, trained to react in a positive or negative way to two different stimuli, is unable to discriminate between the two stimuli, certainly he reacts to the situation in an abnormal way which may be called neurotic. But is this pathologic condition anxiety, or only what may be called "conflictful tension," that is, a general state of hyperirritability due to inability to discharge the tension produced by the stimuli?

I believe that these experimental conditions should not be indiscriminately called experimental anxieties, although many of them actually are so. To consider all these neuroses states of anxiety would be tantamount to subscribing to Freud's earlier theory that anxiety originates whenever a strong impulse was prevented from discharging through the usual motor outlets. Later Freud rejected his "first theory" and adopted the point of view that anxiety is a reaction to a danger signal, that is, a process implying some expectancy or anticipation. Such a state of expectancy is actually present in many experimental situations, for instance those devised by Mowrer (19). Mowrer placed groups of rats on a circular grill, segments of which were charged with a current after the sound of a tone. The expectancy of the shock engendered in the rats a state of anxiety which made it more difficult for them to learn to respond successfully by running from the charged segment of the grill. When the expectancy, and therefore the anxiety, could be reduced by using a regular tone-shock combination, a better learning was obtained. Masserman (18) trained cats to secure food in response to various stimuli. Subsequently, at the moment of food-taking, the animals were subjected to fear-imposing air blasts, so that the act of feeding was "motivationally conflictful." He obtained abnormal states characterized by anxiety, and other neurotic symptoms. It could be that whereas the other neurotic symptoms were due to the conflictful situation, the anxiety was due to the expectancy of the air blasts. Whereas in some of the previous researches there was no danger involved, and the neurotic condition was only due to the inability to discharge the tension, in Masserman's experiments there was not only a conflictful tension, but also the expectancy of danger, which engendered anxiety. Even if we subscribe to the point of view of Masserman himself, that the results he obtained were due to conflictful motivation, one has to admit that his cats were able to *expect* both the air blasts and the feeding. It is true that the cats had to make a choice, but they were also able to expect the result of the choice, that is, the motivation. No matter whether we follow a mechanistic or a teleologic interpretation, the importance of expectation cannot be denied in those animal experiments which engender states of anxiety. We have also to consider the important fact that animals respond with anxiety only to the experimental stimuli, or, to use Masserman's own words, to "configurations previously associated with these stimuli." Although the animal may remain neurotic or maladjusted afterward, the actual state of anxiety is determined by the *presence* of the external stimuli, or of their equivalents. In other words, the reaction of the animal is temporarily tied to the experimental stimulus; the fear of danger always involves the present time or the immediate future. On the other hand, in human anxiety there may be a temporal lapse between the anxiety-precipitating stimulus and the dreaded event, and the anxiety may last even when such external stimulus is removed. This second type of anxiety implies the process of anticipation. The time factor is not the only difference between expectancy and anticipation. Anticipation is probably almost exclusively a mental process, whereas expectation, being at a lower level of integration, may involve also some physiologic changes, muscular or secretory, preparatory for the expected event.

Anticipation, and therefore long-circuited anxiety, are not present in animals. In fact, there is little doubt that animals are unable to foresee the distant future. Although they fear dangerous situations and try to avoid them, they do not fear danger of death because they cannot mentally prospect a distant future. Pre-human species may be called biologic entities without psychic tomorrow. Cattle go to the slaughter house without feelings of anxiety, being unable to foresee what is going to happen to them. This tightness to the present may be proved in the experiments of delayed reactions, which show that cats may delay their reaction for a maximum of only five minutes (14), monkeys for a maximum of two minutes (12), and chimpanzees for a few hours (26). It is true that certain species as low as insects, (ants, bees) display some activities, which seem to imply anticipation of distant future, but in reality these activities are only the expression of instinctual or natively determined behavior.

Anticipation, and therefore long-circuited anxiety, appear in man during the year of life, or anal stage. However, during the first year, or oral stage, expectation and short-circuited anxiety are present. The baby expects the parents, or their substitutes, to relieve him from the tension produced by hunger, thirst, loneliness or other uncomfortable sensations (5). If he is not relieved, because of the parental attitude of letting him cry the discomfort out lest he is spoiled, short-circuited anxiety may be engendered. There is no doubt that babies in the first few months of life *expect* things. They cannot communicate their state of expectation by spoken language, but they may use what Von Domarus called "as if" attitude (25). For instance, the infant cannot verbally express the desire to be in the arms of his parents, but when he sees his mother, he leans toward her and raises his arms "as" he would do "if" she were in the act of picking him up. Von Domarus describes this "as if" attitude in animals, in mute mental defectives, and in the terminal stages of schizophrenia. An elephant in a zoological garden, wishing to obtain a piece of sugar from a visitor, makes with his trunk and snout all the motions that he would make if he would be in the act of obtaining, or had already obtained, a piece of sugar. A very deteriorated patient, who could not speak, ran her fingers through her hair when she saw an attendant, expecting to be combed.

Anticipation originates during the anal period. At this stage of development, the child becomes able to postpone immediate pleasure for some future gratification. In other words, it is at this stage that the "reality principle" originates. The child learns to give up his tendency to relieve the tension of his bowels, and postpone the act of defecation, in order to obtain the immediate or distant approval or love of his parents (5). At this stage, however, his perception of time is still very primitive and inadequate. In the genital and latency periods, the ability to anticipate the future will develop enormously, and in the early part of adolescence, will expand to include all its implications.

In adult age, this future anticipation occupies the greatest part of man's thoughts, and consequently determines the greatest number of man's actions. It is to this process of anticipation that such phenomena or institutions as religion, life insurance, armament, etc., owe their origin and development. When the ontogenetic development of the function of anticipation is completed, the individual is able to revive the past and to anticipate the future; in other words, is able to transport to the only possible subjective or psychologic tense—present—chronologically remote phenomena. Thus, in a certain way, from a psychologic point of view, St. Augustine (2) is right when he states that only the present really is. He says that there are only three times "A present of things past, a present of things present, and a present of things future." "The present of things past is memory, the present of things present is sight, and the present of things future is expectation."

Phylogenetically we may state that anticipation (and, therefore, long-circuited anxiety) appeared at the primordial eras of humanity. Perhaps in some human races, which lived during what was called by Freud the cannibalistic age of humanity, anticipation was not yet possible, or was present to a very limited degree. At that time men were interested mainly in activities like cannibalism and hunting, which are related to the immediate present time. Soon, however, and exactly in what may be called the anal stage of humanity (1), man learned to anticipate the future and to protect himself from distant danger. He protected himself against famine with the habit of hoarding (which is characteristic of this anal stage of humanity (1)) and by experiencing feeling of long-circuited anxiety. Often he tried to protect himself from this anxiety by magic methods (which correspond to the compulsions of the psychoneurotic). Only a few primitives of today seem to be at a stage still preceding the anal or long-anticipatory. The Pitchentara of Central Australia do not hoard, although they live in a land of frequent famine, do not pay attention to the toilet habits of their children and are deprived of anxiety, as shown by their "fatal optimism" (21). More and more as the historical time was approached, anticipation of a more and more distant future was possible to the humans. Bertrand Russell (22) describes well this differential characteristic between what he calls the savage man who is interested only in present problems, and what he calls the civilized man who is able to foresee the future: "The civilized man is distinguished from the savage mainly by prudence, or, to use a slightly wider term, forethought. He is willing to endure present pains for the sake of future pleasures, even if the future pleasures are rather distant. This habit began to be important with the rise of agriculture; no animal and no savage would work in the spring in order to have food next winter, except for a few purely instinctive forms of action, such as bees making honey, or squirrels burying nuts. In these cases, there is no forethought, there is a direct impulse to an act which, to the human spectator, is obviously going to prove useful later on. True forethought only arises when a man does something towards which no impulse urges him, because his reason tells him that he will profit by it at some future date. Hunting requires no forethought, because it is pleasurable; but tilling the soil is labor, and cannot be done from spontaneous impulse." Russell thus describes the shifting from what is psychoanalytically known as the pleasure principle to the reality principle. Although a large literature has been written upon the reality principle, the importance of the process of anticipation for the functioning of this principle has been so far neglected.

The ability to anticipate future events requires a certain degree of intellectual evolution or maturation not yet acquired by the pre-human species, or by the child in the first year of life. To react to a present stimulus, often only a reflex mechanism is necessary. To predict future events, much longer neural circuits are required. It is necessary to be able to connect in a certain sequence a series of events; for instance, phenomenon A (sunset) with phenomenon B (night). For primitive men it is not even necessary to have acquired the abstract concepts of necessity in order to have a mental picture of the future, but only the capacity to expect B a certain lapse of time after A, and to prepare to react to B after experiencing A (long-delayed reaction).

It seems logical to attribute to the frontal lobes the function of anticipation. As a matter of fact, even for the process of expectancy, it was found in rats that a small area of the frontal lobes was necessary (23). Jacobsen (15) has studied the role of the frontal lobes in delayed reactions in monkeys. In a certain sense, the ability to delay reactions may be considered a forerunner of future anticipation, because of the temporal interval between stimulus and response. Jacobsen's monkeys, which had been trained to solve an experimental problem a minute or two after stimulation, were not able to do so after extirpation of the prefrontal areas. Malmo (17), however, in interesting experiments which the author of this article had the privilege of witnessing, ably demonstrated that the frontal lobes are responsible for delayed reaction, not directly, but only inasmuch as they inhibit disturbing secondary stimuli. In fact, by extinguishing lights during the delay period, the prefrontal monkeys were capable of normal delayed reactions. This seems to demonstrate that past experiences are preserved in non-frontal areas, but that prefrontal areas are necessary in delayed reactions, inasmuch as they enable the animal to keep a set in spite of disturbing secondary stimulation. Liberson (16), using electroencephalographic technique, has found functional alterations of frontal lobes during sleep. He plausibly concludes that this functional alteration may explain why in dreams, we live in the present, may remember past events, but do not project ourselves into the future. Although the dream may be the symbolic manifestation of a wish for a future event (9), in the dream the situation is actually lived in the present. Although there may be expectation of events, there is no distant anticipation. In their monograph on Psychosurgery, Freeman and Watts (6) have fully taken into consideration the importance of the frontal lobes for anticipation of the future. Those patients who presented, as fundamental symptom, anxiety about the future showed marked improvement after frontal lobotomy, when there is "an apparent inability to foresee accurately the results of a series of planned acts as they relate to the individual himself." These authors reach the conclusions that the frontal lobes enable the individual to project himself into the future. Thus, after operation, relief is to be expected from those symptoms which require for their occurrence the capacity to foresee.

In the mental activities of the normal adult, this capacity to antici-pate the future plays a tremendous role. Such a role is diminished in some pathologic conditions. We have seen above that the capacity to anticipate is necessary for the engendering of certain psychoneuroses which are characterized by conscious or unconscious long-circuited anx-iety. And yet, paradoxically, many of these psychoneurotics, at a conscious level, do not seem to be concerned so much about the future as about the past. If we ask chronic psychoneurotics the following question, "When you are alone and think, do you think more about the present, past, or future?" it is surprising how many of them answer that they think mostly about the past. Several of my patients, with states of anxiety, gave this question a mathematical answer, "I think 90% about the past, 10% about the present, and zero about the future." How is this to be explained in view of the fact that the engendering of certain human psychoneuroses infers the capacity to anticipate the future? Probably this is an escape mechanism. It is too painful for the patient to think of the uncertain future, in view of the present condition, and he prefers to withdraw into the past which may also have been unhappy, but whose difficulties he somehow managed to overcome. By resorting to the thought of the past, the patient abandons the highest—too difficult—mental mechanism of anticipation, and functionally withdraws—in his conscious life—to a lower level of integration. In reality, anticipation of the future unconsciously remains, as demonstrated by the emotional status and by the actions of the patient. A patient of Freeman and Watts "was uncomfortable if her Christmas shopping was not completed by Thanksgiving time." In some elaborated psychoneuroses, for instance, those presenting claustrophobia, it seems as if the dreaded danger were related to the present or immediate future, and that we were dealing more with expectation than anticipation, in spite of the complexity of the phenomenon. It could be that in these cases the long-circuiting neural activities involve mostly the function of unconscious symbolization and not the process of anticipation.

Future anticipation as related to the self is decreased in normal senescence. The aging individual becomes less and less concerned about the future, and when senescence arrives, his interests are practically con-fined to the present time. In my clinical contacts, I found that contrary to what is generally believed, old people are not chiefly interested in the past, but in the present. Although they are still thinking of the past to a considerable extent, their stream of thought is mostly related to the present time. In other words, we have in old age what I call "a restriction of the psychotemporal field." At times, old people have so little interest in the future and their capacity to worry is decreased to such a point that they become slightly euphoric. For instance, fear of approaching death is felt much less intensely by old people than by young adults. Although this may be explained as a philosophic acceptance of the ineluctable laws of nature, I am more inclined to believe that this is due to minor organic changes affecting predominantly the frontal lobes. As a matter of fact, these characteristics are exaggerated in senile psychosis, and cerebral arteriosclerosis. The alteration of the psychotemporal field is, therefore, different in the senile and in the psychoneurotic. In the latter, it is functionally determined, that is, has a protective purpose against too much concern about the future. Inasmuch as the psychoneurotic apparently diverts his attention from the future to the past, we cannot speak of psychotemporal restriction, but of "apparent psychotemporal inversion" which may be more or less pronounced. In the senescent instead, and to a much more marked degree in the senile, we have a real organically determined psychotemporal restriction. In schizophrenia we have also a considerable restriction of the psychotemporal field. The patient withdraws more or less to a narcissistic level, and his temporal orientation becomes also more and more similar to that of the narcissistic period, that is, related to the present time. Balken, in her study of schizophrenia with the thematic apperception test, finds that the schizophrenic does not distinguish between the past, the present and the future. According to her, the schizophrenic, in the attempt "to relieve the tension between the possible and the real" clings "desperately and without awareness to the present." In early schizophrenia, however, when a considerable part of the libido is still fixated to less regressed stages, the patient is still able to concern himself with past and future. In early paranoid forms, where a great quantity of libido is fixated to the anal stage, anticipation of the future is preserved to a considerable degree. Some delusions may involve the future rather than the present. As a matter of fact, for well-organized delusions, the process of anticipation is necessary. The patient must be able to *foresee* the conclusions of his reasoning, because it is the anticipated conclusion which retrospectively directs his train of thought. In other words, in the process of demonstrating something, the patient chooses only those possibilities which lead to the conclusion he has anticipated and wished. For instance, a 49-year-old patient had the delusion that a certain man she knew was going to divorce his wife and marry her. The wife of this man was a respectable, attractive and young blonde woman who had just given birth to a baby. According to my patient, who had an unconscious homosexual attachment for her, this woman was ugly, had already undergone the menopause and had been a prostitute. How could she sustain her beliefs in front of this contradictory evidence? We shall not take into consideration here the obvious fact that she wanted to reject, unconsciously, her homosexual wish, because this is beyond the purpose of this article. We are interested here only with the formal mechanism of her delusional ideas. Consciously, the patient needed to reach the conclusion that the man was going to divorce this woman and marry her. She needed to believe that this woman was unworthy of the love of this man. According to the patient, she was, therefore, extremely ugly, but being a prostitute, she had learned to dissemble her appearance, as all the prostitutes do. As a matter of fact, this woman was a brunette, but had bleached her hair. She had already undergone the menopause, but she had been visiting a famous obstetrician who had given her hormone therapy, so that she could conceive. As a matter of fact, she (the patient) had seen this woman two or three times walking in the same street where this obstetrician resided. It is obvious that the patient could anticipate the deduction of her thoughts, because it was the conclusion itself (impossibility for the man to love that woman) which retrospectively directed and consequently distorted her reasoning. To repeat, we are considering here only the formal mechanism of the delusion, not the unconscious cause or motivation which was the rejection of a homosexual desire. It seems logical to assume, then, that well-organized delusions, as those of the cited example, cannot exist without the process of anticipation. In the course of the illness, however, the delusions undergo changes in their content and in their formal mechanism. The early paranoid who has delusions of persecution or of jealousy, is able to foresee the future and direct his thought in logical, chronological patterns which lead to the foreseen delusional deduction. He retains a great emotional capacity attached to his complexes, and at times is so apparently logical as to be considered lucid. Later he becomes less logical, less able to foresee the future and the deductions of his reasoning; his delusions become related to the present time and not to the future, their content is not persecutory but more or less grandiose, and their emotional tone is shallower. Later, he becomes even more illogical, his thinking presents definite scattering, his delusions are connected with the immediate present, and are of definite expansive type, "I *am* a millionaire; I *am* the King of Egypt." He accepts his delusions as indisputable, immediate reality, without caring any longer to demonstrate logically their validity. As a matter of fact, he would not be able to do so. Many authors have emphasized this shift of the type of delusions from persecutory in the initial stage of the illness to grandiose in more advanced stages. However, to my knowledge, the fact has been neglected that the delusions of grandeur are generally related to the present time, and are accepted by the patient without necessity of an apparently logical explanation or deduction.

Occasionally, in advanced stages of the hebephrenic and paranoid types, delusions seem to imply anticipation of the future, but it is not really so. For instance, a patient of mine had the delusional idea that for her the calendar was always one day in advance. When for the rest of humanity it was Tuesday, February 13, 1946, for her it was Wednesday, February 14, 1946. This delusion is only superficially connected with anticipation of time, and has on the other hand narcissistic implications.

If the therapeutic mechanism of frontal lobotomy is, as Freeman and Watts think, due to acquired inability to project oneself into the future, it seems that the best results should be obtained in those patients who had retained the ability to foresee. If the restriction of the psychotemporal field is so pronounced that only the narcissistic present time is left, no improvement is to be expected. Non-regressed and nongrandiose paranoids who retain a relatively large psychotemporal field, should be in the schizophrenic group, those who respond better to frontal lobotomy. However, the best results among psychiatric patients, in general, should be obtained in anxiety neuroses. This conclusion has only a theoretical value and should by no means be interpreted as though the author of this article would advocate this type of treatment which produces only symptomatic results (inability to foresee future) when psychologic treatment would attack the real core of the problem (fear connected with future anticipation).

Paranoiacs and paranoids who do not deteriorate show a spontaneous improvement when they reach old age. They become less antagonistic, less unsatisfied, more sociable, less worried about what is going to happen and less concerned about their persecutors. It could be that this improvement is due to the organic cerebral changes, involving also the frontal lobes. No improvement occurs, however, in senescent catatonic, hebephrenic or deteriorated paranoids.

REFERENCES

1. ARIETI, S.: Primitive habits in the preterminal stage of schizophrenia. *Journal of Nervous and Mental Disease*, 102:367, 1945.
2. ST. AUGUSTINE: Quoted by Bertrand Russell.
3. BALKEN, E. R.: A delineation of schizophrenic language and thought in a test of imagination. *J. Psychol.*, 16:239, 1943.
4. CLAUDE, H. and LÉVY-VALENSI, J.: *Les états Anxieux.* Paris: Librarie Maloine, 1928.
5. ENGLISH, O. S. and PEARSON, G. H. J.: *Emotional Problems of Living. Avoiding the Neurotic Pattern.* New York: W. W. Norton & Co., 1945.
6. FREEMAN, W. and WATTS, J.: *Psychosurgery.* Baltimore: Charles C. Thomas, 1942.
7. FREUD, S.: *The Problem of Anxiety.* New York: W. W .Norton & Co., 1936.
8. ——: *A General Introduction to Psychoanalysis.* Tr. by J. Riviere, Garden City Publishing Co.
9. ——: *The Interpretation of Dreams.* New York: Modern Library, 1938.
10. GANTT, W. HORSLEY: Quoted by Hilgard and Marquis (13).
11. GILHAUSEN, H. C.: The use of vision and of the antennae in the learning of crayfish. *Univ. California Publ. Physiol.*, 7:73, 1929.
12. HARLOW, H. F., WEHLING, H., and MASLOW, A. H.: Comparative behavior of primates. Delayed reaction tests on primates. *J. Comp. Psychol.*, 13:13, 1932.
13. HILGARD, E. R., and MARQUIS, D. G.: *Conditioning and Learning.* New York: D. Appleton-Century Co., 1940.
14. HUNTER, W. S.: The delayed reaction in animals and children. *Behav. Monog.*, 2:86, 1913.
15. JACOBSEN, C. F.: Studies of cerebral function in primates. *Comp. Psychol. Monog.*, 13, No. 63, 1936.
16. LIBERSON, W. T.: Problem of sleep and mental disease. *Digest Neurol. & Psychiat.*, 13:93, 1945.
17. MALMO, R. B.: Interference factors in delayed response in monkeys after removal of frontal lobes. *J. Neurophysiol.*, 5:295, 1942.
18. MASSERMAN, J.: *Behavior and Neurosis.* Chicago: Univ. of Chicago Press, 1943.
19. MOWRER, O. H.: Anxiety-reduction and learning. *J. Exper. Psychol.*, 27:497, 1940.
20. PAVLOV, I. P.: *Conditioned Reflexes and Psychiatry.* New York: International Publishers, 1941.
21. ROHEIM, R.: *The Riddle of The Sphinx.* London: Hogarth Press, 1934.
22. RUSSELL, B.: *A History of Western Philosophy.* New York: Simon & Schuster, 1945.
23. STELLAR, S., MORGAN, C. T., and YAROSH,, M.: Cortical localization of symbolic processes in the rat. *J. Comp. Psychol.*, 34:107, 1942.
24. TINKLEPAUGH, O. L.: An experimental study of representative factors in monkeys. *J. Comp. Psychol.*, 8:197, 1928.
25. VON DOMARUS, E.: The specific laws of logic in schizophrenia. In *Language and Thoughts in Schizophrenia.* By J. S. Kasanin. Berkeley and Los Angeles: University of California Press, 1944.
26. YERKES, R. M. and YERKES, D. N.: Concerning memory in the chimpanzee. *J. Comp. Psychol.*, 8:237, 1928.

21

The Microgeny of Thought and Perception

Thoughts and perceptions go through several unconscious stages before they reach consciousness. This paper, published in 1962, constitutes the nucleus of many subjects and ideas expanded in my book The Intrapsychic Self. *It shows how the existence of these unconscious stages is revealed by inference by the study of pathological conditions, such as acute and chronic cases of schizophrenia, some psychoneuroses, aphasias, agnosias, and brain injuries.*

MICROGENY, as defined by Werner (79), is the sequence of the necessary steps inherent in the occurrence of a psychological phenomenon. Microgeny is thus the immediate unfolding of the phenomenon. For instance, in the act of reaching a judgment or simply of perceiving something, the subject goes through different stages which lead to that judgment or that perception.

These stages occur in a very short period of time, often small fractions of a second, and generally without the subject being aware of them. Most of the time the subject is aware of the stimulus or of the initial and terminal steps, but not of what takes place between them. The S-R formula, or a psychology predominantly oriented toward this formula, tends to neglect microgenetic processes. As we have already mentioned, most of these processes are deprived of subjective experience: As a matter of fact many of them seem to reproduce those primary processes which Freud attributed to the unconscious (26). We know that most neurophysiological processes are unconscious, that is, they do not confer a sense of subjective experience. As I have expressed elsewhere (11), by demonstrating that some psychic processes are unconscious Freud actually

277

implied that some of the functions of the nervous system lose this quality of consciousness and become more similar to the rest of the functions mediated by the nervous system.

The study of microgeny presents unusual difficulties because of several facts: 1) Neurophysiology has not yet reached a degree of development which permits an accurate correlation with psychological phenomena; 2) inasmuch as the phenomena cannot be observed, nor in most instances subjectively experienced, we can only infer their occurrence from clues gathered from various fields; 3) methods for controlling or measuring variables are lacking or inadequate. Nevertheless, pessimism is not justified, for we are already in possession of many pertinent facts. An increasing number of experimental works are coming from psychologists (16, 17, 58). The ego psychologists of the orthodox Freudian school have made many excursions into this field (32, 33, 64), but they seem to me to have almost confined their investigation to the study of energetics. Energetics is only one aspect of microgeny, and according to some neurophysiologists (47), not even a necessary one. Some orthodox psychoanalytic contributions, like the one by Linn (48), are very important. As a group, however, general psychiatrists and psychoanalysts have for several decades relatively neglected the field of cognition, focusing their interest on other areas, for instance on the study of motivation. The study of cognition in psychopathology may present unusual difficulties at first, but once the initial efforts have been made, new avenues of understanding present themselves and promising possibilities of research emerge.

The framework of the present study is fairly explicit. First, we shall be directed by a principle underlying the writings of Werner (80, 81)—that microgeny reproduces (but not repeats) phylogeny and ontogeny. Then, following the procedures of Werner's comparative developmental approach, we shall coordinate forms of behavior observed in animal psychology, child psychology, psychopathology, and theoretical as well as clinical neurology. Both forms of regression will be studied. This approach is also guided by the increasingly convincing point of view that psychological phenomena occurring at various levels of integration, for instance perception, thinking, and basic patterns of behavior, although manifesting emerging new traits, still follow fundamental laws which apply to all levels.

This approach perhaps may be seen as the application of a general system theory (72): one, however, limited to psychological functions. Although perception is deemed to be a simpler phenomenon than thinking, thought will be taken into consideration first, since I have more personal material available on this subject.

An attempt will not be made to review the whole topic or refer to all the pertinent literature. For these purposes the reader is referred to the excellent article by Flavell and Draguns (25). The main aim of the present paper is to interrelate the isolated observations of many workers with my own psychiatric research in order to give new significance to the available data and to attempt a systematization of them.

THINKING

It is obvious that thinking does not consist only of searching for data in the storage of our memories. If memory were like a record, long as life is, on which experiences are indited, it would take a long time to retrieve a particular experience from its point in the record. There must be some kind of organization which makes it possible to retrieve quickly the past experience.

Thinking consists of the processes by which past experiences are properly stored, organized, recalled, reorganized in new ways, and verbalized. The study of microgeny tries to trace these various steps, those processes which the Würzburg workers designated with the name *Bewusstseinslage,* meaning "experiences which cannot be closely analyzed" (54).

Primary Aggregation and Fragmentation

The first level of thinking organization is what may be called *primary aggregation.*

Werner (81) has written that, "Wherever development occurs it proceeds from a state of relative globality and lack of differentiation to a state of increasing differentiation, articulation and hierarchic integration." In the case of thinking, this relative globality refers to a group (or as Linn (48) says, a cluster) of stored images or of simple concepts. In the concept formation the concept belongs first to a cluster or to a general, undifferentiated, or "primary aggregation" of connected ideas. How clusters are formed it is difficult to say: Contiguity and primitive, not better defined, organization or contiguous experiences may be responsible.

In pathological conditions, as they occur in regressed schizophrenics or in organically brain-injured patients, especially aphasics, we have an arrest at this stage. For instance, a regressed schizophrenic of whom I asked, "Who was the first President of the United States?" replied, "White

House." Actually George Washington never lived in the White House, but *White House* was an element of a primary aggregation of concepts which had to do with Presidents of the United States. Another schizophrenic patient, reported by Cameron (18), said that he had "three menus" when he meant three meals. Similarly in aphasic patients Bouman and Grunbaum (15) considered the basic change as "an arrest at an earlier stage of development of a mental process, which normally proceeds in the direction from amorphous total reaction toward differentiated and definite forms." Conrad (19) described this as an arrest at a pre-Gestalt level.

Werner (79), following Lotmar (50), speaks of a level where "spheres of meaning" rather than specific concepts are apprehended. Sphere-like forms of cognition in normal and pathological cases would precede more specific levels. Werner is fundamentally correct, but some clarification is necessary. The "sphere of meaning" is recognized by us because of what we infer from the utterances of the patient. The patient is not aware of it. For instance, if the patient says "White House" when he is supposed to say "George Washington," we infer that "the sphere" has to do with Presidents of the United States.

Actually what the patient undergoes when his thinking is arrested at the primitive level is a fragmentation of the "sphere." The sphere becomes a primary aggregation of loosely connected elements. Any element, or fragment, may reach the level of consciousness. The fragment is almost always not the right one, but is more or less related to the right one because every element of the aggregation is related. It is as if each element were identified with (or become equivalent to) any other element with which it is associated in the primary aggregation.

Formation of Primary Classes and Primary Responses

The fragmentation, however, is not arbitrary. At a higher level the element of the primary aggregation which is selected for emergence to the state of consciousness may be recognized as belonging to a class to which the correct thought or response would belong. For instance, to the question, "What city is the capital of France?" organic and also some of the regressed schizophrenic patients have given such a reply as "London." Although the answer is incorrect, it is not haphazard, but related to the right one. Obviously the patient has an inner class or category of capitals" or "European capitals." But the thought is arrested at this level, before all the capitals are microgenetically scanned and the right one is selected. An organic patient reported by Linn called her wheelchair a "chaise longue." Hughlings Jackson was one of the first authors to report similar examples in aphasics (36). In other writings I have suggested that this primitive formation of classes centers around "a releasing element" (14). All members containing the "releasing element" form a primary class. In Linn's patient, who said "chaise longue" for wheelchair, or in the patient who said London for Paris, the implied classes are logical classes. In fact, the releasing element (chair or European capital) corresponds to what appears to us a logical concept. In many other instances, however, the classes are more primitive, the releasing element being a secondary quality or predicate, which generally does not lead to formation of customary classes. For instance, a schizophrenic patient considered herself to be the Virgin Mary "because she was virgin like the Virgin Mary." Each member of the class "being virgin" becomes equivalent to the Virgin Mary. Another schizophrenic considered the doctor the father of all the patients, "because the doctor was in a position of authority like the fathers of many children." At this level identification occurs because the releasing element (a common predicate) is present in the different members of the class.

Here thinking follows the paleologic principle of Von Domarus according to which subjects are identified because they have a common predicate. The common predicate leads to formation of classes whose members are identifiable (5-10, 73). Such arrest at the level of paleologic or of primitive classes may not be general. As a matter of fact, in schizophrenia as a rule it occurs only when the complexes of the patient are involved. For instance, the patient who considered herself to be the Virgin Mary, "because she was a virgin," would not consider another virgin woman to be the Virgin Mary. When the patient thinks about the other woman the thought processes are not influenced by her psychodynamic difficulties and are not allowed to remain fixated at a primitive level (see following section on psychodynamic factors). *At the level of primary classes members of the classes become equivalent.*

The important mechanisms of displacement and primary symbolization, as described by Freud (28), are from a cognitive point of view to be interpreted as manifestations of the formation of the primary categories.

The problem of the primary categories seems to me related to the problem of equivalent stimuli studied by Klüver (42, 43). Klüver calls equivalent all stimuli which are capable of eliciting the same response. He found out that pronounced changes in the stimulus often left the response unaltered. What seem to the observer heterogeneous stimuli (for instance a meshed wire, a floor brush, a live rat, a toothpick, etc.) elicit from certain Cebus monkeys the same response. Klüver, in attempting to specify the factors repsonsible for particular types of equivalence, often was able to define the factors only negatively (43). In other words, after eliminating one factor after another, he demonstrated that "various common properties or sets of properties found in a given group of equivalent stimuli play no role in bringing about the same behavior." In abnormal conditions, for instance in monkeys who underwent surgery of the temporal lobes, the range of equivalence was even increased (44).

Klüver feels that the common property is not necessarily responsible for the same response. But, of course, we have to remember that by common property we do not necessarily mean, in these experimental cases, a property of various stimuli which affects our human senses or intellect in the same way. It may be a multitude of factors which at a primitive level of nervous integration are experienced in the same way. At a primitive level a priori categories may not be Kantian categories.

Any conclusion is premature. At any rate the following hypotheses (which I have elaborated elsewhere (14)) are suggested: 1) The psychological origin of logic is to be found in the fact that the organism responds in the same way to some stimuli (generalization-induction-class formation); 2) a class, at a primitive, prelogical, or paleologic level, is formed by the similarity of the response to some stimuli.

In certain stages of the evolution of the nervous system, an increasing selectivity in the ability to respond sets in. In microgeny probably the nervous system repeats the range of class formation from the most to the least primitive. Probably related to the same category of phenomena are the observations made by several authors (45, 46, 77, 78) that some individuals respond to different stimuli with a fixed patterning or some hierarchy of responses of the autonomic nervous system.

Are responses at certain levels coincident or congruous with thoughts? In the most primitive levels of human cognition, probably yes. For instance, the schizophrenic patient believed that she was the Virgin Mary and acted out (that is, responded to herself) as if she were the Virgin Mary.

The brain-injured patient who says London instead of Paris believes he has given the correct answer, contrary to the distracted student who in a similar situation may catch himself in error and correct himself.

Discrepancy Between Categories of Thought and Categories of Response

In some conditions of less pathological degree than those mentioned in the previous sections, for instance in psychoneuroses, there is no identification of stimuli which belong to primary categories, but there is an identification of responses. That is, the patient is forced to respond *as if* an identification of different, although related, stimuli would take place. The word "splitting" between various functions of the psyche, which is generally used in reference to schizophrenic conditions, seems more appropriate to this psychoneurotic process. At times this discrepancy between cognition and response is referred to as lack of emotional understanding in presence of intellectual understanding, or as a symptom which is not egosyntonic.

For instance, let us take as an example a patient who has become aware of the fact that he reacts with anger, irritation, and unfair discourtesy toward red-haired, elderly women. He does not know why. Finally he remembers that when he was a child his mother, a widow, had to go to work and, when there was no school because of vacation, would leave him in the custody of an aunt who happened to be red-haired. This aunt resented taking care of him and was unkind to him. Apparently here, the way the patient felt toward the aunt was extended to the whole category of elderly, red-haired women. Contrary to what is suggested in many psychoanalytic reports, the memory of the early experiences with the aunt is not repressed or unconscious. What is unconscious is the connection between the present behavior and the origin of such behavior. This unawareness is due to the fact that there is a discrepancy between the cognitive apprehension of elderly, red-haired women and the response to them. That is, the patient recognizes that the women are not his aunt, but his response is equivalent to that he once had toward the aunt. He responds as if these women belong to a primary class of equivalent members. The response has become a neurotic basic pattern of behavior, or a parataxic distortion, as Sullivan would say (69).

In the phenomenon of "imprinting" as described by Lorenz (49), we have perhaps a similar phenomenon. A gosling learns to react to a man as it would react to its mother goose. This seems to be brought about by the fact that at a certain period in the development of the gosling this man disclosed maternal qualities and released filial instinct. This behavior of the gosling becomes imprinted, that is, becomes a basic pattern of behavior which is irreversible. An important aspect of the phenomenon is that the gosling does not learn to respond in this way to a special man, who takes care of him, but "to Man, with a capital, as a species . . . The irreversible imprint refers to the species and not to the individual. We have no explanation of this at all" (49). The response is to a primary class which had the releasing element (maternal attitude), but this primary class of response does not include all objects with maternal attitudes (because in that case geese too would be included). It includes another less primitive class but a wrong one. Perhaps something similar occurs in human homosexuality or other sexual deviations.

In phobias (or anxiety hysterias) a somewhat related situation occurs (12). Threatening situations (or situations containing phobic elements, such as threatening interpersonal relations) ostensibly no longer elicit fear. Fear is elicited by a specific concrete situation, such as the sight of a horse. Whereas the category of abstract threatening situations tends to enlarge in persons suffering from phobias, the response characterized by the experience of fear is evoked only by a certain stimulus. The stereotyped reaction is the response to one of the most concrete and primitive stimuli containing the phobic elements.

We have so far taken into consideration several arrests at various levels during the microgeny of thought. As we shall see in greater detail in the following section, the arrests are engendered, or at least predisposed, by various factors. Fortunately, however, in the majority of cases, thought reaches the terminal and specific level appropriate to the situation. Whereas to the question, "What is the capital of France?" a regressed schizophrenic may reply, "La Marseillaise," and a brain-injured patient "London," the normal person will reply "Paris."

Perhaps what we have so far illustrated would be better understood by resorting to an example from engineering. Suppose a small town or village has a limited number of telephones with only two exchanges, A and B, followed by three-figure numbers. For instance, two typical numbers would be A315 and B702. Let us assume that something goes wrong with the telephone equipment and that after a person has dialed the exchange A, any phone which has an A exchange could reply. This situation in a certain way corresponds to the stage of primary aggregation. The phones whose exchange is B would automatically be excluded, but any number from A000 to A999 could answer. Any number would be an element or a fragment of the "primary aggregation" A.

But suppose that the trouble starts after the telephoning person has dialed the first two letters A3. Then it is obvious that any number from A300 to A399 could answer. This corresponds to the stage of primary category. Again let us assume that the trouble starts after the person has dialed A31: Then it is obvious that any number from A310 to A319 could answer. Again this is a substage of primary category.

Lest the reader be frightened by the simplification of this model, I hasten to emphasize that this example illustrates metaphorically only one aspect of the microgeny of thought. That things are much more complicated will appear evident from the following section.

Dynamic Factors

Among other important questions which remain to be answered are the following: Why, in pathological cases, does the microgenetic process remain arrested at one of the earlier stages, and why at one rather than another? Furthermore, why does the arrested thought assume a certain content instead of another? For instance, why, to the question, "What city is the capital of France?" did the patient reply "London" rather than Rome or Madrid?

Nondynamic factors may provide a partial explanation in some cases. For instance, in the case of aphasic or other brain-injured patients, one may postulate that the high centers where the ultimate scanning or discrimination occurs are organically impaired. We may also state, in agreement with the principles of Hughlings Jackson, that when the higher levels are impaired the lower reemerge—for instance, the levels of the primary categories or of the primary aggregation.

But within a given level other factors may determine the specific content: for instance, familiarity. London may be a more familiar concept to the patient than Rome or Madrid. At times the primitiveness of certain elements or their being "words-of-action" (80) exerts a pulling force. Some aphasics, especially those suffering from aphasia nominorum, retain the use of verbs. A patient who was asked to name a key which was shown to him, replied, "Open—to open."

There is no doubt, however, that in many cases the selection of the element, especially within a certain level, is determined by primitive wishes. This point has been emphasized by Linn and by Weinstein and Kahn (75, 76). In the instance of Linn's patient who said "chaise longue" instead of "wheelchair," her defect did not permit her to find the right word, but the uttered word followed the wish to deny her illness. Weinstein and Kahn have also emphasized the underlying wish of organic patients to deny their illness as well as other covert wishes. For instance, instead of calling the hospital a hospital, a patient called it "church."

Churches like hospitals help people, but the patient preferred to be helped as one is in a church rather than a hospital.

Linn and Weinstein and Kahn, following the mechanisms illustrated by Freud in *Psychopathology of Every Day Life* (27), have shown how the apparent indeterminacy can be disposed of by assuming that the primitive wish has a determining influence. This point is well taken. It applies, of course, even more to functional conditions. Thus the mentioned schizophrenic girl arrests her thought at a level where she and the Virgin Mary could form a primary category of interchangeable members. She is a girl who considers herself unappealing to men, unloved and unlovable, a nonentity. The anxiety-provoking effect of this evaluation of herself is so disturbing that her thought processes are impaired and the primitive wish to escape from this situation, or even to compensate it with an opposite one, emerges and makes her arrest her thinking at a level where her being a virgin is exploited in the most primitive way. Important here is not only the fact that the patient calls herself the "Virgin Mary" and that she responds to herself as to the Virgin Mary, but that she thinks she is the Virgin Mary. As I could elaborate in greater detail in other writings, the arrest of this level of thinking may be formulated as following adualism (13), paleologic, or the principle of Von Domarus (5-9).

Let us take now an example from a less primitive level, the level of discordance between thought and response. Let us consider again the patient who behaves in peculiar ways in the presence of elderly, red-haired women. Obviously there is a formation here of a primary class to which all elderly, red-haired women belong, but why is the behavior of this patient fixated at this level? Let us remember that contrary to what happens in most cases of schizophrenia the identification is in the response only, not in the object. We can give only hypothetical answers. First of all, the trauma inflicted on the patient by the aunt must have been rather serious, so that there was a great deal of emotionality which could extend easily to the whole primary category of red-haired women. Secondly, there is a wish to deny that the aunt is responsible for his behavior, or that he is rejected by the aunt, or that he deserves to be rejected by the aunt. In order to be able not to react in an unpleasant fashion only to the aunt he will react in the same way to the whole category, that is, he acquires a pattern of response which tends to become permanent.

The primitive response may have not only a negative aim—avoidance of unpleasantness—but also a positive one, such as quick attainment of pleasure. For instance, if a gosling can obtain quick mothering from a man he may be "imprinted" to respond to every man as to a goose. If a boy at an early age of his sexual development receives strong stimulation and gratification from another boy or man, he may learn to respond at a homosexual level, instead of overcoming this fixation and moving toward heterosexuality. Additional factors in the family constellation may facilitate this fixation.

The psychodynamic factors involved in phobias have already been alluded to in the previous section. The aim here is to remove the abstract fear from many threatening situations and restrict it to one member of a primary class.

If these intermediary stages, or battle of wishes, are overcome, as it happens in normal cases, and the subject reaches levels of thinking which follow Aristotelian logic, that is, levels which will obtain consensual validation, the course of thought nevertheless continues to be motivated almost always in more than one direction, so that the battle of the wishes continues to go on. Let us take for instance the example of a normal subject who is asked to answer the following question: "According to you, who is the greatest President of the United States?" If our subject were a regressed schizophrenic he could give—as we have already seen—an answer like, "White House" or "Monroe Doctrine," that is, his response would be a fragment of a primary aggregation. If the subject were a brain-injured patient he could reply with the name of any president, even one whom no historian would recognize as a great president, but a president, let us say, who happens to be born in the same hometown as the subject.

However, our healthy subject has already overcome all these stages without even being aware of them, and has come down mentally to a few possible answers: George Washington, Thomas Jefferson, Abraham Lincoln, and perhaps Franklin Roosevelt. At this point he is aware of a strong urge: the urge to answer "Franklin Roosevelt." He rejects the urge, however, and finally says, "Thomas Jefferson."

Now, we should know about our subject that he is a staunch Democrat, who has taken an active role in local politics during the presidency of Franklin Roosevelt. He had a strong desire to reach the conclusion that Roosevelt was the greatest President not only because he was better acquainted with the deeds of Roosevelt, but also because he supported them in his political activities.

At the same time that he was thinking in this way our subject became aware of his tendencies, perhaps of his prejudices, and attempted to correct them and found himself answering "Jefferson," another Democratic president. It may be that historians will reach the same conclusion as that of our subject; the fact remains that the subject's conclusion was not exclusively the result of his cognitive processes, but was to a large extent determined by the concomitant underlying battle of the wishes.

These concepts, of course, are not new. The work of the Würzburg group long ago put in evidence the *Aufgabe* of thought. In the United States, Sells (68) reported that in making syllogistic conclusions "the atmosphere effect" is very important. Janis and Frick (37) also found that the attitude of aggeement or disagreement of the subject predisposed toward acceptance or rejection of some of the offered conclusions in judging logical validity of syllogisms.

The following conclusions seem thus warranted: 1) In the mechanism of thought the subject has *potentially* available a vast range of processes, the primary ones as well as the secondary and most advanced; 2) which stage, or which one of the various processes will be the terminal one depends on factors, including the general state of health or disease, which potentially permit or inhibit the sequence of the various steps; 3) the motivation plays a very important role because it not only determines whether thought should advance or retrogress to a given stage but also selects the content within a given stage. An underlying battle of wishes always exists.

The last of the three statements seems the most confusing and almost impossible of actualization. In fact, it would seem that the conclusion which the person has not yet reached and the accompanying affect which cannot yet have been experienced have already influenced the preceding steps leading to that conclusion. This seems indeed a bizarre phenomenon to explain.

We may advance the following hypotheses:

1. Each stage of the thinking process is accompanied by an emotion or affective change. This hypothesis is susceptible of neurophysiologic interpretation. In fact every neopallic engram or network may be associated with an archipallic or limbic network (51, 52, 59).

2. Each stage, before becoming conscious, goes through a very brief period of unconsciousness.

3. In many cases it is the unconscious affect which will determine whether a given stage of thinking will become conscious or not.

Even the Würzburgers had realized the importance of unconscious processes. Ach (1) stated, "The activity of the determining tendencies is brought to fulfillment in the unconscious. The determination is effective without conscious memory of the task." Messer (55) too spoke of an unconscious machinery underlying the conscious process of thought.

Some objections to these hypothetical constructions may be raised by some, because contrary to popular belief, Freud did not believe in the existence of unconscious affect, but only in the existence of unconscious ideas or cognitive processes (26). According to Freud, an affect may not be experienced because the idea which elicits or accompanies that affect may be repressed. Freud states that emotion exists "only in the act of being felt." This point of view is a confusing one and for practical purposes has not been followed either by Freud or by his pupils (56), but it has been retained in theoretical formulations. But how could that be? If we speak of unconscious wish or of unconscious motivation we imply unconscious affect. A motivation cannot be a purely cognitive process. As a matter of fact, the point of view held by many other workers is just the opposite: It is the accompanying affect which changes a cognitive process into a motivational one.

In other publications (11, 14), I have described how even "sensations" may not be accompanied by subjective experience and remain "physiological processes." Some "physiological sensations" are never felt; other sensations may lose the subjective element in some pathological conditions (53, 57). I have suggested that the same loss of the subjective element may occur in emotions too. They may exist without being felt. They may be experienced only at a subliminal level.

Of course, not all unpleasant emotions are prevented from becoming unconscious. As a matter of fact, their "purpose" in evolution seems to be that of being felt. By being felt they give the indication to the person who experiences them that he has to alter his behavior in such way as to bring about the removal of the causes of the unpleasant emotions, and thus enhance survival. But with the complication of the cognitive equipment of man most emotions come to be consequences of cognitive processes, that is, not as responses to stimulation coming directly from the external world, but as responses to the extremely complicated, potentially endless, cognitive elaboration of these stimuli (11).

Thus became available to the human being another mechanism by which it is possible to avert or correct some emotions—the mechanism that Freud described in pathological conditions and for which he used the word *repression*. Actually, we cannot be sure that an active process of repression, that is, of "submerging into the unconscious," takes place: Rather, what seems to occur is a process by which the subliminal impulse is not allowed to become liminal and is then diverted.

Complications

No matter how complicated the microgenetic process has so far appeared, more complications can be found the more we study the phenomenon. Here are some of them:

1. When we talked of stages of thinking it is impossible to separate thinking from language, because it is almost exclusively through language or concepts expressed verbally that we can acquire a "conceptual" knowledge.

2. In pathological conditions there may be not only an arrest to primitive forms of thinking but something even more primitive than this arrest: an actual transformation of thought into perception, actions, or other psychosomatic activities. For instance, dreams and hallucinations are partial or total transformations of thoughts into perceptions (5, 8-10). These phenomena, although of great importance, are beyond the scope of this paper.

3. A complicating aspect occurring in pathological conditions, especially but not exclusively in schizophrenia, is the fact that when thinking has been arrested at a primitive level, the higher level has not ceased to exist: on the contrary, it is the higher abstract level which assumes a retrograde direction and acquires a more archaic or primitive form. This important topic, dealt with elsewhere (9, 10, 13), will be entirely omitted in this paper. It must be recognized, however, that it is an important complicating characteristic, so that "pure primitive levels" are seldom seen in psychopathological conditions.

4. Some experimental work cannot escape from this impinging of the higher levels. I shall mention in this regard the extremely interesting work by Werner (82) and Kaplan (39). Inasmuch as only a brief summary can be given here, the reader is referred to the original reports of this important investigation. Kaplan and Werner tried "the technique of line schematization" in order to reproduce primitive cognition. For instance, they instructed their subjects to draw lines to express such sentences as "He catches a fly," "He catches a lion," "He catches a criminal." The first sentence was expressed generally as a smooth upward line which turns finally so as to incorporate a small subject. The second was expressed as a line consisting of many small spirals finally ending upward with a big loop. The third sentence was expressed in a more complex way. The authors report that the concepts were fused in one or two lines. For instance, the same phrase "he catches" occurred in all the three

sentences, and yet the three lines were completely different. (There was no special line or part of the line to express "he catches.") The whole meaning was fused in a primitive, syncretic way. The authors are correct in saying that line drawing is a much more primitive symbolic medium than language, but could they really assert that they found a medium in which primitivity expresses itself in pure culture? Obviously not. First of all, the subject is confronted with three articulated and highly sophisticated sentences (He catches a fly; he catches a lion; he catches a criminal), and somewhat like the schizophrenic, he must impinge the high level (of which he is not deprived, but on the contrary of which he is aware) into the low medium. Secondly, contrary to the schizophrenic, the low medium does not reemerge spontaneously. The subject is forced to make a voluntary and not at all primitive effort to express a sophisticated complex in a given medium. No stage of primary aggregation can thus be reproduced in pure culture. These remarks should not be interpreted as a criticism of the work by Werner and Kaplan, which, on the contrary, I consider very valuable and which, in an indirect way, may lead us to understand better the process of secondary primitiveness and of the artistic process (14).

5. Some complicated phenomenon could on the contrary actually be explained by the proposed theory. The phenomenon of *déjà vu*, which so far has defied every interpretation, is susceptible now of understanding. In unconscious mechanisms, or in a primitive phenomenon such as dreams, the sense of time is altered and an occurrence which took place just a fraction of a second ago may seem to have occurred a long time ago. Now it could be that in the *déjà vu* phenomenon, the occurrence which seems to have been already experienced has been experienced in the short previous unconscious stage, before becoming conscious, and that in some people, especially epileptics but also normal subjects, for unclear reasons, a vague remembrance of the unconscious stage is retained.

PERCEPTION

Many of the observations that we have made in relation to thinking could be repeated about the microgeny of perception. Does perception go through a stage of primary aggregation or fragmentation? I shall start by describing some of my findings in the most acute and severe cases of schizophrenia (13).

I have proposed the term "awholism" for a phenomenon to my knowledge not previously described in schizophrenics. The very acutely ill patient goes through periods during which he is unable to perceive wholes. This disintegration of wholes is gradual. At first the patient must divide big or complex wholes into smaller unities. For instance, patients looking at nurses, attendants, physicians, cannot see them as persons, but perceive only parts of them—a nose, right or left eye, arm, etc. A female patient, who had undergone an acute episode with dangerous excitement, described in detail to me the experiences she had while she was in a seclusion cell. She remembered that she could not look at the whole door of the cell. She could only see the knob or the keyhole or some corner of the door. The wall too had to be fragmented into parts. Some other patients who were able to remember the acute episode told me how at first wholes or big unities were divided into the smaller units of which they were composed. Later, however, as the psychomotor excitement increased, even the smaller unities were divided into smaller fragments. Similar pronounced fragmentations probably occur in states of acute confusion such as some toxic-infective deliria, and in some bizarre, almost entirely forgotten dreams of normal people. One of the reasons why the phenomenon has not been described in the literature in reference to schizophrenia is the difficulty most patients encounter in remembering it. These amnesias are at least partially determined by the fact that disintegrated wholes or fragments have no names or do not correspond to schemata of previous experiences, similarly perhaps to what according to Schachtel (67) occurs in childhood amnesias.

Many years ago (1941-1945) I noticed the fragmentation of wholes in drawings of very regressed patients. At that time I did not understand the phenomenon and unfortunately did not preserve those drawings, with one exception, which was reproduced elsewhere (8).

In this case, whereas, prior to her illness, the patient was able to draw very well, from the beginning of the psychosis her drawings started to show the usual schizophrenic bizarreness. Later, when the illness was very advanced, the disorganization became very marked. For instance, when she wanted to draw a profile she could not finish it. Parts of the profile were disconnected; furthermore, some of these parts were repeated several times, conferring a confusing appearance to the whole drawing.

Some patients have reported to me that during the acute episode they were aware that they were losing perception of wholes and were making conscious efforts to reconstruct these wholes, but the attempts were only partially successful. At times the filling parts which were replaced for the missing ones were not appropriate and distorted wholes resulted.

Can this difficulty of the very ill schizophrenic be interpreted as a return to a primitive stage of perception, perhaps to a stage of "primary aggregation" in which wholes are not yet organized and in which elements of fragments may reappear in isolation?

There is presumptive evidence, coming from various sources, that it is so. Von Senden's classic book, which has just been translated into English 28 years after its original appearance, is of great help (74). Von Senden reported that study of the congenitally blind who later underwent cataract surgery and acquired eyesight disclosed that visual part-perception precedes perception of wholes and is additive. Riesen's studies on chimpanzees raised in darkness add further weight to this hypothesis (65). Melanie Klein's psychoanalytic concept of part-objects as very early introjections in newborn babies seems also confirmed (40, 41). Hebb's theoretical formulations also postulate that part perception precedes perception of wholes (34).

Impressive evidence comes also from neurologists who have studied cases of visual agnosia. The literature is abundant but, according to my own knowledge, no report is so accurate, and pertinent to the present topic as that by Alexandra Adler on the disintegration and the restoration which occur in visual agnosia (2, 3). Adler described, among other things, the alteration in visual perception which occurred in a 22-year-old woman who was injured in the famous fire of the Coconut Grove night club in Boston on Nov. 28, 1942. At first she was totally blind; after two days she could distinguish white from dark but could not recognize colors. She presented also a picture of a pure subcortical visual alexia, Wernicke type. The diagnosis of lesion of the brain, probably caused by carbon monoxide fumes, was made. After her injury this woman was no longer able to perceive wholes. She had to add part by part in order to reconstruct wholes and recognize objects. Often the patient recognized parts and guessed the rest. She could not recognize the figures 2, 3, 5, 6, 8, and 9 because she could not recognize the direction of the curves of which these figures were composed, but she was able to recognize 1, 4, and 7 during the second week of her illness because she could guess where a straight line was going. Since this patient recognized objects "by tracing the contours, by adding the parts and by making conclusions from all she had perceived, she had to take more time than did the normal person, who recognizes all the parts, in the main, simultaneously" (quoted verbatim from Adler (2) except for change from present to past tense).

Some neurologists [Brain; Nissl von Mayendorf; Poppelreuter, cited by Adler (2)] had suggested that a patient's inability to perceive the whole might be caused by a defect in the visual fields. Some controversy for instance, arose in the interpretation of a famous case, described by Goldstein and Gelb (31), of a man whose brain was injured during combat in World War I. This man lost the capacity of recognizing by a simultaneous act of visual perception the whole of a figure or the Gestalt. Goldstein (29, 30) and Adler herself (4), supported by observations made by other authors (38, 83, 84), could disprove that interpretation. The conclusion reached is that in certain pathological conditions wholes cannot be perceived, only parts. A tendency exists, however, to reconstruct wholes, at times inappropriate ones, only loosely related to the original.

Important corroboration can also be obtained from the experimental works of Pritchard, Hebb, and Heron (62, 63). Following previous works by Ditchburn (21) and Riggs (66), they confirmed that movements of the eyeballs are necessary for normal perception.* If the eye movements are made impossible and an image is thus stabilized on the retina, an abnormal, presumably primitive form of perception occurs. Pritchard and associates have attached to the eyeball itself a special device consisting of a contact lens and an optical projector. With this device the image remains fixed on the retina and does not move with the movements of the eyeball. The authors found that with this procedure a complex image, such as the profile of a face, may vanish in fragments with one or more of its parts fading independently. Some fragments remain in perception. This fragmentation seems to correspond to the original part-perception and, if we compare perception to thinking, to the fragmentation of the primary aggregation. For some fleeting periods of time parts may remain aggregated but do not form wholes. In tachistoscopic and other subliminal experiments often parts only are registered (79). Some parts, which in subliminal experiments were apparently not perceived, were registered instead, as demonstrated by the fact that they appeared in subsequent dreams. Fisher and his associates (22-24) have done interesting work in this respect by continuing and expanding work originally devised by Pötzl (60, 61).

Another important phenomenon appears in all these situations—acute schizophrenia, tachistoscopic experiments, visual agnosias, stablized images, etc. When the primary aggregation is broken and fragmented, there is a spontaneous effort on the part of the subject to reaggregate and possibly to reform wholes. If we want to anthropomorphize, we could say

---

* Eye movements seem also necessary for the occurrence of dreams (20).

that it is almost as if these parts or fragments were searching for wholes to which to belong.

But the new wholes (whether they appear in experimental perceptions or in dreams, as in Pötzl's and Fisher's experiments) are wrong or only loosely associated wholes, and correspond to the primary categories which we have described in the microgeny of thought. We cannot talk of categories, however, in the phenomenon of perception, which is probably precategorial. An appropriate name for this phenomenon may be "primary awholism."

This new formation of wholes may give some encouragement to the gestaltists, who may see in it an urge toward a Gestalt. The phenomenon may be called "primary Gestalt." Let us remember, however, that this phenomenon is secondary to the primary aggregation and follows mechanisms similar to those occurring in the formulation of the primary categories.

In schizophrenia, we have seen the formation of distorted wholes. Adler (2, 3) has described the reading and perceiving of related words in her patient suffering from visual agnosia, and similar phenomena have been reported in many aphasias. Pritchard (62), too, with his method of the stabilized image, reported that when entire words were presented to the subject, the partial fragmentation of letters caused different words to be perceived (for instance, the word *Beer* was perceived, *Peer, Peep, Bee, Be*).

In the microgeny of thought we have given paramount importance to affective factors in the determination of the primary categories. It is much more difficult to do so in the case of perception. Here we would have to take into consideration, instead of emotions, the pleasantness or unpleasantness of subliminal perception. The time is premature for such study both at a psychological and at a neurophysiological level.

SUMMARY

Thoughts and perceptions go through several unconscious stages before they reach consciousness.

The existence of these microgenetic stages is revealed by inference by the study of pathologic conditions, such as acute and chronic cases of schizophrenia, some psychoneuroses, aphasias, agnosias, and brain injuries. Some experiments dealing with subliminal perception or with the method of the stabilized image have also provided much relevant material.

In these pathologic or experimental conditions thoughts and perceptions tend to become conscious before they have completed their microgenetic development. It is possible to differentiate the stages of "primary aggregation" and of the "formation of primary categories" in thought processes. At times these stages of thought are congruous or syntonic with the behavior they elicit (as in psychoses), at other times they are not (as in psychoneuroses).

Perceptions go through the stages of "primary aggregation" and of primary formation of wholes (pre-Gestalt stages).

REFERENCES

1. ACH, N.: *Analyse des Willens.* Berlin: Urban & Schwarzenberg, 1935. Quoted by Humphrey (35).
2. ADLER, A.: Disintegration and restoration of optic recognition in visual agnosia. *Arch. Neurol. Psychiat.,* 51:243-259, 1944.
3. ADLER, A.: Course and outcome of visual agnosia. *J. Nerv. Ment., Dis.,* 111:41-51, 1950.
4. ADLER, A.: The concept of compensation and overcompensation in Alfred Adler's and Kurt Goldstein's Theories. *J. Individ. Psychol.,* 15:79-82, 1959.
5. ARIETI, S.: Special logic of schizophrenic and other types of autistic thought. *Psychiatry,* 11:325-338, 1948.
6. ARIETI, S.: Autistic thought: Its normal mechanisms and its relationships to schizophrenia. *J. Nerv. Ment. Dis.,* 111:288-303, 1950.
7. ARIETI, S.: Primitive intellectual mechanisms in pyschopathological conditions: Study of the archaic ego. *Amer. J. Psychother.,* 4:4-15, 1950.
8. ARIETI, S.: *Interpretation of Schizophrenia.* New York: Robert Brunner, 1955, Fig. 2, p. 334.
9. ARIETI, S.: Schizophrenic thought. *Amer. J. Psychother.,* 13:537-552, 1959.
10. ARIETI, S.: Schizophrenia: The manifest symptomatology, the psychodynamic and formal mechanisms. In *American Handbook of Psychiatry,* Vol. 1. Edited by S. Arieti. New York: Basic Books, Inc., 1959, pp. 455-484.
11. ARIETI, S.: The experiences of inner status. In *Perspectives in Psychological Therapy.* Edited by B. Kaplan and L. Wapner. New York: International Universities Press, Inc., 1960.
12. ARIETI, S.: A reexamination of the phobic symptom and of symbolism in psychopathology. *Amer. J. Psychiat.,* 118:106-110, 1961.
13. ARIETI, S.: The loss of reality. *Psychoanalysis,* 48:3-24, 1961.
14. ARIETI, S.: *The Intrapsychic Self. Feeling, Cognition and Creativity in Health and Mental Disease.* New York: Basic Books, 1967.
15. BOUMAN, L. and GRUNBAUM, A. A.: Experimentell-psychologische untersuchungen zur aphasie und paraphasie. *Zbl. Ges. Neurol. Psychiat.,* 96:481-538, 1925. Quoted by Werner (79).
16. BRUNER, J. S.: Going beyond the information given in contemporary approaches to cognition; symposium. Cambridge: Harvard University Press, 1957.
17. BRUNER, J. C., GOODNOW, J. J., and AUSTIN, G. A.: *A Study of Thinking.* New York: John Wiley & Sons, Inc., 1956.
18. CAMERON, N.: Reasoning, regression and communication in schizophrenics. *Psychol. Monogr.,* 50:1, 1938.
19. CONRAD, K.: Über den begriff der vorgestalt und seine bedeutung für die hirnpathologie. *Nervenarzt,* 18:289-293, 1947.

20. DEMENT, W.: Experimental and studies of sleep and dreaming. Lecture delivered at the Association for the Advancement of Psychotherapy. New York, May 19, 1961.
21. DITCHBURN, R. W.: Report to the experimental pyschology group. University of Reading, Reading, England, 1957. Quoted by J. S. Brunner, in *Sensory Deprivation*. Edited by P. Solomon and others. Cambridge: Harvard University Press, 1961.
22. FISHER, C.: Dream and perception: The role of preconscious and primary modes of perception in dream formation. *J. Amer. Psychoanal. Asso.*, 2:380-445, 1954.
23. FISHER, C.: Subliminal and supraliminal influences on dreams. *Amer. J. Psychiat.*, 116:1009-1017, 1960.
24. FISHER, C., and PAUL, J. H.: The effect of subliminal visual stimulation on images and dreams: A validation study. *J. Amer. Psychoanal. Asso.*, 7:35-83, 1959.
25. FLAVELL, J. H., and DRAGUNS, J.: A microgenetic approach to perception and thought. *Psychol. Bull.*, 54:197-217, 1957.
26. FREUD, S.: *The Unconscious* (1915). In *Collected Papers*, Vol. 4. New York: Basic Books, Inc., 1959, pp. 98-136.
27. FREUD, S.: Psychopathology of everyday life. In *The Basic Writings of Sigmund Freud*. Edited by A. A. Brill. New York: Modern Library, Inc., 1938, pp. 33-178.
28. FREUD, S.: *The Interpretation of Dreams*. Edited by J. Strachey. New York: Basic Books, Inc., 1960.
29. GOLDSTEIN, K.: *The Organism*. New York: American Book Company, 1939.
30. GOLDSTEIN, K.: Some remarks on Russel Brain's articles concerning visual object agnosia. *J. Nerv. Ment. Dis.*, 98:148-153, 1943.
31. GOLDSTEIN, K. and GELB, A.: Psychologische analyse hirnpathologischer fälle, Vol. 1. Leipzig: J. A. Barth, 1920, pp. 1-143.
32. HARTMANN, H., KRIS, E., and LOWENSTEIN, R. M.: Comments on the formation of psychic structure. *Psychoanal. Study Child*, 2:11-38, 1946.
33. HARTMANN, H., KRIS, E., and LOWENSTEIN, R. M.: Comments on the Formation of psychic structure. *Psychoanal. Study Child*, 2:11-38, 1946.
34. HEBB, D. O.: *The Organization of Behavior*. New York: John Wiley & Sons, Inc., 1949.
35. HUMPHREY, G.: *An Introduction to Its Experimental Psychology*. New York: John Wiley & Sons, Inc., 1951.
36. JACKSON, J. H.: On afflictions of speech from disease of the brain. In *Selected Writings of John Hughlings Jackson*, Vol. 2. Edited by J. Taylor. London: Hodder and Stoughton, 1932, pp. 184-204.
37. JANIS, I. L. and FRICK, F.: The relationship between attitudes toward conclusions and errors in judging logical validity of syllogisms. *J. Exp. Psychol.*, 33:73-77, 1943.
38. JOSSMAN, P.: Zur psychopathologie der optischagnostischen störungen. *Mschr. Psychiat. Neurol.*, 72:81-149, 1929.
39. KAPLAN, B.: Some psychological methods for the investigation of expressive language. In *On Expressive Language*. Edited by H. Werner. Worcester: Clark University Press, 1955.
40. KLEIN, M.: *Contributions to Psycho-Analysis*. London: Hogarth Press, Ltd., 1948.
41. KLEIN, M., HEIMANN, P., and MONEY-KRYLE, R.: *New Directions in Psychoanalysis*. New York: Basic Books, Inc., 1955.
42. KLÜVER, H.: *Behavior Mechanisms in Monkeys*. Chicago: University of Chicago Press, 1933.
43. KLÜVER, H.: The study of personality and the method of equivalent and non-equivalent stimuli. *Character Personality*, 5:91-112, 1936.
44. KLÜVER, H.: Functional differences between occipital and temporal lobes. In

Cerebral Mechanisms of Behavior. Edited by L. A. Hoffress. New York: John Wiley & Sons, Inc., 1951.

45. LACEY, J. I., BATEMAN, D. E., and VAN LEHN, R.: Automatic response specificity: An experimental study. *Psychosom. Med.,* 15:8, 1953.

46. LACEY, J. I. and LACEY, B. C.: Verification and extension of the principle of autonomic responsestereotopy. *Amer. J. Psychol.,* 71:50, 1958.

47. LASHLEY, K. S. and COLBY, K. M.: An exchange of view on psychic energy and psychoanalysis. *Behav. Sci.,* 2:230-240, 1957.

48. LINN, L.: The discriminating function of the ego. *Psychoanal. Quart.,* 23:38-47, 1954.

49. LORENZ, K. Z.: Comparative behaviorology, in discussions on child development, Vol 1. Proceedings of the WHO study group on the psychobiological development of the child, Geneva, 1953. New York: International Universities Press, Inc., 1956.

50. LOTMAR, F.: Aus kenntnis der erschwerten worfindung und ihrer bedeutung für des denken des aphasischen. *Schweiz. Arch. Neurol. Psychiat.,* 5:206-239, 1919.

51. MacLEAN, P. D.: The limbic system ("visceral brain") and emotional behavior. *A.M.A. Arch. Neurol. Psychiat.* 73:130-134, 1955.

52. MacLEAN, P. D.: In *Handbook of Physiology, Section One: Neurophysiology, Vol.* 3. Edited by J. Field, Washington, D. C.: American Physiological Society, 1960, pp. 1723-1744.

53. MAGEE, K. R., SCHNEIDER, S. F., and ROSENZWEIG, N.: Congenital indifference to pain. *J. Nerv. Ment. Dis.,* 132:249, 259, 1961.

54. MARBE, K.: Experimentell-psychologische untersuchungen über das urteil. Leipzig 1901. Quoted by Humphrey (35).

55. MESSER, A.: Experimentelle psychologische untersuchungen über das denken. *Arch. Ges. Psychol.,* 8:1-224, 1906.

56. NUNBERG, H.: *Principles of Psychoanalysis: Their Application to the Neuroses.* New York: International Universities Press, Inc., 1955.

57. OGDEN, T. E., ROBERT, F., and CARMICHAEL, T. E.: Some sensory syndromes in children: Indifference to pain and sensory neuropathy. *J. Neurol. Neurosurg. Psychiat.,* 22:267-276, 1959.

58. OSGOOD, C. E.: A behavioristic analysis of perception and language as cognitive phenomena, in contemporary approaches to cognition; symposium. Cambridge: Harvard University Press, 1957.

59. PAPEZ, J. W.: A proposed mechanism of emotion. *Arch. Neurol. Psychiat.,* 38:725-743, 1937.

60. PÖTZL, O.: Experimentell erregte traumbilder in ihren beziehungen zum indirekten sehen. *Z. Neurol. Psychiat.,* 37:278-349, 1917.

61. PÖTZL, O., ALLERS, R., and TELER, J.: Preconscious stimulation in dreams, associations, and images. *Psychol. Issues,* 11:3, 1960.

62. PRITCHARD R. M.: Stabilized images on the retina. *Sci. Amer.,* 204:72-78, 1961.

63. PRITCHARD, R. M., HERON, W., and HEBB, D. O.: Visual perception approached by the method of stabilized images. *Canad. J. Psychol.,* 14:67-77, 1960.

64. RAPAPORT, D.: Toward a theory of thinking in organization and pathology of thought. Edited by D. Rapaport. New York: Columbia University Press, 1951.

65. RIESEN, A. H.: The development of visual perception in man and chimpanzee. *Science,* 106:107-108, 1947.

66. RIGGS, L. A. and TULUNAY, S. U.: Visual effects of varying the extent of compensation for eye movements. *J. Optic Soc. Amer.,* 9:741-745, 1959.

67. SCHACHTEL, E. G.: *Metamorphosis.* New York: Basic Books, Inc., 1959.

68. SELLS, S. B.: The atmosphere effect: An experimental study of reasoning. *Arch. Psychol.,* 1936, p. 200.

69. SULLIVAN, H. S.: *Conceptions of Modern Psychiatry.* New York: W. W. Norton & Company, Inc., 1953.
70. VINACKE, W. E.: *The Psychology of Thinking.* New York: McGraw-Hill Book Company, Inc., 1952.
71. VINACKE, W. E.: Relations between motivational conditions and thinking, fundamentals of psychology: The psychology of thinking. *Ann. N.. Acad. Sci.,* 91: 76-93, 1960.
72. VON BERTALANFFY, L.: General system theory. In *General Systems Yearbook of the Society for the Advancement of General Systems Theory.* Edited by L. Von Bertalanffy and A. Rapaport. Ann Arbor: University of Michigan Press, 1956.
73. VON DOMARUS, E.: The specific laws of logic in schizophrenia. In *Language and Thought in Schizophrenia: Collected Papers.* Edited by J. S. Kasanin. Berkeley: University of California Press, 1944, pp. 104-114.
74. VON SENDEN, M.: Space and and light: The perception of space and shape in congenitally blind patients before and after operation. London: Methuen & Co., Ltd., 1960.
75. WEINSTEIN, E. A. and KAHN, R. L.: *Denial of Illness: Symbolic and Physiological Aspects.* Springfield: Ill., Charles C. Thomas, Publisher, 1955.
76. WEINSTEIN, E. A. and KAHN, R. L.: Symbolic reorganization in brain injuries. In *American Handbook of Psychiatry,* Vol. 1. Edited by S. Arieti. New York: Basic Books, Inc., 1959, pp. 964-981.
77. WENGER, M. A., ENGEL, B. T., and CLEMENS, T. L.: Studies of autonomic responses patterns: Rationale and methods. *Behav. Sci.,* 2:216, 1957.
78. WENGER, M. A., CLEMENS, T. C., COLEMAN, D. R., CULLEN, T. D., and ENGEL, B. T.: Autonomic response specificity. *Psychosom. Med.,* 23:185-193, 1961.
79. WERNER, H.: Microgenesis and aphasia. *J. Abnorm. Soc. Psychol.,* 52:347-353, 1956.
80. WERNER, H.: *Comparative Psychology of Mental Development.* New York: International Universities Press, Inc., 1975.
81. WERNER, H.: The concept of development from a comparative and organismic point of view. In *The Concept of Development.* Edited by D. B. Harris. Minneapolis: University of Minnesota Press, 1957.
82. WERNER, H. and KAPLAN, B.: The developmental approach to cognition: Its relevance to the psychological interpretation of anthropological and ethnolinguistic data. *Amer. Anthropologist,* 58:866-880, 1956.
83. WILBRAND, H. and SANGER, A.: *Die Neurologie des Auges,* Vol. 7. Wiesbaden: J. F. Bergmann, 1917, pp. 393-446.
84. WOLPERT, L.: Die simultanagnosie—störung der gesamtauffassung. *Ztschr. Ges. Neurol. Psychiat.,* 93:397-415, 1924.

22

Toward a Unifying Theory
of Cognition

Inspired by the newly emerged science of general systems, this paper illustrates structural similarities or isomorphics in the different forms of cognition and discusses the biological origin of knowledge in the cosmos known to man.

THE AIM OF THIS PAPER is to illustrate structural similarities or isomorphics in the different forms of cognition.

Can general principles be found which apply to such different levels as perception, recognition, memory learning, simple ideation, language, conceptual thinking, arithmetic, etc.? Moreover, if such principles are found, will they be so generic that nothing will be added to our common knowledge?

The author's answer to these questions is that such inquiry is worth being pursued, first, because what appears simple may imply much more; second, because principles found at a certain order of generality do not exclude that each subsumed level has an organization of its own. For instance, thinking may have some properties which are not inherent in learning, and learning may have some characteristics which are not inherent in perception.

In other words, following the method of von Bertalanffy (18), we shall pursue a general system theory, although one which can be applied only to cognition, not to the whole universe. However, inasmuch as cognition plays such an important role in the understanding of the universe, any presentation of this kind has implications that transcend cognition itself.

In our attempt we cannot follow a neurophysiological approach, as we do not yet have the necessary knowledge for it, in spite of the fact that great progress has been made [for instance, through the work of Eccles

300

(13, 14)] and daring working hypotheses have been advanced [for instance, by Hebb (15)]. The author will adhere to a psychological approach. In what follows a few new ideas and a considerable number of old ones will be presented. The old ones, however, will be considered in a new and larger context. Actually what we are going to adopt is the inductive method. From several instances, occurring at different levels of cognition, we shall infer general rules.

SENSORY ORGANIZATION AND PERCEPTION

Sensory-perceptual data undergo some kind of organization as soon as they are experienced. We shall take into consideration here those senso-perceptions which do not remain predominantly experiences of the inner status of the organism (like pain, hunger, thirst, etc.), but those which become parts of the field of cognition (4). These psychological phenomena seem to us to follow three types or modes of organization.

The first mode of organization is *contiguity*. Sense-data experienced together tend to be reexperienced together, if they produced *one* effect in the organism by the fact of being together. The effect in its turn connects more firmly together the sense-data.

Let us assume that the four components of Figure 1, which we shall call a, b, c, d, produce an effect E in the perceiving organism. The effect E binds together a, b, c, d. Obviously the qualities which a, b, c, d must have in order to produce E vary with each case, but what is important is that a, b, c, d must be experienced together. Only those elements will be perceived together which are retained together by the feed-mechanism of the effect. When we state that the elements should be experienced together we do not mean it in an absolute sense. We mean that the perception of them is either simultaneous or overlapping or contiguous in time or space. The organismic effect, important in segregating perceptual wholes from the infinity and indefiniteness of the universe, varies with the level of organization and evolution. At first it may be a not-felt chemical change; later a not-conscious nervous change; still later a felt change, etc. With the evolution of cognition, however, the immediate effect loses importance and what counts more and more is the externalization of the perception, more or less independently of the effect. In Figure 1 the four elements by being contiguous constitute a form, reminiscent of a human face; but sensory-data may be experienced together even when they do not form a definite whole, or a definite Gestalt, but just a group.

In Figure 2 the nonsensical lines are seen as forming one "group" of lines.

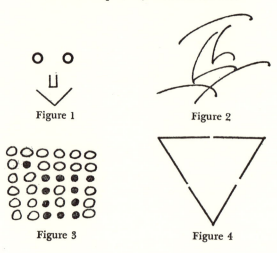

Figure 1   Figure 2

Figure 3   Figure 4

The mode of operation by *contiguity*, which seems at first so simple, is something which instead requires the solution, through evolutionary mechanisms of a difficult problem which we have discussed elsewhere: response to a part versus response to a whole (6, 10). We shall not repeat here this important subject. In normal conditions, whole-perception wins out and the mode of contiguity generally applies to the contiguity of the various parts which form differentiated wholes.

The second mode of operation is the mode of *similarity*. Figure 3 contains dots of different shapes and colors. Alike dots tend to form a separate group or to be perceived together. Here similarity and contiguity reinforce one another. Elements which are similar or identical associate very well.*

The mode of operation by similarity applies to both part-perception and whole-perception.

The third mode of operation is *pars pro toto*. The perception of a part has upon the organism an effect which is equivalent to that of the perception of the whole.

If we look at Figure 4 we see a triangle, in spite of the fact that there are three gaps in the picture, which technically therefore is not a triangle. The followers of the Gestalt school call this way of perceiving "closure."

---

* Advertisers know very well the effect of this reinforcement. Operators of newsstands often display the cover of the same magazine many times. The increase-effect is not merely due to the repetition of the advertisement, but to the fact that when similar elements are together they reinforce one another.

According to them the closure, as a principle of organization, permits the perception of the whole; the small gaps are filled in. This tendency to close a gap is considered by them the expression of a fundamental principle of brain functioning. Tension is supposed to be built up on both sides of the gap, like the tendency of an electric current to jump a small gap in the electric circuit. This tendency eventually would close the gap.

Let us give another look at Figure 4. The gaps are *never* closed. We continue to see the interruptions; but *in spite* of the gaps we perceive a triangle. The triangle of Figure 4 is not a whole triangle, but *stands for* a whole triangle. The Gestaltists speak of closure because they have taken into consideration especially experimentally devised stimuli with small gaps. Actually very little in nature is perceived totally. More often than it seems at first impression, we perceive parts which stand for wholes. For instance, I see only a crescent in the sky and I know I see the moon; I see only a side of the table and I know I see the table; I see only the facade of a cathedral and I know I see the cathedral. This phenomenon is not the simple phenomenon of closure of the Gestaltists, but a much more general faculty of the psyche, which permits a part to stand for the whole. As we shall see later in this paper, it is on this third mode of organization that the whole phenomenon of symbolism is based. Let us remember, however, that except for a few optic illusions, purposely arranged, the whole is not experienced at a sensory level. The whole is filled in by our responses (inasmuch as we react as to wholes), or by our memories (of parts being generally associated with their respective wholes), or by symbolic processes.

At this point we must recognize that we have hit on important, apparently paradoxical facts. In other writings, we have determined how important the biological struggle is between part and whole, and how pathological or anti-evolutionary it is for the organism to confuse the part with the whole (1-7). Now on the contrary, we come to the realization that the third mode of operation on which (as we shall see later) the highest levels of our cognition are based, actually consists of the ability of a part to stand for the whole. The whole seems again broken up and a part or a few parts together seem to resume importance. Often what is perceived is a *clue* or a *sign*, which stands for a whole. It could be that this facility with which a part can stand for the whole is somehow based on that ancient property of the organism of responding to parts rather than to wholes (5, 6, 10).

LEARNING

We shall consider now a different level of cognition, learning, and its relation to the same three modes of operation which we have outlined in reference to perception. By learning is generally meant a change in behavior as a result of individual experience.

There is no doubt that there is a strong relation between the mode of contiguity, or first mode of operation, and learning. Some learning theories, like those of Thorndike, Guthrie, and Pavlov, regard contiguity the most important factor in learning. According to these theories, an association (that is, a relationship based on temporal or spatial contiguity) occurs between stimulus and response. For instance, in conditioning, the dog learns to salivate in response to the ringing of a bell. But during the learning period the bell is rung shortly before or at the same time that food is seen. There is thus a temporal contiguity between food (unconditioned stimulus) and ringing of the bell (conditioned stimulus). In this type of learning a congenital response is extended to a stimulus which ordinarily would not elicit that congenital reaction. This type of learning is relatively simple. Nothing new has been added to the repertory of the dog's responses. The animal learns only to extend to a different context what its organism was already capable of doing.

It is beyond the purpose of this paper to evaluate all the ways in which the mode of contiguity operates in learning. The numerous psychological books on learning deal with this subject. It is beyond the purpose of this paper also to evaluate why, out of all possible associations, only some actually occur. This evaluation would require a study of the law of effect, reinforcement, etc. (10, Ch. 4).

Although the mode of contiguity plays a tremendous role in learning, and is probably the mode on which the other two are founded, it is difficult to subsume all types of learning under that mechanism. What psychologists call "transfer" may be viewed as an application at the level of learning of the second mode of operation, or mode of *similarity*. An acquired response is extended to many or all similar situations. For instance, if I have learned to avoid certain insects, like wasps, I may extend my avoidance reaction to similar insects, like bees. Learning by transfer is based on the fact that similar situations have identical elements. The learning is based on the identity or equivalency of certain elements (10, Ch. 7). Learning by the mode of similarity requires a power of abstraction, just as does perceptual organization by the mode of similarity. Although generally useful, learning by similarity may lead to errors when the identity of a few elements do not warrant the same response (1, 2, 3, 6, 7, 8).

The third mode of operation, *pars pro toto*, operates in all types of learning, even the simplest. For instance, in conditioning, when the dog secretes gastric juice in response to the buzzing of the bell, the buzzing of the bell may be seen as a part which stands for a whole (buzzing of the bell plus sight of food).

At a neurophysiological level too, the whole process of learning can be seen as an application of the third mode of operation. The activation of certain neuronal elements through the stimulus brings about the arousal of the whole neuronal circuit or patterns involved in that given learning situation (11). The phenomena which Gestalt psychologists attribute to insight may be viewed as based on the concomitant application of the second and third modes of operation. The "insight" is due to the fact that the organism responds as it would to a previous situation because of the presence of identical elements in the old and new situation. The *identical elements* stand for the total situations.

Since these three modes of operation are mixed together in learning, the possibility which one may prospect is that even these three modes may be synthesized or unified into just one mode. In learning, we could be tempted to reduce the whole process to the fact that reactivation of a part leads to the reactivation of the whole. However, we have to assume that prior to this reactivation the modes of contiguity and similarity have already been in operation.

MEMORY

We shall take into consideration only two mechanisms of memory: recognition and recall; and only in relation to the three general modes of operation.

Recognition is the simplest of the two and exists, at a more or less elaborate degree, in most animals. It means that a perception A^1, occurring now, is compared automatically or unconsciously with a past experience A, and found to be eliciting the same response of A. A^1 is then considered similar or identical to A. The first mode of operation, contiguity, differentiates perception A from the manifold of experiences. A will remain as a differentiated memory trace. The first mode of operation will later differentiate A^1 too. The mnemonic trace of A and the perception of A^1 are connected by the second mode of operation, similarity.

How this is possible at a neurophysiological level must remain the object of speculation. Perhaps the perception of A^1 sends several "echoes" throughout the nervous system, but the only echo which is absorbed is the one received by the engram of A. The engram A thus becomes associated with and reinforces the perception of A^1 and also confers the feeling of recognition. The perception of A^1, however, does not bring about the reactivation of A only, but also of many things formerly associated with A. We have thus again a *pars pro toto* mechanism.

Recall is a much more complicated mechanism. It differs from recognition inasmuch as it is not brought about by an external perception, but by a voluntary effort to reproduce stored images. However, images once recalled, organize also according to the three modes of operation that we have described.

SIMPLE IDEATION OR ASSOCIATIONS OF IDEAS

It is difficult to individualize all the cognitive forms which enter into the process of thinking. Simple ideation is a form of thinking which is organized by the simple laws of association. Simple ideation, however, although possible through sensory images, generally consists of verbal symbols. Nevertheless, for expository reasons, we shall postpone to the next section of this paper the discussion of language in relation to the three modes of operation.

The study of associations of ideas goes back to Aristotle. In the past 50 years this study has been discredited by people who have repeatedly pointed out that the laws of association are too simple, mechanical, and cannot explain the whole field of cognition. Of course, any attempt to explain the whole field of cognition by the laws of association is indicative of an extreme reductionistic approach. On the other hand, the phenomenon of association of ideas must be acknowledged and recognized as *one* of the foundations of the high levels of cognition. To discredit this phenomenon because it is insufficient to explain the whole human psyche is an excessive and inappropriate attitude.

The first law of associations of ideas, the law of contiguity, is another expression of the mode of contiguity. This law states that when two mental processes have been active together or in immediate succession, one of them on recurring tends to elicit the recurrence of the other. For instance, if I think of my grandmother I may also think of the house where she lived when I visited her in my childhood. The mode of contiguity which existed even in low animal forms now acquires an evocative and representational status.

The second law (or law of similarity) is another expression of the second mode of operation. It states that if two mental representations resemble each other, that is, if they have one or more characteristics in common, the occurrence of one of them tends to elicit the occurrence of the other. For instance, I visualize the Eiffel Tower and I may think of the Empire State building, because they are both very tall constructions. If I think of Beethoven, I may start to think of Brahms and Mozart, because the three were great composers.

A third law, mentioned in old books of psychology, is the law of contrast. For instance, the idea of white brings about the idea of black, its opposite. In normal mentation, actually, contrast plays a secondary role and may be subsumed under the second law (for instance, black and white are both similar, inasmuch as they are both "colors"). However, in primitive and schizophrenic thinking, association of opposites plays an important role, for reasons which cannot be discussed in this paper (10, 16).

Our third law, which is not mentioned in any book of psychology, corresponds to our third mode of operation: *pars pro toto*. This third law is actually inherent in the concept of association. The few ideas which are associated by contiguity and similarity stand for a whole constellation of ideas and tend to bring about the whole constellation. For instance, the idea of my grandmother may stand for my whole childhood and bring about many memories of my childhood.

This is also, in a certain way, *thinking by cue*. A small cue may arouse a complex pattern. A fragment of a situation may evoke the total situation; a member of a series may evoke the whole series.

High levels of cognition cannot be easily distinguished from one another. Some functions which appear different are based on the same fundamental processes. We shall try to avoid repetitions as much as we can.

HIGHER LEVELS OF COGNITION

In language, a sound (the word) becomes connected with an object or meaning by the mode of contiguity. It becomes applied to all the members of the class by the mode of similarity and may stand for the denotation or connotation of one or more members of the class or for the whole class (*pars pro toto*).

We can repeat approximately the same things for concept formation. The mode of contiguity is used to collect and connect the data which form the concept. The mode of similarity will make us extend the concept to all the members of a class. Finally, by virtue of the mode of *pars pro toto*, the concept will stand for the whole class.

In induction, the mode of contiguity makes us associate A and B because we have observed that B has followed A many times. The mode of similarity will make us associate all A's with all B's. The mode *pars pro toto* will make us extend to the whole series of A's and B's what we have observed in just a segment of that series. This apparently unwarranted generalization has worried philosophers since Hume. Just because we have noticed that B follows A a certain number of times, we are not entitled to infer that B will always follow A. Although the philosophers may be right in an absolute sense, life can exist only on such presuppositions as the one mentioned, that B would always follow A. Life is possible as long as the observed uniformities of sequences will recur. Let us examine again the conditioned reflex. If the sight of food is preceded by the ringing of a bell, the ringing of a bell (A) after a few exposures will make the experimental dog secrete gastric juice (B). The organism of the dog follows *induction*. The only difference between us, as conscious beings, and the organism of the dog (or even our organism), is that in us induction is accompanied by awareness, whereas in the organism of the dog it is an automatic mechanism. Most probably the same basic mechanism operates in us and in the conditioned dog; but in us, who are endowed with self-consciousness (or reflected activity), the mechanism has become subjectivized to a degree which includes a consciousness of it. The philosophers are right in stating that it does not follow that just because B has followed A several times, B should always follow A; but without such assumption life mechanisms cannot be understood. When we say assumption we actually anthropomorphize; we mean expectation which, although it is a human faculty, perhaps can be conceived as a property of life, a certain type of memory and preparation for similar events, which may exist in every protoplasm.

Life would not be possible without the living organisms functioning in an inductive way. Only the organism which can perform inductively and transmit genetically this inductive form of functioning can survive. Although induction may be based on something which cannot be proved philosophically, life depends on it.

In *deduction* the whole membership of the series is included in the big premise, for instance: All men are mortal. The big premise is made possible by the fact that the mode of contiguity (which connects "men" and "being mortal") is used together with the mode of similarity, which together extend the concept to the whole series (all men). The third mode (*pars pro toto*) is also applied in the big premise inasmuch as the symbol "all men" stands for the whole class (all past, present, and future men). The second premise (Socrates is a man), by following the mode of similarity, makes us attribute to Socrates membership in the series of men. The inference which we shall be able to make, using again the mode of similarity, will apply to Socrates the characteristics of the members of the class of men.

About deterministic causality we could more or less repeat what we have said about induction: an association is made between B and A (mode of contiguity). The association is extended to all the sequences A → B. Inasmuch as this law will be applied to all similar data in the cosmos, it will follow the *pars pro toto* mode.

The three modes apply, of course, to arithmetical thinking also. Although all numbers imply the three modes, we could say that in number one the mode of contiguity predominates. In fact, by the contiguity of parts, a unity is formed which is separated from the rest of the world and will be later recognized as being one (10). Number two uses predominantly the mode of similarity. In fact, unless objects are at the same time seen as distinct and similar, no concept of two or of any subsequent plurality is possible. The properties of 1 and 2 and of 1 and 2 together are then applied by *pars pro toto* to the whole series of positive integer numbers.

UNIFYING HYPOTHESES

At this point we can perhaps conclude that the three basic modes of operation determine and structure our knowledge of the world.

The first mode determines *what is and what is not*. What is, is a unity.

The second mode *identifies*, by discovering similarity, or identity, and permitting class formation.

The third mode *infers* the not given from the given.

These three modes could really be considered three basic pre-experiential categories. We can, however, represent the general process of cognition with a different formulation and say that it is based on two fundamental characteristics: progressive abstraction and progressive symbolization.

The first mode abstracts unities and groups from the manifold of the universe. The second mode abstracts the similarity between different unities. The third mode abstracts (that is, infers) the not given from the given.

Abstraction, as important as it is, does not comprehend the whole cognitive process. Symbolization has to be added.

If we include both signs and symbols under the general process of symbolization, we can say that even a perception is a symbol, inasmuch as it stands for the perceived thing. Images, endocepts, paleosymbols, verbal symbols, preconceptual and conceptual, are different forms of progressive symbolization (9).

The ideal symbol is the symbol which, although different from the thing it represents, has the same properties of the represented thing. The symbol which comes closer to this ideal is not the onomatopoetic symbol or an iconic symbol, but the number. Although the number is not the thing that it represents, it has the numerical properties of the represented things. For instance, the symbol 15, although a symbol, has all the numerical properties of the group of 15 integer objects. Although 15 is an abstract symbol it retains its concrete numerical qualities. At the same time it is independent of its concrete embodiments and other concrete qualities, so that it permits the best possible identity with any of its embodiments.*

We could therefore say that abstraction includes all the modes of operation, whereas symbolization is a different name for the third. Although there may be some merit in visualizing cognition in this way, this writer's preference is for retaining the formulation of the three modes of operation. It seems to come closer to a unifying theory of cognition.

The question may be asked whether these three modes of operation rule the other important areas of the psyche, for instance, the experiences of inner status (sensations, feelings, emotions). The answer is that if we separate feelings from their cognitive associations it will be very difficult to apply to them the basic modes. Unity of feeling as feeling is at most hazy. Moreover, if for instance, a feeling like a pain is recognized as similar to a previous feeling, this act of recognition is a cognitive act. Feelings do not have the finiteness, nor the potential symbolic infinity of acts of cognition, unless associated with acts of cognition. They have, however, the power to transform or determine cognitive processes.

THE BIOLOGICAL ORIGIN OF KNOWLEDGE AND THE MESOCOSMIC REALITY

It would seem thus that the basic principles of cognitive organization are responsible for the way we interpret reality. That is tantamount to advocating a biological origin of our knowledge.

Let us re-examine briefly some of our basic concepts. In other writings, we have shown how the possibility of perceiving wholes and parts eventually led to the distinction of subjects and predicates. The ability to recognize, or to respond in the same way to similar or/and identical

---

* We could approximately repeat the same things for algebraic symbols; *n* is independent of any embodiment and yet retains all its algebraic qualities.

things, led to the formation of classes and, incidentally, to the laws of Aristotelian logic. The excluded middle, or the third law of thought of Aristotle, represents the victory of identifying by wholes rather than by parts. Our process of induction is nothing else but the subjectivization of the inducting capacity of the animal organism.

We must add something to which we have not yet made reference: space perception. Three-dimensional or Euclidian space is based not so much on our visual perceptions, as some people believe, but on our vestibular apparatus with its three semicircular canals. It is not due to chance that we perceive space as we do: we have no choice.

Thus, our whole interpretation of nature is imposed on us by the biological origin of our cognition. Moreover, it would seem that *the psyche brings to awareness what was already implied in the living matter.*

Does this mean that in our understanding of the world we use a priori categories? Are, for instance, the three basic modes of operation that we have described a priori categories? We think they are, but not in the Kantian sense, because we believe that the animal organism, through evolutionary mechanisms, has assimilated them from the external world. They are a priori as far as the individual is concerned. However, they are a posteriori if we consider evolution as a whole. Evolution has to "learn" them from the external environment and transmit them from generation to generation.

These *biologicogenic* categories, however, permit us to conceive the universe in a frame of reference which seems to reflect the Euclidian-Newtonian-Kantian universe. Thus, in a certain way, they seem antiquated in a world which is viewed today in Einsteinian-Heisenbergian terms. To give just two examples of fundamental importance: 1) we perceive space as three dimensional, but modern non-Euclidian geometry considers it more appropriate to consider space as non-three dimensional; 2) we have seen how not only our cognition but life itself is based on the reliability of induction. And yet we know that according to Heisenberg's principle of indeterminacy, the ideas of exceptionless repetitions, induction, and strict causality have to be abandoned.

Reichenbach (17) and Capek (12) made it clear that modern physics does not deny the validity of the Euclidian-Newtonian-Kantian world. It only restricts it to the mesocosm, a world of middle dimensions. For the macrocosm (a world larger than solar systems) the Einsteinian-Heisenbergian physics applies.

But life exists in the mesocosm. In order to originate and evolve it had to incorporate mesocosmic laws. Without such incorporation life could not exist. On the other hand, the fact that life exists proves that there is some order in the mesocosm. Perhaps it is an order which applies only to the mesocosm, but in its restricted dimensions it exists and has to be taken into account. If a man would be deprived of his three semicircular canals and consequently of equilibrium and space-perception, he could not survive for more than a few days unless helped by others. If the principle of induction would not apply to life, the living world would be transformed into chaos.

The order which we, as animal forms, have incorporated is then re-externalized or projected into the external world from where it originated. What Euclid, Newton, and Kant did was to increase our awareness of mesocosmic categories and to enlarge our understanding of the mesocosmic reality of which we are the products. These categories represent what we have acquired from mesocosmic reality through a process of evolutionary adjustment. It would have been unnatural for Euclid to describe a non-three dimensional space.

We often read criticisms of Freud because he would have viewed the human psyche in the restricted Euclidian-Newtonian-Kantian world. Alas! This is not the error of Freud. The psyche itself, the whole life, as it is known to us, is based on the Euclidian-Newtonian-Kantian world. If some aspects of life follow mesocosmic categories, neither Freud nor anybody else could demonstrate this fact at the stage of our knowledge. The error Freud made was to apply to the psyche, especially in relation to the libido theory, concepts which pertain only to physics and economics, by-passing general biology and neurophysiology. Einsteinian-Heisenbergian notions, which are usually derived from the physical world, would be equally inappropriate if transplanted in the original form to the study of the psyche. The same thing would be repeated for more modern types of economics.

To our statement that the order of cognition derives from the order of the mesocosm we have to add important qualifications. At least one aspect of psychological life does not seem to derive from the mesocosmic environment: awareness, or subjectivity. As far as we know, only animal life is endowed with awareness. Automatic cognition can be seen as existing outside of the animal kingdom, and not exclusively in modern computers made by men. For instance, a solar system can be viewed as a machine which reflects a cosmic order—a machine, however, which in spite of its immensity is not, as far as we know, aware of its existence. Cognition acquires a human flavor when it is accompanied by awareness, and thus leads to the possibility of making choices and of *willing*.

Does the fact that our knowledge is mesocosmic in origin deny us access to the understanding of a macro- and microcosmic reality or of an absolute or noumenal reality? Adventurous excursions into these other segments of reality are difficult and contrary to our present understanding of the biological nature of man. That is why they have occurred so late in history. Nevertheless, they are possible, as modern physics shows. My belief (or, perhaps, wish!) is that our mesocosmic knowledge (again applying the *pars pro toto* mode of operation) will permit men to understand not only the microcosm and the macrocosm but realms of reality now unimaginable and unthinkable. In fact, the *pars pro toto* mode implies that if a little order exists a big order also exists. But in believing so I have made an unwarranted generalization. I have applied to the unknown the inductive method which I know may be valid only in the mesocosm. My belief, thus, must remain a belief.

REFERENCES

1. ARIETI, S.: Special logic of schizophrenic and other types of autistic thought. *Psychiatry*, 11:325, 1948.
2. ——: *Interpretation of Schizophrenia.* New York: Brunner, 1955.
3. ——: Schizophrenic thought. *Am. J. Psychotherapy*, 13:537, 1959.
4. ——:The experiences of inner status. In: B. Kaplan and S. Wapner (Eds.), *Perspectives in Psychological Theory.* New York: Intern. Univ. Press, 1960.
5. ——: The loss of reality. *Psychoanalysis*, 48:3, 1961.
6. ——: The microgeny of thought and perception. *Arch. Gen. Psychiatry.* 6:454, 1962.
7. ——: Studies of thought processes in contemporary psychiatry. *Am. J. Psychiatry*, 120:58, 1963.
8. ——: The rise of creativity: From primary to tertiary process. *Contemporary Psychoanalysis*, 1:51, 1964.
9. ——: Contributions to cognition from psychoanalytic theory. In: J. Masserman (Ed.), *Science and Psychoanalysis,* Vol. VIII. New York: Grune and Stratton, 1965.
10. ——: *The Core of Man* (in preparation).
11. BUGELSKI, R.: *The Psychology of Learning.* New York: Holt, 1956.
12. CAPEK, M.: The development of Reichenbach's epistemology. *Review of Metaphysics*, 9:42, 1957.
13. ECCLES, J. C.: *The Neurophysiological Basis of Mind.* Oxford: Oxford Univ. Press, 1953.
14. ——: *The Physiology of Nerve Cells.* Baltimore: Johns Hopkins Press, 1957.
15. HEBB, D. O.: *The Organization of Behavior.* New York: Wiley, 1949.
16. KAPLAN, B.: On the phenomena of "opposite speech." *J. Abnormal Social Psychol.,* 55:389, 1957.
17. REICHENBACH, H.: *The Rise of Scientific Philosophy.* Berkeley and Los Angeles: Univ. of Calif. Press, 1951.
18. VON BERTALANFFY, L.: General system theory. *General Systems*, Vol. I, 1, 1956.

23

Cognition and Feeling

Cognition transcends cognition. This paper shows that most human emotions could not exist without a cognitive substratum. This is actually the premise on which most of my studies on depression and schizophrenia are based.

AS A PSYCHIATRIST, I must preface my paper with the statement that emotions and feelings have played a very ambiguous role in psychiatric theory. It is true that the psychiatric literature has constantly reaffirmed the importance of emotion, motivation and feeling. As a matter of fact, in psychodynamic interpretations it is assumed that we discuss the emotional forces which consciously or unconsciously determine the individual's overt or hidden behavior. However, when we deal with a theoretical presentation of this matter, we promptly discover a state of utter confusion. In my opinion, one of the reasons for this lack of clearness can be found in the fact that most psychiatrists, classical psychoanalysts as well as experimental psychologists, have tried to pattern all levels of psychological organization in accordance with what they have learned from the study of the simplest physiological and emotional levels. Undoubtedly, the states of hunger, thirst, fatigue, the need for sleep, the sexual urges, the fear about one's physical survival, are powerful dynamic forces and require much additional study. However, they do not include all the psychological factors that affect man favorably or unfavorably.

Modern civilization has in many countries increased the opportunities for physical comfort, adequate nourishment, and sexual gratification. And yet, clinical evidence—although not yet validated by reliable statistical analysis—seems to indicate that mental illness and psychological malaise have increased and not decreased in these countries. It should thus be relatively easy to infer that problems belonging to the higher levels of the psyche are to a large extent responsible for man's psychological difficulties. For this reason, comparative studies of animals, although elucidat-

314

ing basic psychological mechanisms, do not enlighten us on many aspects of human psychopathology.

In my opinion, the factors responsible for these difficulties have to do directly or indirectly with cognition; and cognition has not received adequate consideration in psychiatric and psychoanalytic studies. Perhaps historians of science will find deeply rooted cultural reasons for this neglect. They may interpret it as part of an overall anti-intellectual cultural climate which started toward the end of the nineteenth century and continued into the twentieth. More specifically, psychologists and psychiatrists may justifiably be inclined to believe that the behavioral school, with its emphasis on overt behavior, and classical psychoanalysis with its emphasis on psychic energy or libido, have not been well-disposed, and perhaps even intolerant of studies of cognition. In my opinion, this neglect of cognition has hindered the study of human feelings and emotions.

FIRST-ORDER EMOTIONS OR PROTOEMOTIONS

In other writings I have described what I think are the relations between simple feelings like pain, hunger, etc., and emotions (1). All of them are "felt experiences" or experiences of the inner status of the organism. The main characteristic which justifies the inclusion of feelings and emotions in the category of experiences of inner status is the fact that they occur when an intraorganismic state is subjectively experienced. It is thus not without reason that in English the word *feeling* has a connotation so vast as to include simple sensation as well as high-level affects. It refers to all experiences of inner status. From all of these experiences we can abstract the subjective qualities of pleasantness and unpleasantness. These experiences become motivational factors because the awareness of what is pleasant elicits behavior aimed at searching for or retaining of pleasure. On the other hand, the awareness of what is unpleasant elicits behavior which tends to avoid or discontinue the experience.

Such awareness of pleasantness and unpleasantness is an experience which may not be accompanied by higher cognitive processes. Let us see, however, what happens in emotional experience. In previous writings I have divided emotions into three orders. The first order includes the simplest, which I have called protoemotions or first-order emotions. They are of at least five types: (a) *tension*—a feeling of discomfort caused by different situations, like excessive stimulation and obstructed physiological or instinctual response; (b) *appetite*—a feeling of expectancy which accompanies a tendency to move toward, contact, grab, or incorporate an almost immediately attainable goal; (c) *fear*—an unpleasant, subjective state, which follows the perception of danger and elicits a readiness to flee; (d) *rage*—an emotion which follows the perception of danger to be overcome by fight; that is by aggressive behavior, not by flight; and (e) *satisfaction*—an emotional state resulting from the gratification of physical needs and relief from other emotions.

In a general sense we can say that protoemotions: (a) are experiences of inner status which cannot be sharply localized and which involve the whole or a large part of the organism; (b) either include a set of bodily changes, mostly muscular and humoral, or retain some bodily characteristics; (c) are elicited by the presence or absence of specific stimuli, which are perceived by the subject as related in a positive or negative way to its safety and comfort; (d) become important motivational factors and to a large extent determine the subject's type of external behavior; (e) have an almost immediate effect; if they unchain a delayed reaction, the delay ranges from a fraction of a second to a few minutes; (f) require a minimum of cognitive work in order to be experienced. For instance, in fear or rage a stimulus must be promptly recognized as a sign of present or imminent danger.

The last two characteristics require further discussion. Protoemotions are not experienced instantaneously like simple sensations. They presuppose some cognitive work. However, this cognitive work is of very short duration, presymbolic, or in some cases, symbolic to a rudimentary degree. Presymbolic cognition includes perception and some learning. It also includes the sensorimotor intelligence described by Piaget (2) in the first year and a half of life. The learning required at this level is very simple. It deals with the immediately given, that is, with either direct stimuli or with signals and not symbols. Signals (or signs) indicate things. Some of them may actually be parts of the things they indicate, though that is not always the case. Like the ringing of the bell for the conditioned dog, signals announce something that is about to occur.

An organization at the protoemotional level is very simple. It is, indeed, extremely important from the point of view of man, but does not include what is most pertinent to the field of psychiatry. In fact, we must go to the second-order emotions to find such psychological experiences as anxiety, anger, wish, security.

SECOND-ORDER EMOTIONS

Second-order emotions are not elicited by a direct or impending attack on the organism or by a threatened immediate change in homeostasis, but by cognitive symbolic processes. The prerequisite learning does not deal only with immediate stimuli, or with signals, but also with symbols; that is, with something that represents stimuli, something that stands for the direct sense-data.

These symbols may vary from very simple forms to the most complicated and abstract cognitive representations. I shall start with considering the simplest: the image, that psychological phenomenon which has been so badly neglected in psychology and psychiatry. We know that an image is a memory trace which assumes the form of a representation. It is an internal quasi-reproduction of a perception which does not require the corresponding external stimulus in order to be evoked. Although we cannot deny that at least rudimentary images occur in animals, there seems to be no doubt that images are predominantly a human characteristic. The child closes his eyes and visualizes his mother. The mother may not be present, but her image is with him; it stands for her. He may lie peacefully in bed and that image will be with him until he falls asleep. By being represented by her image, the mother acquires a psychic reality not tied to her physical presence. Image formation is actually the basis for all higher mental processes. It enables the human being not only to recall what is not present, but to retain an affective disposition for the absent object. The image thus becomes a substitute for the external object. It is actually an *inner object,* although it is not well organized. When the affective associations to the image are pleasant, it reinforces our longing or appetite for the corresponding external object. The image thus has a motivational influence in leading us to search out the actual object, which in its external reality is still more gratifying than the image. The opposite is true when the affective associations to the image are unpleasant: we are now motivated to keep from exchanging the unpleasant inner object for the corresponding external one, because that is even more unpleasant.

Now, let us see how images may increase the emotional gamut. Anxiety is the emotional reaction to the expectation of danger. The danger is not immediate, nor is it always well defined. Its expectation is not the result of a simple perception or signal, as it is in the case of fear. Images may enable a man to anticipate a future danger and its dreaded consequences, even though he does not expect it to materialize for some time. In its simplest forms, anxiety is fear mediated by images, it is image-determined fear. However, as we shall see shortly, the danger is often represented by sets of symbols that are more complicated than sequences of images.

The same remarks apply to another second-order emotion: anger. In its simplest form, anger is image-determined rage, that is, rage elicited by the images of the stimuli which generally elicit rage. While rage usually leads to immediate motor discharge, generally directed against the stimulus which elicits it, anger tends to last longer, although it retains an impelling character. The prolongation of anger is possible because it is mediated by symbolic forms, just as anxiety is. If rage is useful for survival in the jungle, anger was useful within the first human communities to maintain a hostile-defensive attitude toward the enemy, whether the latter was present or not.

Wishing is an emotional state that has received little consideration in the literature, except when it has been confused with appetite. While appetite is a feeling accompanied by a preparation of the body for approach and incorporation, wishing means a pleasant attraction toward something or somebody, or toward doing something. Contrary to appetite, wishing is made possible by the recall of the image or other symbols of an object whose presence is pleasant. The mnemic image of an earlier pleasant experience—for instance, of the satisfaction of a need—evokes an emotional disposition which motivates the individual to replace the image with the real object of satisfaction. A search for the real object is thus initiated, or at least contemplated. This search may require detours, since a direct approach is often not possible.

Security is the last second-floor emotion. It has played an important role in the theoretical framework of the psychiatrist, Harry Stack Sullivan (3). It is debatable whether such an emotion really exists or whether the term indicates only the absence of unpleasant emotions or else a purely hypothetical concept. We may visualize the simplest form of security, an image-determined satisfaction. That is, images permit the individual to visualize a state of satisfaction not only for today but also for tomorrow.

Much could be said about the somatic processes that accompany these second-order emotions and how they have changed to adapt to less immediate situations; for instance, how anxiety differs somatically from fear. But in this paper I must limit myself to deal with the connection of feelings and emotions with cognition. Thus far, I have discussed second-order emotions in their relation to images. Images are analogous symbols —a relation of likeness between the image and the represented thing is established .The brain can be compared to an analog computer in its use of images. With the advent of language, however, the nervous system becomes more like a digital computer. A system of arbitrary signs is now capable of eliciting the emotions which before could be aroused only by external stimuli or images.

Up to this level of development, emotions seem to be experiences of inner status which are involved only with the organism itself, its immediate surroundings, or the image of the immediate surroundings. Emotions, *qua* emotions, *qua* experiences of inner status, are not symbolic. They stand only for themselves. They do not go beyond the boundaries of the organism. However, when they become connected with symbols, they partake of the infinity of the universe. I shall come back to this point later. Here, however, I want to emphasize that second-order emotions can be elicited by a preconceptual type of cognition. Phylogenetic, ontogenetic and microgenetic studies by Werner (4) and many other authors, including myself, have revealed that before reaching a mature intellectual level (what in psychoanalysis is called secondary process thinking, and in logic Aristotelean thought) the psyche goes through various levels of symbolic prelogical thinking variously designated as primary process, paleologic, paralogic, etc.

I cannot go into this matter now; but what I want to say is that at a developmental level where only first-order emotions are possible, the animal remains within the boundaries of a limited psychological reality, but is indeed a realist. The animal is capable of a nonsymbolic reality-bound type of learning. He interprets signs in the light of past experience. When man starts to use symbols, especially preconceptual symbols, he opens his eyes toward the infinity of the universe, but also toward an infinity of errors and toward the realm of unreality. For instance, anxiety may be inappropriate because it is based, not on a realistic appreciation of danger, but on danger which is based on inaccurate or arbitrary symbolization. Psychiatry offers numerous examples of this possibility. For instance, some psychiatric patients tend to revert to the level of first-order emotions, as in developing a phobia, which is an abnormal fear. The patient changes his anxiety into fear, though the fear is groundless. Thus a patient, who is anxious about serious psychological problems he has to face in life, becomes afraid of dogs or horses. He goes into a state of panic at the sight of them.

THIRD-ORDER EMOTIONS

With the development of language, the gradual abandonment of preconceptual levels and the development of conceptual levels, third-order emotions occur, as I have described in other writings. In conjunction with first-and second-order emotions, these offer to the human being a very complex and diversified emotional repertory. In third-order emotions, language plays a greater role. The temporal representation is enlarged both toward the past and toward the future. Emotional experience has only one temporal dimension: the present. When it becomes connected with cognitive structures, it remains an experience in the present, but an experience which may be involved with a distant past or a distant future. A person may be disturbed now by what happened long ago or may happen in the future.

Third-order emotions, although capable of existing even before the advent of the conceptual level, expand and are followed by even more complex emotions at the conceptual level. Important third-order emotions are depression, hate, love and joy. To discuss adequately even what we know about them—which is little in comparison to what remains to be known—would fill many books. In the remaining time I shall make some comments about depression, and finally, I shall say a few words about hate.

Before the psychoanalytic era, depression received even more consideration by psychiatrists than anxiety. For the purpose of this paper, I shall make no distinction between depression, melancholia, sadness, anguish, mental pain, etc.

As a subjective experience, depression is difficult to define or even describe. It is a pervading feeling of unpleasantness, often accompanied by bodily symptoms. In depression, contrary to what happens in anxiety, there is no thought that a dangerous situation is about to occur. The dangerous event has already taken place; the loss has been sustained. Indeed, not only the present but the future seems affected by this loss. Whatever happened to make the individual feel depressed seems to him to have an impact on the future, too.

Thus it is evident that depression follows cognitive processes, such as evaluations and appraisals which require verbal expression. For example, a person is told of the sudden death of a friend. He evaluates the news and understands what it means to his dead friend and to him, too, as the survivor, who will be deprived of his friend's company. All these processes would not be possible without language. Linguistic forms evoke surprise, evaluation and an unpleasant feeling called sadness or depression. This feeling tends to linger. Some people may compare this feeling to apparent similar ones which occur in the newborn when the mother leaves, or even in animals, like dogs, when the master leaves and they are left alone. These feelings in newborn babies and in animals are unpleasant, but should more properly be called deprivation, discomfort, tension, because they are not based upon anticipation of the future. Depression seems to me to be accompanied by complex and elaborate cognitive processes. However, in many cases, particularly in psychiatric conditions, the feeling of depression is so powerful that it drowns out the idea that actually aroused the depression—which then is said to have been produced by unconscious causes. At times, the idea has an inappropriate symbolic value and so engenders a depression that seems incongruous.

Although at first sight depression appears to have no purpose it has protective value, just as anxiety has. Like other unpleasant sensations and emotions, it is useful because it stimulates the person to nonacceptance of the emotion, that is, to its removal. How can depression be removed? Let us take again the person saddened by the death of someone close to him. For a few days, all thoughts connected with the beloved departed will bring about a painful, almost unbearable feeling. Any thought even remotely related to him will arouse depression. The survivor cannot adjust to the idea that the deceased is no longer alive. But since the deceased was so important to him, many of the survivor's thoughts or actions are directly or indirectly connected with the deceased and so elicit an unpleasant reaction.

Nevertheless, after a certain period of time, the survivor becomes adjusted to the idea that the deceased is no longer present. The unpleasant, unacceptable sadness is removed because it has forced the survivor to reorganize his thinking, to regroup his thoughts into different constellations, to search for new directions. He especially had to rearrange the ideas connected with the departed. This rearrangement can be carried out in several ways, according to a person's mental predisposition. He may no longer consider the deceased indispensable; he may associate the image of the beloved dead mainly with the qualities he had that brought joy, so that the memory no longer brings mental pain; or he may think of his friends's life as not really ended but as being continued either in another world, or in this world through the lasting effects of his actions. Those who try to console the survivor do so by helping him to rearrange his thoughts. Whatever the ideational rearrangement, it does not mean moving away from a physical source of discomfort, as in pain, or from the source of threat, as in fear and some forms of anxiety. The moving away is only from depressive thoughts. The escape from depression can only occur through cognitive means.

The cognitive means I have mentioned above are very common, but they are not the only ones. A few people make different cognitive rearrangements. They do not try to change their thought pattern nor do they try to persuade themselves that the unacceptable is acceptable. They end up by accepting the unacceptable. This acceptance of mental pain or sadness as a fact of life adds a new dimension to experience, for the enigma of man's position in the universe and the mysterious order of things is forcibly brought to his attention. Such acceptance of pain may actually decrease or even dissolve the depression.

These remarks should not be interpreted as meaning that man should make no effort to remove or change the sources of pain. But when he is faced with the immutable, he may learn to accept it; and he can do this only through the media of cognitive processes. As a matter of fact, we know of cultural trends toward making an apotheosis of melancholia. One such trend started in the Italian Renaissance with Marsilio Ficino (1433-1499), Lorenzo the Magnificent (1449-1492), and Iacopo Sannazzaro (1456-1530). As we know, this trend expanded to other countries and to other media, as seen, for instance, in the art of Albrecht Dürer (1471-1528).

I must resist the urge to go deeper into these cultural trends, and mention instead that *hate* is the third-order emotion which corresponds to the second-order emotion *anger* and to the first-order emotion *rage*. The three together constitute hostility, but hate is the only one among the three which has the tendency to become a chronic emotional state sustained by special thoughts. Thus a feed-back mechanism is established between these sustaining thoughts and the emotion. Hate leads to calculated action, and at times to premeditated crimes. Some authors in the fields of psychology and ethology have a tendency to reduce every form of hostility to rage and aggression, as is the case in animals. This can be done only when the role of cognition is minimized.

The emotions I have mentioned (as well as others I have not mentioned) may combine in many ways. With the ontogenetic and cultural development of man, cognition and affect have an increasing reciprocal influence. Cognitive processes create more and more motivational and therefore emotional factors, and emotions become the propelling drives toward further cognitive processes. By accompanying any cognitive process, emotions transcend the boundaries of the organism and, like human symbolic processes, may become involved with the whole universe known to man. If man studies complicated mathematical problems or looks at the distant stars, or thinks of things that occurred in the remote past or are expected to occur in the distant future, not only does he attempt to reflect on events regardless of space and time, not only does he search for a coherent relationship among the apparently unrelated parts of nature, but his inner self, his inner status, his highest level homeostasis is altered as a result of endeavors. Thus every cognitive process becomes an inner experience. He who looks on all time and all existences is touched in his inner being by every time and every existence. Whatever is conceived touches the core of man. The process called internationalization in psychoanalysis comes about not just because a portion of the ordered external world has become an enduring part of the knower but rather because it has been transformed into an emotional experience.

REFERENCES

1. Arieti, S.: The intrapsychic self: Feeling, cognition and creativity in health and mental illness. New York: Basic Books, 1967.
2. Piaget, J.: La naissance de l'intelligence chez l'enfant. Neuchatel: Delachaux and Niestle, 1936.
3. Sullivan, H. S.: The interpersonal theory of psychiatry. New York: Norton, 1953.
4. Werner, H.: Comparative psychology of mental development (rev. ed.). New York: Follett, 1948.

24

The Structural and Psychodynamic Role
of Cognition in the Human Psyche

*Cognition is not only necessary for the emotional life of the
human being; in its conscious and unconscious forms it constitutes the inner reality of the individual. The psychodynamic
role of the various cognitive stages is described in this paper.*

INTRODUCTION

A STRONG DESIRE TO EMULATE chemistry and physics and to strive toward
the unity of science has predisposed many researchers in the fields of
psychology and psychiatry to adopt a positivistic, operationalist approach.

Most of these researchers insist in viewing the psyche mainly as a
complex apparatus that permits and enhances animal species to adapt to
environmental reality. In the human being, this apparatus is viewed as
having reached a degree of complexity that leads to an increasing understanding and mastery of the world.

This methodology has led to an accumulation of significant data and is
responsible for outstanding progress in our knowledge of certain aspects
of the psyche, especially by disclosing how previous external influences
affect objective behavior. Nevertheless, if it is not complemented by different types of inquiry, this point of view ignores other parts of the
psyche—actually those that matter most within a psychiatric and psychoanalytic frame of reference. To be specific, an exclusively empirical, opera-
tionalistic approach first minimizes the role that subjectivity plays in
psychological processes; second, it deals almost exclusively with that part
of the psyche that makes contact with the surrounding world by perceiving, reacting, and approaching. In infrahumans, this part constitutes
almost the whole psyche, but in human beings another important part

324

acquires prominence; in the various terminologies this has been called "inner life," "inner reality," "psychic reality," "intrapsychic self," "intrapsychic life," "endopsychic structure," "proprium," "core of man," and the like.

Inner life, or inner reality, may represent, substitute, distort, enrich, or impoverish the reality of the external world. Although this inner reality too has many exchanges with the environment, it has an enduring life of its own. It becomes the essence of the individual. Its organization is what we call the "inner self."

Inner reality is the result of a constant reelaboration of past and present experiences. Its development is never completed throughout the life of man, although its greatest rate of growth occurs in childhood and adolescence. It is based on the fact that perceptions, thoughts, feelings, actions, and other psychological functions do not cease completely to exist once the neuronal mechanisms that mediated their occurrence have taken place. Although they cannot be retained as they were experienced, their effects are retained as various components of the psyche. Freud wrote that in mental life nothing that has once been formed can perish.

From approximately the ninth month of life the child internalizes: he retains as inner objects mental representations of external objects, events, relations, and the feelings associated with these psychological events. Inner objects acquire a relative independence from the correspondent external stimuli that elicited them. They progressively associate and organize in higher constructs.

This chapter illustrates some major elements of inner reality, giving particular consideration to the role of cognition in its development, structure, and psychodynamics.

PSYCHOANALYTIC VIEWS OF INNER REALITY

Whereas some schools (behavioristic, behavior therapy, conditioned response, aversion therapy, and so forth) are interested in studying and altering man's behavior and capacity for adaptation, most psychoanalytic and psychotherapeutic schools are interested in studying and changing the inner self, even if it is more difficult to do so. The premise of psychoanalysis and psychodynamic psychotherapy is that if you change the inner self, sooner or later a change, and a more reliable one, will occur also in the external behavior and capacity for adaptation.

As Guntrip (18) has pointed out, historically psychoanalysis is the first science to illustrate the existence of a psychic reality that is distinct from the reality of the external world. It is one of Freud's great achievements to have demonstrated the existence of this psychic reality as an entity in its own right, an entity that is alterable, but at the same time highly resistant to change. Other points of view, advanced by Freud, are still open to debate: 1) whether the psyche is nearly formed by the age of four or five; 2) whether its only or most important dynamic components are instinctual forces; 3) whether its only conflicts derive from the desire, on one hand, to satisfy instinctual drives and, on the other hand, to abide with the restrictions imposed by society; 4) whether it can be divided into three parts—id, ego, and superego.

Some neo-Freudian schools of psychoanalysis, as well as the existentialist school of psychiatry, criticize Freudian theory as being too biological, for minimizing that part of man that transcends or even negates nature by not wanting to adapt to the imposition, limitation, or restriction of nature. We can add to this criticism that man, as he is seen by classic Freudian theory, is not even a full biological man: he is fundamentally a hypothalamic organism. The hypothalamic functions of sex and rage dominate all others. All the structures above the hypothalamus are seen predominantly as restricting or controlling or sublimating the functions of the hypothalamus and related organs.

The cultural and interpersonal schools of psychoanalysis have tried to enlarge this view of man. They have rightly stressed that one becomes a person mainly by virtue of relations with other human beings and not predominantly by virtue of inborn instinctual drives. What they do not indicate, however, is that the sequence of external influences is integrated by intrapsychic mechanisms, so that it becomes personal history and part of the inner self. What these cultural-interpersonal schools fail to point out is that the individual is not passively molded by these environmental influences: he does not just react; he acts autonomously. Whatever is above the hypothalamus meets, assimilates, transforms, expands what comes from the external world as well as from within or below the hypothalamus. The integration of all these intrapersonal factors opens up a new universe, the universe of symbols. Merely from the point of view of survival, symbolic function is not so important as hypothalamic regulation; but from the specific point of view of human psychology and psychopathology, it is much more important.

Some psychoanalytic schools have tried, although not very successfully, to include in their theoretical framework the psychodynamic and psychostructural aspects of high symbolism. Melanie Klein (20), for instance, recognizes that internalized object relations become permanent features of inner life. For her, however, these mental incorporations correspond to oral incorporation. She sees the formation of the psyche in a theoretical framework that retains Freud's oral, anal, and genital stages. She believes that these stages unfold much earlier in life than Freud had postulated, and therefore even more than Freud she is compelled to neglect cognitive forms that develop after the first year of life. Klein repeatedly refers to unconscious fantasies, but does not indicate the cognitive features or the media that sustain these fantasies. It is difficult to visualize how in the three-month-old baby they can consist of ideas, thoughts, images, feelings of hopelessness, abandonment, and so forth. Although Klein has correctly stressed the importance of man's inner world, she has been quite nebulous in her description of the structure and functioning of this inner world. Fairbairn (14), too, stressed the importance of the endopsychic structure and its relevance to object relations, but did not examine the cognitive elements of this structure. The classic psychoanalytic school has studied internalization, but with a few recent exceptions has studied them predominantly from the energetic or economic point of view.

SIMPLE FEELINGS AND PRESYMBOLIC ORGANIZATION

Although the main aim of this chapter is to discuss the cognitive forms that enter into the constitution of inner reality, we shall at this point give some consideration to feelings and to presymbolic organizations, which are prerequisite to any form of inner reality. Most of these functions start at birth or in the first few months of life and remain throughout the life of the individual.

Feeling is a characteristic unique to the animal world and is the basis of psychological life. Feeling is unanalyzable in its essential subjective nature and defies any attempt toward a noncircular definition. Synonyms of "feeling," which are often used, are "awareness," "subjectivity," "consciousness," "experience," "felt experience." Although each of these terms stresses a particular aspect, all refer to subjective experience.

Transmission of information from one part of the organism to another exists even without subjective experience. For instance, the important information transmitted through the spinocerebellar tracts never reaches the level of awareness. As long as information is transmitted without awareness, the organism is not too different from an electronic computer or a transmitter or transformer of data. When any change in the organism is accompanied by awareness, a new phenomenon emerges in the cosmos—experience. Awareness and/or experience introduced the factor psyche.

As Freud clarified, and as we shall consider later in this chapter, some psychological functions lose the quality of awareness and become unconscious. However, if in phylogeny some functions had not become endowed with awareness, the psyche would not have emerged and the physiology of the nervous system would consist only of unconscious neurological functions.

The most primitive forms of felt experiences are simple sensations and perceptions, such as pain, temperature perception, hearing, vision, thirst, hunger, olfaction, taste. These sensations and perceptions can be considered in two main ways: 1) as subjective experiences that occur in the presence of particular somatic states, for instance, a specific state of discomfort, which we call pain; 2) as functions mirroring (or producing analogs of) aspects of reality.

We encounter here a basic dichotomy. On one hand is the awareness of a particular state of the body or part of the body: that is, the awareness of an inner status of the organism, the experience as experience. On the other hand is the function of mirroring reality, a function that generally expands into numerous ramifications that deal with cognition. The importance of these two components varies a great deal in the various types of perceptions. The experience of inner status is very important in the perception of pain, hunger, thirst, temperature and less important in other perceptions, such as touch, taste, smell. In auditory and visual perceptions, the experience of a change of inner status plays a minimal role. These perceptions make the animal aware of what happens in the external world and become the foundation of cognition.

Elsewhere (8) I have described the various experiences of inner status (sensations, perceptions, physiosensations, such as hunger, thirst, fatigue, sleepiness, sexual urges, other instinctual experiences) and how from all of them we can abstract feelings of pleasure and unpleasure. Motivation becomes connected with the awareness of what is pleasant (and to be searched for) and what is unpleasant (and to be avoided).*

I have also tried to show how not only the simple experiences of inner status, such as sensations, but all emotions or affects can be included in the category of feeling. They are experienced within the organism. They are felt experiences. From all of them the motivational characteristics

---

* For the intricate relation between feeling, causality, and motivation see Chapter 2 of reference 8.

of pleasure and unpleasure can be abstracted. It is not without reason that in English the word "feeling" has a connotation so vast as to include simple sensations as well as high-level affects.

Emotions can be divided into several ranks or categories. The simplest (protoemotions or first-order emotions) are of at least five types: 1) tension—a feeling of discomfort caused by different situations, such as excessive stimulation, hindered physiological or instinctual response; 2) appetite—a feeling of expectancy that accompanies a tendency to move toward, contact, grab, or incorporate an almost immediately attainable goal; 3) fear—an unpleasant, subjective state, which follows the perception of danger and elicits a readiness to flee; 4) rage—an emotion that follows the perception of a danger to be overcome by fight, not flight; 5) satisfaction—an emotional state resulting from gratification of physical needs and relief from other emotions.

In a general sense, we can say that protoemotions 1) are experiences of inner status that cannot be sharply localized and that involve the whole or a large part of the organism; 2) either include a set of bodily changes, mostly muscular and humoral, or retain some bodily characteristics; 3) are elicited by the presence or absence of specific stimuli, which are perceived by the subject as related in a positive or negative way to its safety and comfort; 4) become important motivational factors and to a large extent determine the type of the external behavior of the subject; 5) in order to be experienced require a minimum of cognitive work. For instance, in fear or rage, a stimulus must be promptly recognized as a sign of danger. The danger is present or imminent.

What we have described under the headings of simple sensations, physiological and instinctual functions, perception, nonsymbolic learning, and protoemotions enable the animal organism (human or infrahuman) to survive and adjust to the environment. The effect of all these functions tends to be immediate or almost immediate. If they unchain a delayed reaction, the delay ranges only from a fraction of a second to a few minutes. Protoemotions are not experienced immediately, as are such simple sensations as pain or thirst. They require some cognitive work. However, this cognitive work is presymbolic or, in some cases, symbolic to a rudimentary degree. Presymbolic cognition includes perception and simple learning that have been intensely investigated by experimental psychologists. It also includes the sensorimotor intelligence, which has been accurately studied by Piaget in the first year and a half of life.

The motivational organization, based on the physiological, instinctual, or elementary emotional states we have mentioned, unchains in man, too, powerful dynamic forces, but it does not include all the psychological factors that affect him favorably or unfavorably. Because of the impact of symbolic cognition, man's needs, desires, purposes, and conflicts go far beyond physiologic-protoemotional motivation.

Most of the functions mentioned in this section do not lead to the formation of inner constructs unless associated with other psychological mechanisms. However, it would be inaccurate to state that they have no role in the making of inner reality. In the human being the memory and recall of these experiences becomes connected with higher level functions, especially after the acquisition of language. Feelings and protoemotions are also part of inner reality as long as they are experienced.

Protoemotions have even a greater role as potentialities, in that they remain as affective or primary predispositions toward a given type of personality, when they are not well balanced by other emotions. There are some human beings in whom fear (later changed into anxiety) is the predominant emotion. Depending on its interaction with other emotions and on the prevailing type of their interpersonal relations, these people may eventually become either detached (that is, prone to withdraw from frightening stimuli) or compliant (prone to placate the source of fear). People in whom rage prevails tend to become aggressive and hostile. People in whom appetite is the principal emotion tend to become hedonistic. When tension predominates, the individual is likely to be hypochondriacal and more interested in his body than in the external environment. When satisfaction is the principal protoemotion, the person's predominant outlook is conservative, centered on the status quo.

Presymbolic types of learning and a relating to other members of one's species predispose to specific styles of behavior and of personality. Comparative psychologists have reported that when animals are kept together in a certain environment some assume a dominant and some a submissive role. Presumably this role is determined by a preponderance of a protoemotion and by the learning of a type of behavior that fits the environmental circumstances. Among these environmental circumstances, the type of behavior of the other animals and consequent interplay are very important. The preponderance of a protoemotion and of some kinds of presymbolic learning and ways of relating constitute the temperament.

The characteristics and functions that we have described, unless followed by others, constitute a primordial self. Inner reality is still rudimentary. More mature levels or organization of the self are possible because toward the end of the first year of life the human being acquires symbolic cognition. Symbolic cognition is not simply a system of intellectual mechanisms or a content dynamically neutral or conflict free. It permits emotions and emotional states that could not exist without symbolic functions. It introduces new motivations as powerful as those originated at lower levels and establishes the ground where human conflicts originate. Gratification of the self or the self-image (and not of one's physiological or instinctual needs) will eventually become the main motivation.

For expository reasons, we have so far made no reference to evolvement in time and to interpersonal relations. Actually the presymbolic stage of childhood can be divided into many substages. In the first six to eight weeks of life, the infant is predominantly a bundle of proprioceptive and enteroceptive sensations. Then he becomes more and more involved with sensory perceptions and the simplest forms of learning. First the presence of mother, as the overpowering environmental object, and second, the development of locomotion, help the little child to shift the focus of his awareness from his body to his immediate environment.

THE THREE CATEGORIES OF SYMBOLIC COGNITION

The development of new media—imaginary and language—changes enormously the child's relation with his environment. Although at this level of maturation the cortical centers of language are ready to begin to function, it is necessary for the child to be in contact with a human environment to transform his babbling and environmental sounds and noises into meanings. He learns to connect them with things, events, or special states of the organism. That's why children who are deaf or without human contacts cannot learn symbolic processes in normal ways. Consensual validation, that is, the recognition that a given sound has the same or a related effect on the mother and on himself, is an absolute necessity to trigger off verbal symbolization in the child. When the function of language is chiefly denotative, consensual validation is easy; this is "daddi" and this is "mamme." From the very beginning, however, language goes beyond its purely denotative functions. In the course of evolving toward maturity, language and other symbolic functions can be classified as pertaining to three categories of cognition: primary, secondary, and tertiary.

The designations primary and secondary derive, respectively, from Freud's (16) original formulation of the primary and secondary processes, made in Chapter 7 of *The Interpretation of Dreams* (1901). To quote Jones (10):

Freud's revolutionary contribution to psychology was not so much his demonstrating the existence of an unconscious, and perhaps not even his exploration of its content, as his proposition that there are two fundamentally different kinds of mental processes, which he termed primary and secondary. . . .

Freud gave the first description of these two processes but tried to differentiate the particular laws or principles that rule the primary process; primary because, according to him, it occurs earlier in the ontogenetic development and not because it is more important than the secondary. Freud elucidated very well two mechanisms by which the primary process operates: namely the mechanisms of displacement and condensation. However, after this original breakthrough, he did not make other significant discoveries in the field of cognition. This arrest of progress is to be attributed to several factors. First, Freud became particularly interested in the primary process as a carrier of unconscious motivation. Second, inasmuch as he interpreted motivation more and more in the function of the libido theory, the primary process came to be studied predominantly as a consumer of energy.

The Freudian school, as a rule, has continued to study the primary process almost exclusively from an economic point of view. Its main characteristic would be the fact that it does not bind the libido firmly, but allows it to shift from one investment to another (11). Some Freudians, however, for instance, Schur (26), reassert the preponderantly cognitive role of the primary process.

I am also particularly concerned with the cognitive functions of the primary process; namely what I call "primary cognition." I have described primary cognition in numerous publications, but to maintain the continuity of the exposition, I will repeat briefly some of the main concepts.

Primary cognition prevails for a very short period of time early in life as a normal aspect of development. In most cases, it is almost immediately overlapped by secondary cognition, so that it is difficult to retrieve it in pure forms, even in the young child. Primary cognition also prevails and is easier to detect in those mental mechanisms 1) that are classified in classic psychoanalysis as belonging to the id. The dream work to a large extent follows primary cognition; 2) in the early stages of what Werner (33) called the "migrogenetic process"; and 3) in psychopathological conditions. Its most typical forms occur in advanced stages of schizophrenia (1, 2, 3, 4). Some theorists (especially those belonging to the self-actualization schools, such as Fromm, Rogers, &

Maslow) do not include in their system anything pertaining to primary cognition. Their omission is in some respects diametrically opposite to that of the Freudian school. Consequently, their contributions, although offering numerous important insights about some aspects of man and about mild psychopathology, is of much less value in understanding severe psychopathology and dream work.

Secondary cognition consists predominantly of conceptual thinking; most of the time it follows the laws of logic and inductive and deductive processes. Tertiary cognition occurs in the process of creativity and most of the time consists of specific combinations of primary and secondary forms of cognition. The important topic of tertiary cognition cannot be dealt with in this essay, and the reader is referred to other writings of mine (7, 8).

In what follows, I shall describe some developmental aspects of cognition. I shall not follow the usual approaches to cognition, not even Piaget's. The contributions of this Swiss author (22, 23, 24, 25) reveal very well the process of cognitive maturation and adaptation to environmental reality and disclose the various steps by which the child increases his understanding and mastery of the world. Although they are very important, they do not represent intrapsychic life in its structural and psychodynamic aspects.

In what follows, we shall give particular consideration to the formation in childhood of various forms of primary cognition, namely to imagery, endocept, and preconceptual thinking. Although for didactical purposes we may divide early childhood in stages or in a hierarchy of levels, generally these levels occur in combination, with one or the other predominating at a certain time.

THE PHANTASMIC STAGE OF INNER REALITY

At first psychological internalization occurs through images (8, Ch. 5). An image is a memory trace that assumes the form of a representation. It is an internal quasi-reproduction of a perception that does not require the corresponding external stimulus in order to be evoked. The image is indeed one of the earliest and most important foundations of human symbolism, if by symbol we mean something that stands for something else that is not present. Whereas previous forms of cognition and learning permitted an understanding based on the immediately given or experienced, from now on cognition will rely also on what is absent and inferred. For instance, the child closes his eyes and visualizes his mother.

She may not be present, but her image is with him; it stands for her. The image is obviously based on the memory traces of previous perceptions of the mother. The mother then acquires a psychic reality that is not tied to her physical presence.

Image formation is actually the basis for all higher mental processes; it starts in the second half of the first year of life. It introduces the child into an inner world that I have called "phantasmic" (8). It enables the child not only to reevoke what is not present, but to retain an effective disposition for the absent object. For instance, the image of the mother may evoke the feelings that the child experiences toward her.

The image thus becomes a substitute for the external object. It is actually an inner object, although it is not well organized. It is the most primitive of the inner objects, if, because of their sensorimotor character, we exclude motor engrams from the category of inner objects. When the image's affective associations are pleasant, the evoking of the image reinforces the child's longing or appetite for the corresponding external object. The image thus has a motivational influence in leading the child to search out the actual object, which in its external reality is still more gratifying than the image. The opposite is true when the image's affective associations are unpleasant: the child is motivated not to exchange the unpleasant inner object for the corresponding external one, which is even more unpleasant.

Imagery soon constitutes the foundation of inner psychic reality. It helps the individual not only to understand the world better, but also to create a surrogate for it. Moreover, whatever is known or experienced tends to become a part of the individual who knows and experiences. Thus, cognition can no longer be considered only a hierarchy of mechanisms, but also an enduring psychological content that retains the power to affect its possessor, now and in the future.*

The child who has reached the level of imagery is now capable of experiencing not only such simple emotions as tension, fear, rage, and satisfaction, as he did in the first year of life, but also anxiety, anger, wish, perhaps in a rudimentary form even love and depression, and, finally, security. Anxiety is the emotional reaction to the expectation of danger, which is mediated through cognitive media. The danger is not immediate, nor is it always well defined. Its expectation is not the result of a simple perception or signal. At subsequent ages, the danger is represented by complicated sets of cognitive constructs. At the age level

---

* For a study of the phenomenology of images and the formations of their derivatives —paleosymbols—see Chapter 5 of reference 8.

that we are discussing now, it is sustained by images. It generally refers to a danger connected with the important people in the child's life, mother and father, who may punish or withdraw tenderness and affection. Anger, at this age, is also rage sustained by images. Wish is also an emotional disposition, which is evoked by the image of a pleasant object. The image motivates the individual to replace the image with the real object satisfaction. Sadness can be felt only at a rudimentary level at this stage, if by sadness we mean an experience similar to the one the sad adult undergoes.* At this level, sadness is an unpleasant feeling evoked by the image of the loss of the wished object and by the experience of displeasure caused by the absence of the wished object. Love, at this stage, remains rudimentary. For the important emotion, or emotional tonality, called after Sullivan's security, the author must again refer the reader to another publication (8).

The child does not remain for a long time at a level of integration characterized exclusively by sensorimotor behavior, images, simple interpersonal relations, and the simple emotions that we have mentioned. Higher levels impinge almost immediately, so that it is impossible to observe the phantasmic level in pure culture. Nevertheless we can recognize and abstract some of its general characteristics.

Images, of course, remain as a psychological phenomenon for the rest of the life of the individual. At a stage, however, during which language does not exist or is very rudimentary, they play a very important role. Unless initiated, checked, or corrected by subsequent levels of integration (secondary process), they follow the rules of the primary process. They are fleeting, hazy, vague, shadowy, cannot be seen in their totality, and tend to equate the part with the whole. For instance, if the subject tries to visualize his kitchen, now he reproduces the breakfast table, now a wall of the room, now the stove. An individual arrested at the phantasmic level of development would have great difficulty in distinguishing images and dreams from external reality. He would have no language and could not tell himself or others, "This is an image, a dream, a fantasy; it does not correspond to external reality." He would tend to confuse psychic with external reality, almost as a normal person does when he dreams. Whatever was experienced would become true for him by virtue of its being experienced. Not only is consensual validation from other people impossible at this level, but even intrapsychic or reflexive validation

---

* Correcting the text of this paper, as it was originally published, I use the term "sadness" here in reference to a normal and perhaps adaptive emotion, "depression" in reference to a pathological and maladaptive emotion.

cannot be achieved. The phantasmic level of young children is characterized by what Baldwin (12) called "adualism," or at least by difficult
dualism: lack of the ability to distinguish between the two realities, that
of the mind and that of the external world. This condition may correspond to what orthodox analysts, following Federn (15), call "lack of ego
boundary."

Another important aspect that the phantasmic level shares with the
sensorimotor level of organization is the lack of appreciation of causality.
The individual cannot ask himself why certain things occur. He either
naïvely accepts them as just happenings or he expects things to take
place in a certain succession, as a sort of habit rather than as a result of
causality or of an order of nature. The only phenomenon remotely connected with causation is a subjective or experiential feeling of expectancy,
derived from the observation of repeated temporal associations.

THE ENDOCEPT

The endocept is a mental construct representative of a level intermediary between the phantasmic and the verbal. At this level, there is a
primitive organization of memory traces, images, and motor engrams (or
exocepts). This organization results in a construct that does not tend to
reproduce reality, as it appears in perceptions or images: it remains non-
representational. The endocept, in a certain way, transcends the image,
but inasmuch as it is not representational, it is not easily recognizable.
On the other hand, it is not an engram (or exocept) that leads to prompt
action. Nor can it be transferred into a verbal expression; it remains at a
preverbal level. Although it has an emotional component, most of the
time it does not expand into a clearly felt emotion.

The endocept is not, of course, a concept. It cannot be shared. We
may consider it a disposition to feel, to act, to think that occurs after
simpler mental activity has been inhibited. The awareness of this construct is vague, uncertain, and partial. Relative to the image, the endocept involves considerable cognitive expansion; but this expansion occurs
at the expense of the subjective awareness, which is decreased in intensity.
The endocept is at times experienced as an "atmosphere," an intention, a
holistic experience that cannot be divided into parts or words—something similar to what Freud called "oceanic feeling." At other times, there
is no sharp demarcation between endoceptual, subliminal experiences
and some vague protoexperiences. On still other occasions, strong but
not verbalizable emotions accompany endocepts.

For the evidence of the existence of endocepts and for their importance in adult life, dreams and creativity, the reader is referred else-where.* In children, endocepts remain in the forms of vague memories that will affect subsequent periods of life. In adult life, they often evoke memories expressed with mature language, which was not available to the child when the experiences originally took place.

Endoceptual experiences exist even when the child has already learned some linguistic expressions—expressions, however, that are too simple to represent the complexities of these experiences. To avoid misinterpretations, I wish to repeat at this point that the acquisition of language (that is, the verbal level) overlaps the endoceptual, phantasmic, and, to a small degree, toward the end of the first year of life, even the sensorimotor (or exoceptual) level (8).

PRECONCEPTUAL LEVELS OF THINKING

It is beyond the purpose of this essay to study the child's acquisition of language and the experience of high-level emotions, which presuppose verbal symbols. I am referring to the mature experience of depression, hate, love, joy, and derivative emotions (8, Ch. 7). From the acquisition of language (naming things) to a logical organization of concepts various substages follow one another so rapidly and overlap in so many multiple ways that it is very difficult to retrace and individualize them. These intermediary stages are more pronounced and more easily recognizable in pathological conditions.

Some of the stages, which some authors call "prelogical" and which I call "paleological" (or following ancient logic) (1, 2), use a type of cognition that is irrational according to our usual logical standards. However, paleologic thinking is not haphazard, but susceptible of being interpreted as following an organization or logic of its own. A considerable aspect of paleologic thinking can be understood in accordance with Von Domarus' principle (31), which (in a formulation I have slightly modified) states: Whereas in mature cognition or secondary cognition identity is accepted only on the basis of identical subjects, in paleologic thinking identity is based on the basis of identical predicates. In other publications (6, 8), I have illustrated the relations among part perception, paleological thinking, and some psychological mechanisms reported by ethologists, for instance, Tinbergen (28).

Paleologic cognition occurs for a short period of time early in child-hood, from the age of one to three. It is difficult to recognize because it

---

* Especially Chapter 6 of reference 8.

is, in most instances, overlapped by secondary cognition. Here are a few examples: An eighteen-month-old child is shown pictures of different men. In each instance he says, "Daddy, daddy." It is not enough to interpret this verbal behavior of the child by stating that he is making a mistake or that his mistake is owing to lack of knowledge, inadequate experience of the world, or inadequate vocabulary. Obviously, he makes what we consider a mistake; however, even in the making of the mistake, he follows a mental process. From perceptual stimuli, he proceeds to an act of individualization and recognition. Because the pictures show similarities with the perception of his daddy, he puts all these male representations into one category: they are all daddy or daddies. In other words, the child tends to make generalizations and classifications, which are wrong according to a more mature type of thinking. Obviously, there is in this instance what to the adult mind appears a confusion between similarity and identity. Children tend to give the role of an identifying or essential predicate to a secondary detail, attribute, part, or predicate. This part is the essential one to them either because of its conspicuous perceptual qualities or because of its association with previous very significant experiences. Levin (21) reported that a twenty-five-month-old child was calling "wheel" anything that was made of white rubber, as, for example, the white rubber guard that was supplied with the little boys' toilet seats to deflect urine. The child knew the meaning of the word wheel as applied, for example, to the wheel of a toy car. This child has many toy cars whose wheels, when made of rubber, was always of white rubber. It is obvious that an identification has occurred because of the same characteristic, namely, white rubber.*

Young children soon become aware of causality and repeatedly ask why. At first, causality is teleological: events are believed to occur because they are willed or wanted by people or by anthropomorphized forces.

We should not conclude that young children must think paleologically: they only have a propensity to do so. Unless abnormal conditions (either environmental or biological) make difficult either the process or maturation or the process of becoming part of the adult world, this propensity is almost entirely and very rapidly overpowered by the adoption of secondary-process cognition. Moreover, they may still deal more or less realistically with the environment when they follow the more primitive type of nonsymbolic learning, which permits a simple and immediate

---

* This confusion between identity and similarity reacquires prominence in some psychopathological conditions. It has been studied intensely in schizophrenia by Von Domarus (31) and later by Arieti (1, 2).

understanding. In secondary-process cognition the individual learns to distinguish essential from nonessential predicates and develops more and more the tendency to identify subjects that are indissolubly tied to essential predicates.

THE IMAGE OF MOTHER AND THE SELF-IMAGE

The randomness of experience is more and more superseded by the gradual organization of inner constructs. These constructs continuously exchange some of their components and increase in differentiation, rank, and order. A large number of them, however, retain the enduring mark of their individuality. Although in early childhood they consist of the cognitive forms that we have described (images, endocepts, paleologic thoughts) and of their accompanying feelings (from sensations to emotions), they become more and more complicated and difficult to analyze. Some of them have powerful effects and have an intense life of their own, even if at the stage of our knowledge we cannot give them an anatomic location or a neurophysiological interpretation. They may be considered the very inhabitants of inner reality. The two most important ones in the preschool age, and the only two that we shall describe herein, are the image of mother and the self-image.

Before proceeding, we must warn the reader about a confusion that may result from the two different meanings given to the word "image" in psychological and psychiatric literature. The word "image" is often used, as we did in a previous section of this chapter, in reference to the simple sensory images that tend to reproduce perceptions. This word also refers to those much higher psychological constructs or inner objects that represent whatever is connected with a person: for instance, in this more elaborate sense, the image of the mother would mean a conglomeration of what the child feels and knows about her. From the context, the reader will easily realize which of the two denotations we refer to.

In normal circumstances the mother as an inner object will consist of a group of agreeable images: as the giver, the helper, the assuager of hunger, thirst, cold, loneliness, immobility, and any other discomfort. She becomes the prototype of the good inner object. The negative characteristics of mother play a secondary role that loses significance in the context of the good inner object. In pathological conditions, the mother becomes a malevolent object, and an attempt is made to repress this object from consciousness (9, 10).

Much more difficult to describe in early childhood is the self-image. This construct will be easier to understand in later developmental stages.

At the sensorimotor level, the primordial self probably consists of a bundle of relatively simple relations between feelings, kinesthetic sensations, perceptions, motor activity, and a partial integration of these elements. At the phantasmic level, the child raised in normal circumstances learns to experience himself not exclusively as a cluster of feelings and of self-initiated movements, but also as a body image and as an entity having many kinds of relations with other images, especially those of the parents. Inasmuch as the child cannot see his own face, his own visual image will be faceless—as, indeed, he will tend to see himself in dreams throughout his life. He wishes, however, to be in appearance, gestures, and actions like people toward whom he has a pleasant emotional attitude or by whom he feels protected and gratified. The wish tends to be experienced as reality, and he believes that he is or is about to become like the others or as powerful as the others. Because of the reality value of wishes and images, a feeling results that in psychoanalytic literature has been called a "feeling of omnipotence."

In the subsequent endoceptual and paleologic stages, the self-image will acquire many more elements. However, these elements will continue to be integrated so that the self-image will continue to be experienced as a unity, as an entity separate from the rest of the world. The psychological life of the child will no longer be limited to acting and experiencing, but will include also observing oneself and having an image of oneself.

In a large part of psychological and psychiatric literature, a confusion exists between the concepts of self and of self-image. In this section, we shall focus on the study of self-image.* Also in a large part of the psychiatric literature the self and the consequent self-image are conceived predominantly in a passive role. For instance, Sullivan has indicated that the preconceptual and first conceptual appraisals of the self are determined by the relationships of the child with the significant adults. Sullivan (27) considers the self (and self-image) as consisting of reflected appraisals from the significant adults: the child would see himself and feel about himself as his parents, especially the mother, see him and feel about him. What is not taken into account in this conception is the fact that the self is not merely a passive reflection. The mechanism of the formation of the self cannot be compared to the function of a mirror. If we want to use the metaphor of the mirror, we must specify that we mean

---

* The vaster concept of the self will be more accurately dealt with in the last section of this chapter.

an activated mirror that adds to the reflected images its own distortions, especially those distortions that at an early age are caused by primary cognition. The child does not merely respond to the environment. He integrates experiences and transforms them into inner reality, into increasingly complicated structures. He is indeed in a position to make a contribution to the formation of his own self.

The self-image may be conceived as consisting of three parts: body image, self-identity, and self-esteem. The body image consists of the internalized visual, kinesthetic, tactile, and other sensations and perceptions connected with one's body. The body is discovered by degrees and also the actions of the body on the not-self are discovered by degrees. The body image eventually will be connected with belonging to one of the two genders. Self-identity, or personal identity or ego identity, depends on the discovery of oneself not only as continuous and as same, but also as having certain definite characteristics and a role in the group to which the person belongs.

Self-esteem depends on the child's ability to do what he has the urge to do, but is also connected with his capacity to avoid doing what the parents do not want him to do. Later it is connected also with his capacity to do what his parents want him to do. His behavior is explicitly or implicitly classified by the adults as bad or good. Self-identity and self-esteem seem thus to be related, as Sullivan has emphasized, to the evaluation that the child receives from the significant adults. However, again, this self-evaluation is not an exact reproduction of the one made by the adults. The child is impressed more by the appraisals that hurt him the most or please him the most. These partial salient appraisals and the ways they are integrated with other elements will make up the self-image.

For a better understanding of the nature of personal images and other complex mental constructs, we must study how these inner objects are formed. Not only early in childhood but throughout the life of the individual experiences of inner and external origin are processed in two different mechanisms, which for didactical purposes I have called spontaneous or protopathic organization and epicritic organization (or organization that tends toward higher forms of rationality).

Both ways tend to transform experiential conglomerations into structures and syntheses that aim at pseudo or real consistency. In structures formed by spontaneous organization, any experience may add to a construct, either by contiguity, conditioned reflex mechanisms, repetition, and so forth, or because an overpowerful emotion or motivation affects all mental processes. For instance, if a person is experienced by the individual as very frightening, any action of this person, even a benevolent one, will be interpreted or experienced as frightening. Every relation with that person may thus accrue to the original negative image. Similarly, an overpowering sexual or aggressive motivation may be reinforced by any stimulus whatsoever emanating from the source of that motivation.

In epicritical organization, the experiences do not accrue by the simple mechanisms that I have mentioned. First, every experience retains a separate existence, even though associated with others. Second, the symbolic processes that we shall study in the following sections and more complicated ones will lead to various degrees of abstraction and inference and will restructure experiences in accordance with high schemata offered by culture or created by the individual himself. In those ages and conditions in which the primary process prevails, spontaneous organization prevails too. And when secondary process prevails so does epicritic organization.

In the psychoneurotic, but especially in the psychopath and in the person who eventually will develop schizophrenia, specific factors contribute to the prevailing of spontaneous organization in the formation of many complex constructs and especially of the self-image (8, 9, 10).

SECONDARY COGNITION: THE CONCEPT

It is beyond the scope of this chapter to describe the stages intermediary between early childhood and mature adulthood. We shall consider only the role of concepts. As Vygotsky (32) has illustrated, conceptual thinking starts early in life, but it is in adolescence that it acquires prominence. Conceptual life is a necessary and very important part of mature life. Many authors (13, 24, 35) have made important studies of the mechanisms involved in the formation of concepts and of concepts as psychological forms. In this chapter I shall instead stress their content. This position is a departure from what I have done in reference to less mature forms of cognition (1, 2). In fact, in psychiatric studies, especially in such conditions as schizophrenia, in which severe pathology is found, it is important to study not only content but also form; it is crucial to understand not only what the individual experiences but how he experiences it. Is he perceiving in terms of parts or wholes? Is he using images, endocepts, or paleologic cognition? How are these cognitive modalities varying during the course of the illness or even during the course of a single therapeutic sesion? What is the meaning of such variety of forms? On the other hand, the psychiatrist's and analyst's main interest in concepts resides in determining how their content psychodynamically affects human life.

In a large part of psychiatric, psychoanalytic, and psychological literature concepts are considered static, purely intellectual entities, separate from human emotions and unimportant in psychodynamic studies. I cannot adhere to this point of view. Concepts and organized clusters of concepts become depositories of emotions and also originators of new emotions. They have a great deal to do with the conflicts of man, his achievements and his frustrations, his states of happiness or despair, of anxiety or of security (6). They become the repositories of intangible feelings and values. Not only does every concept have an emotional counterpart, but concepts are necessary for high emotions. In the course of reaching adulthood, emotional and conceptual processes become more and more intimately interconnected. It is impossible to separate the two. They form a circular process. The emotional accompaniment of the cognitive process becomes the propelling drive not only toward action but also toward further cognitive processes. Only emotions can stimulate man to overcome the hardship of some cognitive processes and lead to complicated symbolic, interpersonal, and abstract processes. On the other hand, only cognitive processes can extend indefinitely the realm of emotions. As I have illustrated elsewhere (8), some very important human emotions could not exist without a conceptual foundation. For instance, depression should not be confused with lower feelings, which require no cognitive counterpart at all or only nonsymbolic learning. I am referring to the state of deprivation, discomfort, and anaclitic frustration of lower animal forms or human babies. Sadness requires an understanding of the meaning of loss (actual or symbolic) and may reach a state of despair (which follows a belief that what is lost cannot be retrieved). The importance of this understanding is not recognized, because it is based on cognitive processes that often become almost immediately unconscious (see below). The conceptual presuppositions to mature love, to symbolic anxiety, to hate (as distinguished from rage or anger) have been described elsewhere (8).

Reification of concepts (that is the assumption that concepts faithfully correspond to external reality) is considered by science an invalid procedure. It is obvious that concepts do not correspond to external reality, nor do they most of the time represent reality adequately. Nevertheless, they do have an enduring psychological life or a reality of their own as psychological constructs. Even more criticized and reputedly unscientific is the reification of emotions or feelings in general.

Certainly, thoughts and feelings do not easily submit to the rigor and objectivity of a stimulus-response psychology. However, to dismiss all studies of thoughts and feelings as mystical is to dismiss most of man as mystical. Thoughts and feelings make up what is most valuable in man. If this essential part of man requires methods of study that do not correspond to those of standardized science, we must be ready to accept unusual methods of inquiry.

Even what I said about the relative lack of importance of concepts as forms needs clarification. Concepts, too, undergo organization of increasing order, rank, and level and become components or organized conceptual constructs, whose grammar and syntax we do not yet know. Undoubtedly, future studies will reveal the structure of these, so far, obscure organizations and configurations.

From a psychiatric and psychoanalytic point of view, the greatest importance of concepts resides in the fact that to a large extent they come to constitute the self-image (6). When this development occurs, the previous self-images are not completely obliterated. They remain throughout the life of the individual in the forms of minor components of the adult self-image or as repressed or suppressed forms. In adolescence, however, concepts accrue to constitute the major part of the self-image. Such concepts as inner worth, personal significance, mental outlook, more mature evaluations of appraisals reflected from others, attitudes toward ideals, aspirations, capacity to receive and give acceptance, affection, and love are integral parts of the self and of the self-image, together with the emotions that accompany these concepts. These concepts and emotions, which constitute the self, are generally not consistent with one another, in spite of a prolonged attempt made by the individual to organize them logically.

The motivation of the human being varies according to the various levels of development. When higher levels emerge, motivations originated at lower levels do not cease to exist. At a very elementary sensorimotor level, the motivation consists of obtaining immediate pleasure and avoidance of immediate displeasure by gratification of bodily needs. When imagery emerges, either phylogenetically or ontogenetically, the individual becomes capable of wishing something that is not present and is motivated in more advanced stages of primary cognition, such as paleological stage. As we have already mentioned, although the motivation can always be understood as a search for, or as an attempt to retain, pleasure and avoid unpleasure, gratification of the self becomes the main motivational factor at a conceptual level of development. Certainly, the individual is concerned with danger throughout his life: immediate danger, which elicits fear, and a more distant or symbolic danger, which elicits anxiety. However, whereas at earlier levels of development this danger is experienced as a threat to the physical self, at higher levels it is many times experienced as a threat to an acceptable image of the self.

Many psychologic defenses are devices to protect the self or the self-image. Here are a few examples: A woman leads a promiscuous life; she feels she is unacceptable as a person, but as a sexual partner she feels appreciated. The hypochondriacal protects his self by blaming only his body for his difficulties. The suspicious person and the paranoid attribute to others shortcomings or intentions that they themselves have. These examples could be easily multiplied. They represent cognitive configurations that lead the patient to feelings, ideas, and strategic forms of behavior that make the self-image acceptable or at least less unacceptable. Neurotic behavior is to a large extent based on these particular defensive cognitive configurations, which often become unconscious and are applied automatically. Often the patient has learned to apply these configurations in situations in which they were appropriate. Later, because of his lack of security or ability to discriminate, he has extended their sphere of applicability. In most cases, important cognitive configurations are completely repressed, because ungratifying or inconsistent with one's cherished self-image. Contrary to what is often believed, repression and suppression from awareness do not apply only to primitive strivings and to the contents of primary cognition, but also to the content of high conceptual ideation.

In some psychoneuroses, such as phobic conditions and obsessive-compulsive syndromes, the self is also, in specific situations, protected by some use of primary cognition. In the schizophrenic psychosis, the self is defended by an extensive use of primary cognition, which is not corrected or counterbalanced by the secondary. Various forms of displacement and transformation of a cognitive construct into another that is less disturbing (such as in regression, fixation, paleologic thinking) occur in dreams and in many pathological conditions.

As described elsewhere, no anticipation of the future is possible without symbolic processes (8). In order to feed his present self-esteem and maintain an adequate self-image, the young individual has, so to say, to borrow from his expectations and hopes for the future. It is when a present vacillating self-esteem cannot be supported by hope and faith in the future that severe psychopathological conditions may develop (9, 10).

Most concepts that affect the individual are learned from others, either private persons or social and cultural institutions. This point has been stressed in the Whorf-Sapir theory of cognition (36). Culture, with its system of knowledge, languages, beliefs, and values, bestows on each person a patrimony of concepts that becomes part of the individual. The acknowledgment of this fact should not induce psychiatrists and psychoanalysts to equate a cognitive approach to an interpersonal-cultural one. Certainly, a cognitive approach is closer to the cultural than to one based on instinctual theories. However, it does not conceive the individual as molded entirely by culture or by interpersonal relations. First, innate functions and structures vary and affect each individual in different ways. Second, temperament and primary cognition have different shaping influences on the individual. Third, the person's various uses of the different modalities of cognition confer on him a certain individuality that is not derivative from cultural factors.

Nevertheless, it is accurate to say that a given culture predisposes the individual to build some self-images rather than others and special patterns of defenses. This topic is too vast to be discussed here. However, it is relevant to mention that even the need to build and retain a self-image that is gratifying is to a large extent culturally determined. In some medieval cultures, for instance, the prevailing philosophy was that of mortifying the self and of depicting the individual as an insignificant entity, a sinner, an individual who is not "his own." This self-effacing cultural attitude should not be confused with individualistic masochistic traits.

We must acknowledge that learning has a very important role in the organization of inner reality. However, we must specify that the content of a learning experience becomes part of inner reality when it becomes integrated with the rest of the psyche and has an effect that transcends the original experience. Undoubtedly, there are intermediary stages between learning experiences and components of inner reality. Generally, but not in an absolute sense, we can state that:

1. The more emotional the effect of the experience, the more it tends to become part of inner reality. On the contrary, the less emotional the experience, the more it may be viewed as a learning process.

2. The more diffuse the effect of the experience (that is, related to many aspects of the life of the individual, such as the interpersonal relation with a parent), the more related to inner life it becomes. On the contrary, the more specific the effect, the more it remains part of learning.

3. The more the experience is seen as particular (that is, as belonging to a specific member of a category: for instance, how to feel and respond in the presence of the family's dog), the more the experience becomes part of the inner self. On the contrary, the more the experience is from the very beginning categorical or universal (for instance, how to respond or feel in the presence of any member of the whole class of dogs), the more it tends to remain a learning experience. This third point has many exceptions that cannot be discussed here. Thus, although many learning experiences accrue the inner reality, many others remain limited or preponderantly connected with specific behavioral problems and patterns.

Table 1 outlines the cognitive and affective components of inner reality, which we have discussed in this chapter.

GENERAL ASPECTS OF THE SELF AND CONCLUSIONS

The comparative developmental approach I have followed is in many respects similar to the one advocated by Werner (35). Probably, insights obtained through new approaches, such as the one introduced by Von Bertalanffy's general system theory (29, 30), will do much to clarify the intricacies of inner reality. I have already referred to the self as an "open system," always related to external reality.

From a general point of view, the self (and in particular, the inner self) can be examined from five different aspects: 1) representational function, 2) subjectivity, 3) potentiality, 4) integration, 5) desubjectivation. These aspects are so interrelated that we cannot understand any of them without taking into consideration the others. For didactical reasons only we shall discuss them separately.

The representational function is the formation of inner constructs that represent objects or events of the external world. These representations are not analogic reproductions of what they stand for. They are mediated by various kinds and ranks of intrapsychic mechanisms and are under the influence of previous experience. Psychologically, they may become more important than external reality.

The second aspect of the self refers to the fact that what is objective or objectivizable becomes subjective, is appropriated by the individual as a subjective experience, acquires a subjective reality, and becomes part of the individual himself. This subjectivization is not adequately accounted for by psychological or psychiatric authors who give exclusive or almost exclusive importance to the environment. This subjectivization is a phenomenon as difficult to understand as the whole mind-body

TABLE 1

Presymbolic Organization

  A. Simple feelings
  B. Immediate (nonsymbolic) learning
  C. Protoemotions
    1. Tension
    2. Appetite
    3. Fear
    4. Rage
    5. Satisfaction

Symbolic Organization

  A. Primary
    1. Phantasmic stage
      a. Images
      b. Second-order emotions
        i. Anxiety
        ii. Wish
        iii. Anger
        iv. Primitive love
        v. Primitive sadness
        vi. Security
    2. Endoceptual stage
      a. Ineffable thoughts
      b. Atmospheric feelings
    3. Preconceptual
      a. Paleologic thinking
      b. Primitive language
      c. Primary generalization
      d. Teleologc causality
      e. Third-order emotions
        i. Sadness (and depression)
        ii. Hate
        iii. Love
        iv. Joy
  B. Secondary
    1. Conceptual
      a. Abstract thinking
      b. Highly connotative language
      c. Deduction and induction
      d. Deterministic causality
      e. High-order emotions
  C. Tertiary
    Creativity

Progressive formation of inner objects ⟶

problem. The intensity of a subjective construct does not correspond to the external objective event or stimulus to which it is related. It depends, as we have already mentioned, on the mechanisms triggered off in its formation, on the selection of other constructs with which it is integrated, and on the processes used in such integration. The subjective aspect is particularly evident when we study sensations and emotions, but emotions accompany and transform cognitive constructs and in their turn are trasformed by them.

The potentiality of the self can be seen: 1) in the way it affects the behavior of the individual in relation to other people, himself, the world in general; 2) it affects itself. In other words, the self feeds on the external world as well as on itself.

The term integration refers to a large number of psychological mechanisms, most of them unknown, by virtue of which all functions of the psyche are related to one another and synthesized into higher ranks of organization.

Desubjectivization is the fifth property and, in a certain way, the opposite of subjectivity. It refers also to a group of phenomena that tend to decrease the private or subjective aspects of the experience. We have seen that in subhuman animals and during the first year and a half of human life the inner self exists only in rudimentary form. In the growing and grown human being, however, it becomes so intense that during the evolution of *Homo sapiens* mechanisms developed that had the purpose of decreasing its intensity and prominence. These various mechanisms have been described, under various terminologies, in psychological, psychiatric, and psychoanalytic literatures. We have already mentioned some of these mechanisms as the adoption of special cognitive configurations or special types of cognition. Others should be considered under the heading of desubjectivization:

1. Decrease of affective or sensuous content, for instance by the mechanisms of denial, reaction-formation, undoing, blunting of affect, depersonalization, alienation, hysterical anesthesia, and so forth.

2. Suppression, or more or less voluntary removal of some psychological content from the focus of attention or of consciousness. This content goes into a state of quiescence, like a language or skill that is not used.

3. Repression, or removal of psychological content, from consciousness. The study of this mechanism is the main topic of psychoanalysis.

These mechanisms alter and complicate but do not eliminate inner life. Desubjectivization is not necessarily a useful procedure. Although, from the point of view of the whole human race, it may have statistically useful survival effects, it often has undesirable consequences on the individual. As a matter of fact, it is the aim of psychoanalysis to make conscious again what became unconscious. According to me and other writers, this psychoanalytic procedure is not therapeutically sufficient in most instances. Therapy must also aim at reintegrating harmoniously with the rest of the self what was restored to consciousness.

The respective role of these five aspects or functions of the self can be appreciated particularly in relation to the self-image. The first aspect is easy to understand, as it is obvious that the self-image is a representation of the self to the self. The second aspect is recognized when we consider that the self-image is not a collection of data, but something that is subjectively experienced and evokes in the individual satisfaction or discomfort, security or anxiety. The self-image has the potentiality of changing the behavior of the individual in order to effect a desirable change in itself. The self-image, of course, is the result of the integration of many data and mechanisms. Finally, the self-image may undergo suppression, repression, or distortions of some parts that are disturbing to the rest of the inner self.

This enumeration of the aspects of the self and the separation of the self from the self-image may seem an unwarranted dissection of something that is experienced and therefore by somebody supposed to exist only as a unity. However, all these separate characteristics and their blending together into a subjective unit appear more clearly in the state of dreaming, which is one of the normal states of the self. When an individual dreams, that part of him that makes the dream is the representational function. The part of him that experiences the dream as a felt experience is the subjectivity. The effect of the dream (assuaging, waking up, sexual arousement, enlightenment, and so forth) is related to the potentiality. The integrative aspect consists of all the mechanisms that made the dream possible as a synthesis of many psychological factors. At first impression, desubjectivization does not seem to occur in dreams. As a matter of fact, the main function of the dream seems to make alive and representational again what was in a state of quiescence. However, often compromises occur in dreams, as Freud (16) demonstrated: events take place after they have been made less unacceptable by the dream work.

What about the self-image? It corresponds to the individual himself, as he sees himself in the dream. What in the state of wake is predominantly a cognitive-affective entity becomes a visual image in the dream.

Thus, in the dream, the representational function is perfectly fused with the subjectivity. At the same time that the dreamer produces an image of himself, he experiences that image as himself. For instance, if he sees himself threatened by a danger or kissed by his sweetheart, he experiences the horror of the threat or the pleasure of the kiss in himself, not in an object of his observation.

REFERENCES

1. ARIETI, S.: Special logic of schizophrenic and other types of autistic thought. *Psychiatry*, 11:325-338, 1948.
2. ARIETI, S.: *Interpretation of Schizophrenia*. New York: Brunner, 1955.
3. ARIETI, S.: Schizophrenia: The manifest symptomatology, the psychodynamic and formal mechanisms. In: S. Arieti (Ed.), *American Handbook of Psychiatry*, Vol. 1. New York: Basic Books, 1959, pp. 455-484.
4. ARIETI, S.: The microgeny of thought and perception. *Archives of General Psychiatry*, 6:454-468, 1962.
5. ARIETI, S.: Contributions to cognition from psychoanalytic theory. In: J. H. Masserman (Ed.), *Science and Psychoanalysis*, Vol. 3. New York: Grune & Stratton, 1965, pp. 16-37.
6. ARIETI, S.: Conceptual and cognitive psychiatry. *American Journal of Psychiatry*, 122:361-366, 1965.
7. ARIETI, S.: Creativity and its cultivation: Relation to psychopathology and mental health. In: S. Arieti (Ed.), *American Handbook of Psychiatry*, Vol. 3. New York: Basic Books, 1966, pp. 722-741.
8. ARIETI, S.: *The Intrapsychic Self: Feeling, Cognition, and Creativity in Health and Mental Illness*. New York: Basic Books, 1967.
9. ARIETI, S.: New views on the psychodynamics of schizophrenia. *American Journal of Psychiatry*, 124:453-458, 1967.
10. ARIETI, S.: The psychodynamics of schizophrenia: A reconsideration. *American Journal of Psychotherapy*, 1:366-381, 1968.
11. ARLOW, J. A.: Report on panel: The psychoanalytic theory of thinking. *Journal of the American Psychoanalytic Association*, 6:143, 1958.
12. BALDWIN, J. M.: Quoted in J. Piaget, *The Child's Conception of the World*. New York: Harcourt, Brace, 1929.
13. BRUNER, J. S., GOODNOW, J. J., and AUSTIN, G. A.: *A Study of Thinking*. New York: Wiley, 1956.
14. FAIRBAIRN, W.: *Psychoanalytic Studies of the Personality*. New York: Basic Books, 1952.
15. FEDERN, P.: *Ego Psychology and the Psychoses*. New York: Basic Books, 1952.
16. FREUD, S.: The Interpretation of Dreams (1900). In: J. Strachey (Ed.), *Standard Edition*, Vol. 4, pp. 1-621; Vol. 5, pp. 687-751. London: Hogarth Press. (Also published as *The Interpretation of Dreams*. New York: Basic Books, 1960.)
17. FREUD, S.: The future of an illusion (1927). In: J. Strachey (Ed.), *Standard Edition*. London: Hogarth Press, Vol. 21.
18. GUNTRIP, H.: *Personality Structure and Human Interaction*. New York: International Universities Press, 1961.
19. JONES, E.: *The Life and Work of Sigmund Freud*. New York: Basic Books, Vol. 1, 1953.
20. KLIEN, M.: *Contributions to Psychoanalysis*. London: Hogarth Press, 1948.

21. LEVIN, M.: Misunderstanding of the pathogenesis of schizophrenia, arising from the concept of 'splitting.' *American Journal of Psychiatry*, 94:877, 1938.
22. PIAGET, J.: *The Child's Conception of the World*. New York: Harcourt, Brace, 1929.
23. PIAGET, J.: *The Child's Conception of Physical Causality*. New York: Harcourt, Brace, 1930.
24. PIAGET, J.: *The Origins of Intelligence in Children*. New York: International Universities Press, 1952.
25. PIAGET, J.: *Logic and Psychology*. New York: Basic Books, 1957.
26. SCHUR, M.: *The Id and the Regulatory Principles of Mental Functioning*. New York: International Universitiesc Press, 1966.
27. SULLIVAN, H. S.: *Conceptions of Modern Psychiatry*. New York: Norton, 1953.
28. TINBERGEN, N.: *The Study of Instinct*. Oxford: Clarendon, 1951.
29. VON BERTALAOFFY, L.: General systems theory. In: L. von Bertalanffy and A. Rapaport (Eds.), *Society for the Advancement of General Systems Theory*. Ann Arbor: University of Michigan Press, 1956.
30. VON BERTALANFFY, L.: General system theory and psychiatry. In: S. Arieti (Ed.), *American Handbook of Psychiatry*, Vol. 3. New York: Basic Books, 1966, pp. 705-721.
31. VON DOMARUS, E.: The specific laws of logic in schizophrenia. In: J. S. Kasamin (Ed.), *Language and Thought in Schizophrenia: Collected Papers*. Berkeley: University of California Press, 1944.
32. VYGOTSKY, L. S.: *Thought and Language*. Cambridge, Mass.: M.I.T. Press, 1962.
33. WERNER, H.: Microgenesis and aphasia. *Journal of Abnormal and Social Psychology*, 52:347-353, 1956.
34. WERNER, H.: *Comparative Psychology of Mental Development*. New York: International Universities Press, 1957.
35. WERNER, H., and KAPLAN, B.: *Symbol Formation. An Organismic-Developmental Approach to Language and the Expression of Thought*. New York: Wiley, 1963.
36. WHORF, B. L.: *Language, Thought and Reality*. New York: Wiley, 1956.

25

Cognitive Components in Human Conflict and Unconscious Motivation

This paper investigates what ideas do to men or what men do to ideas—in other words, how ideas are essential components in human conflict and unconscious motivation.

THE IDEA

IN THE LAST of his writings, "An Outline of Psychoanalysis," Freud (13) wrote, "The symptoms of neuroses are exclusively, it might be said, either a substitute satisfaction of some sexual impulse or measures to prevent such a satisfaction, and are as a rule compromise between the two." In a large part of classic psychoanalytic literature not only neurotic behavior but every kind of behavior, including creative activity, is interpreted as motivated by sexual instincts, aggressivity, and other relatively simple emotional states, or as based on the displacement or sublimation of such states. It is to the merit of other schools of psychoanalysis, especially those which constitute the bulk of the American Academy of Psychoanalysis, to have recognized that the instinctual life and the simple levels of physio-psychological organization do not constitute the only sources of psychogenic motivation, and that the three major psychological phenomena that Freud was the first to illustrate—the unconscious, the intrapsychic conflict, and symbolism—involve many other levels of the psyche.

Even when psychological phenomena originate at instinctual or simple psychophysiological levels, they soon become connected with the cognitive functions of the psyche. To take a very common example, many patients complain of sexual difficulties. But sexual problems become rapidly connected with such concepts as being accepted or rejected, desirable or undesirable, loved or unloved, capable or incapable, normal or abnormal.

If it is true that sexual dysfunctions lead to these concepts and to a state of general anxiety, it is also true that these cognitive appraisals of the self bring about a state of anxiety, which in its turn causes sexual dysfunctions. Sexual gratification, deprivation, and dysfunction are phenomena that affect the whole self-image, and the self-image often affects sexual functions.

It is to the merit of such people as Harry Stack Sullivan, Erich Fromm, Karen Horney, Erik Erikson, and Harry Guntrip, to mention only the major innovators, that new dimensions were added to the Freudian model of the psyche and that the realm of our inquiry was vastly enlarged. And yet even in the authors that I have mentioned, we can recognize two restricting attitudes which have been retained more or less from the classic school. The first is a reluctance in all of them to stress the importance of the idea as an ingredient of the psyche, as a source of conflict and pathology. There has been almost a sense of prudish embarrassment in admitting that ideas count; or to investigate deeply what ideas do to men or what men do to ideas, so that they become disturbing factors. And yet I do not need to point out to anyone that in psychoanalytic therapy we deal with ideas constantly, and that almost all our exchanges with patients occur through ideas, and that it is through ideas that we bring about improvement or cure.* A prevailing cultural anti-intellectualism has caused misapprehensions and distortions even in the field of psychoanalysis. When we stress the importance of ideas, we do not minimize the importance of affective life, or of motivation, conscious or unconscious. On the contrary, we stress a fact which is very seldom acknowledged, namely, that at a human level most emotions would not exist without a cognitive substratum. The expansion of the neocortex and, consequently, of our cognitive functions has permitted an expansion of our affective life also. In a classic paper, published in 1937, Papez (15) demonstrated that several parts of the rhinencephalon and archipallium are not used for olfactory functions in the human being, but for the experience of emotion. In spite of the diminished importance of olfaction, these areas have expanded, not decreased in man, and have become associated with vast neocortical areas. Elsewhere (3) I have shown how in the human being elementary emotions, such as tension, fear, and rage, are changed into higher emotions (anxiety, anger, depression, hate, and so forth) through the intervention

---

* I do not mean to discount nonverbal communications, like the therapist's general attitude, position of the body, tone of voice, sequence of silences; but in the majority of therapeutic situations, these nonverbal signals remain minimal or much less important than the verbal and conceptual.

of complicated cognitive mechanisms. To omit the study of man at a conceptual level is not only a reductionistic approach, it is a transformation of man into a prehuman species, endowed with a simpler life, susceptible only of relatively elementary psychopathology.

Behavior therapy guides the patient to proceed directly from stimulus to response and to bypass the conceptual level with its billions of neurons and infinite number of complications. But we analysts cannot accept this bypassing unless every other attempt has failed to remove the psychiatric condition or its distressing symptoms. Some schools of psychoanalysis are also practicing a different type of bypassing when they ignore or do not acknowledge the role of cognition. I believe that we must face the complexity that has made the human being great and, at the same time, the most vulnerable (the only species that can suffer from schizophrenia and psychotic depression).

The second attitude of most, but not all, of the authors that I have mentioned is the genetic fallacy, the almost exclusive preoccupation with childhood and the primitive. There is no doubt that childhood experiences are extremely important, and generally much more so than experiences occurring in subsequent ages. Nevertheless, we should not make the error of considering them the exclusive determinants of psychological events or of psychopathology.

In the terminology of general system theory, the psyche is not a closed system, but a system open to continuous influences from factors occurring outside the system (Bertalanffy 10). Psychopathological structures are also open systems. They are states of various degrees of improbability which are maintained by negative psychological entropy coming from outside the original system. An open system like the psyche follows the principle of equifinality; the final state is not unequivocally determined by the initial condition.

The reluctance to relinquish the two attitudes that I have mentioned is based on the fact that in psychoanalysis we do not have a theoretical system which takes cognition into proper account and sustains and guides our steps in exploring the psychogenic effect of ideas. We must recognize, on the other hand, that retention of the old theoretical systems is comparable to the use of ancient legal codes and to the practice of habits of behavior which do not fit present eras any longer.

Classic psychoanalysis has dealt with the highest levels of the psyche in its formulation of the ego and superego. The superego is seen as an institution which imposes renunciation by requesting a repression of instinctual life. This formulation does not require an inquiry of cognitive processes, which in Freudian theory are generally attributed to the ego. However, most ego psychologists follow the leadership of Hartmann, Kris, and Lowenstein (14) and Rapaport (16) in considering these processes only as carriers of conflicts which originate elsewhere. As a matter of fact, these authors have called these cognitive functions autonomous and conflict-free areas and do not see them as sources of, or direct participants in, the conflict. For the cognitive school of psychoanalysis, they are not conflict-free, but active participants or generators of conflict (6). In a short presentation like the present one I cannot possibly describe or even enumerate even the major conflicts which originate at higher levels of the psyche. To some extent, I have done so elsewhere (4). I cannot even refer to the cognitive dissonance described by various authors, after Festinger's (12) initial contribution; that is, to the conflict deriving from the desire to find consistency among the various ideas that we entertain and at the same time the wish to retain discordance or actually incompatible and self-contradictory thoughts.

The cognitive school of psychoanalysis also asserts that not only primitive ideations dealing with infantile strivings can become repressed from consciousness, but even highly cognitive structures which use high symbolism. Whenever the patient is unable to face certain conceptual issues, conscious and, much more often, unconscious mechanisms are put into motion which repress, suppress, distort, displace, isolate, ignore these particular issues. It is one of the tenets of the cognitive school of psychoanalysis that in most instances gratification of the self or the self-image (and not necessarily of one's instincts) becomes the main motivational factor at a conceptual level of development. The meaning of one's life is soon connected with the self-image and becomes also a conscious and, more often, an unconscious preoccupation in the psychogenesis of many psychiatric conditions. In the remainder of this paper I shall limit myself to discussing briefly these two clusters of concepts, the self-image and the meaning of one's life, especially, but not exclusively, in reference to the psychogenesis of schizophrenia and of psychotic depression.

THE SELF-IMAGE

What is the self-image? At the sensorimotor level described by Piaget, the self-image consists of relatively simple relations between feelings, kinesthetic sensations, perceptions, motor activity, and a partial integration of these elements. Later the self-image includes also the body image, but toward the end of childhood and throughout adolescence the self-image comes to be constituted more and more of concepts, an enlarging constellation of thoughts which give to the person an understanding of his own identity and of his own attitude toward such understanding. Concepts like inner worth, personal significance, mental outlook, appraisals reflected from others, attitudes towards these appraisals, comparison and competition with others, working ability, attitudes toward ideals, aspirations, capacity to receive and give acceptance, affection, and love, together with the emotions that accompany these concepts, are integral parts of the self-image, or, if one prefers, of one's own identity. To think that these concepts and their concomitant emotions are only displacements or rationalizations which cover more primitive instinctual drives is a reductionistic point of view. We must add that whatever would disturb one's cherished self-image tends to be modified, re-evaluated, denied, or repressed. Whatever might make the individual appear to himself unworth, guilty, inadequate, sadistic, inconsistent with his ideas or ideals, escapist, or not living up to his ideals tends eventually to be removed from consciousness. Indeed, some of these evaluations of the self remain conscious; but even so, what is eliminated from consciousness is much more than the individual realizes. Psychoanalytic practice reveals how many of these cognitive constructs about oneself, and how many of their ramifications, are kept in a state of unconsciousness.

Often repression of the main motivation (protecting the self-image) is achieved with the help of psychological mechanisms that detour consciousness toward other avenues of thought and behavior. Intricate cognitive configurations lead the patient to feelings, ideas, and strategic forms of behavior that make the self-image acceptable or at least less unacceptable. Here are a few of the simplest examples: A woman leads a promiscuous life; she feels unacceptable as a person, but as a sexual partner she feels appreciated. The hypochondriac protects his self by blaming only his body for his difficulties. The suspicious person and the paranoid attribute to others shortcomings or negative intentions that they themselves have.

In many other cases, which range from normal persons to neurotic and even psychotic, cognitive configurations constitute general attitudes, premises, or even philosophies of life that determine the behavior or the individual who is completely unaware of the existence of them. For instance, a man repeatedly becomes involved with women who are sick physically or mentally, or who have been victimized by cruel parents, society, poverty, or from a terrible husband or a former psychopathic fiancé. At first it seems that the patient is motivated only by love, and that the condition in which the woman was found is purely due to chance. Actually, when we analyze the patient, we come to see that the choice was determined by an unconscious constellation or premise that we could call "the savior complex." The patient wants to save a woman from her miserable fate, and can fall in love only with a woman who needs him. At times the patient, in saving the partner, wants to save the neurotic, or fallen part of himself. Most of the time he believes he is great for having saved another person. A deep feeling of inadequacy may be at the bottom of this savior complex. "Only if I save her," he says to himself, "will she love me. I am not worthy of love under any other circumstances." In other words, this patient unconsciously retains the idea that he will not be able to arouse love, but only gratitude, and he hopes that the gratitude will eventually turn into love. In a few of these cases we may recognize an original Oedipal situation.* The partner who wants to save the woman previously had fantasies as a child of how to save or console the mother, who was harassed by the misdeeds of the father. However, even when we find an original Oedipal fixation, we realize that the savior complex could not have developed and would not unconsciously affect the patient's life if he had not had at his disposal cognitive media that allowed him to become aware of women in the position of needing to be saved and of ways by which he could become a "rescuer."

My studies of preschizophrenics and schizophrenics have disclosed that the preschizophrenic, in a period of life which precedes the psychotic break, generally during adolescence or young adulthood, finds himself threatened on all sides, as if he were in a jungle (Arieti, 5). It is not a jungle where ferocious animals are to be found, but a jungle of concepts that remain unconscious until shortly before the onset of the psychosis, or the phase that I have called the prepsychotic panic. The threat is again not to physical survival, but to the self-image. The dangers are concept-feelings, such as those of being unwanted, unloved, unlovable, inadequate, unacceptable, inferior, awkward, clumsy, not belonging, peculiar, different, rejected, humiliated, guilty, unable to find his own way among the different paths of life, disgraced, discriminated against, kept at a distance, suspected, and so forth. Some of these concepts were conscious even in earlier periods of life. What had remained unconscious were their full significance, their ramifications and connections, especially with similar concepts about the self, originated in childhood. When these constellations of concepts are interconnected and become vividly conscious, they

---

* I have retained the term Oedipal not because a sexual attachment to the mother is necessarily implied, but because the situation involves the classic Oedipal triangle—the relation between son, mother, and father.

are experienced as unbearable and undergo drastic changes. At first the patient's distortion is not yet a paranoid projection or a delusion in a technical sense. It is predominantly experienced as anguish, increased vulnerability, fear, anxiety, mental pain. The patient is not able to change his self-image or to discover that his negative appraisal of himself is unfounded. Soon he comes to feel that the segment of the world which is important to him finds him unacceptable. He also believes that as long as he lives, he will be unacceptable to others. He is excluded from the busy, relentless ways of the world. He does not fit. He experiences ultimate loneliness; he does not find himself at home in the universe. At this point he undergoes a conceptual transformation of cosmic magnitude, that is, his way of relating to the whole world goes through a metamorphosis. Rather than to accept his unbearable self-image, he withdraws from the world. It is a major, psychotic withdrawal, an attitude of almost complete detachment, the result of all his previous experiences, of his infinite fear of life, infinite distrust of people, total desire to escape. Often the desire to escape is covered up by the feeling that the world is not worth being looked at, of being contacted, not worth participating in. In an even greater percentage of cases, the clinical picture is not of withdrawal but of projection. A system of false beliefs possesses the patient. Now he sees his surroundings as threatening. The danger is there; the persecutors are plotting in a myriad of possible ways. The dangers are many, and the patient lives them in agonizing ways.

The danger, of course, is an externalization of an inner danger. The patient who, before he became psychotic, had a bad opinion of himself, now tends to believe that the others are possible perpetrators of pain and evil. Whereas he earlier accused and denigrated himself, now he believes that the accusation and the denigration come from the external world. No matter how unpleasant it is to feel that people accuse him and persecute him, it is better than to accuse himself. Although persecuted, he feels his spirit is free. He has succeeded in changing an inner anxiety, which was connected with an original unbearable self-image, into an external danger, which is still objectionable, but with which he can live.

In a minority of cases the psychotic metamorphosis is of a different nature. The patient becomes grandiose, megalomaniac, and immune to any danger. I cannot continue with a detailed analysis of the psychopathology of schizophrenia. I just want to conclude by stressing that through the schizophrenic process an attempt is made to solve a conceptual conflict with a conceptual transformation.

THE MEANING OF ONE'S LIFE

At one time or another every human being thinks about the meaning of life. This may occur in adolescence, but more frequently in youth and adult age. The philosopher or the deep thinker tackles this problem from a universal point of view, in a way which is quite different from the one we are discussing here. We are referring to the conscious conceptualizations and unconscious premises that occur in the psyche of each human being concerning the significance that he himself gives to his own life, and to his own life exclusively. Without even using words, or formulating clear ideas, the individual generally assumes that his life has a purpose and a meaning, at least for him, the owner of that life. There is no more depressing thought, or deeper state of despair, than the one derived from the conclusion that one's own life either has no meaning, has lost meaning, or has become something which signifies nothing. Poets have been able to express this feeling at a conscious level, with the most striking metaphorical representations. Let us reconsider the following well known passage from Shakespeare:

> . . . Out, out brief candle!
> Life's but a walking shadow, a poor player
> That struts and frets his hour upon the stage,
> And then is heard no more; it is a tale
> Told by an idiot, full of sound and fury,
> Signifying nothing . . . .

I was urged to quote these verses by the fact that many seriously depressed patients have reported to me dreams in which their life was symbolized by a brief candle soon to be extinguished, or by a walking shadow, or a poorly played performance, or a tale told by an idiot. The metaphorical images that a great poet is able to rediscover sojourn in some recesses of our psyche, where concepts have become unconscious or transformed into dark visions. Of course, we know that Shakespeare attributes this negative definition of life not to the average denizen of the earth, but to Macbeth, a hero ef evil, certainly not a man whom we should listen to as a master of life. Macbeth defines life in this way when he has realized that the meaning he gave his life—obtaining power by means of crime—was a false meaning, discordant with the basic principles of human nature. Thus his life became a tale told by an idiot, which signified nothing.

Since Shakespeare's passage has such a profound impact on all of us, we must assume that the poet does not speak only about Macbeth's life, but about the life of all of us, even though we have not committed

Macbeth's crimes. The poet tells us that our life, too, can become a shadow, a poor player, a tale told by an idiot, unless we find a meaning in it—and it must be a proper meaning.

The person who becomes psychotically depressed is certainly not one who has committed crimes, although at times he feels as guilty as if he had committed crimes. He has reached a stage in his life in which he feels his existence has no meaning, or no worthwhile meaning, or if such meaning once existed, it has been lost. Such realization produces a sense of hopeless, irretrievable loss, because what has been lost is the meaning of what one is. The patient is unable to formulate such thoughts in words. The depression has, among others, the functions of repressing, especially of repressing the constellation of thoughts which led to the depression itself. Only the mood of depression, in its greatest possible intensity, remains conscious.

In other publications (1, 2, 7, 8) I have described in detail how the cognitive structures and patterns of living which led to psychotic forms of depression started early in life. In many cases these cognitive structures and patterns compelled the patient to live not for himself, but for the sake of another person, whom I have called the dominant other (Arieti 1962, 1974c). The dominant other is represented most often by the spouse, less frequently by the mother, a lover, an adult child, a sister, the father. The dominant other may be represented, through anthropomorphism, by the firm where the patient works, or a social institution, a class of people. Another large category of depressed patients seems to live for the pursuit of an inaccessible aim, which I have called the dominant goal. The dominant goal may not be unethical like that of Macbeth. It may be very ethical, but unsuitable or destructive for the patient.

When the patient realizes the failure of his pattern of living, he also recognizes that he is unable to change it. He realizes that the meaning he has given to his life is false or unworthy; but if he renounces that meaning, his life sustains the greatest possible loss: it becomes meaningless. The patient finds himself in a state of helplessness and hopelessness. A frequent example is that of a woman who used to consider her husband a dispenser of love and affection, a protector, a friend, a partner in every respect. Now she sees him as an authoritarian person who imposed his rule, at times in a subtle, hardly visible way, at other times in a manifest manner. The patient's own life, at first believed devoted to love and affection, is seen now as not genuine. By doing always what the husband wanted and denying her wishes, she has not been true to herself; as a matter of fact, she has betrayed herself.

Life seems meaningless also to the category of patients who realize they have failed to reach the dominant goal and cannot escape from the self-imposed predicament. The patient knows now that he is not going to be a great doctor, lawyer, politician, writer, actor, industrialist, lover, musician, and so forth. But without the dominant goal, life appears worthless. If the patient wanted to be a great conductor, a Toscanini, now he has to face the fact that he is not a Toscanini, that he is himself, John Doe. But he has no respect for John Doe, as he should. He believes John Doe is nothing. There is some tangential and partial justification in the patient's assessing himself in a negative way because he spent so much of his thoughts in being Toscanini; and his psychological life without this overpowering fantasy seems empty. The limitations of the patient, determined by his rigidity and adherence to an inflexible pattern of life, do not provide him with alternatives.

I must stress once more that when the patient has reached the stage of psychotic depression, he has lost awareness of the cognitive structures which led to his sorrow. Even before he became depressed, although he might have been aware of the importance of certain mental constructs, he was unaware of their origin, of how much they involved, of all the ramifications, assumptions, presuppositions, and feelings connected with them. Moreover, he was unaware of his inability to search for alternatives. Whereas another person would try to escape from the blind alley and search for solutions, he finds himself in a state of hopelessness. His loss thus appears irreplaceable and, therefore, immense, and immense is his sorrow. With special techniques, described elsewhere (8; Arieti and Bemporad, in preparation), we can help restore to consciousness the psychogenetic ideation, provided we are also able to present the prospect of alternative ways of living and offer the understanding, the hope, and the attitude necessary for their realization.

REFERENCES

1. Arieti, S: Manic-depressive psychosis. In: S. Arieti (Ed.), *American Handbook of Psychiatry*, First ed., Vol. 1. New York: Basic Books, 1959, pp. 419-454.
2. Arieti, S.: The psychotherapeutic approach to depression. *Amer. J. Psychother.*, 16:397-406.
3. Arieti, S.: *The Intrapsychic Self: Feeling, Cognition and Creativity in Health and Mental Illness*. New York: Basic Books, 1967.
4. Arieti, S.: The structure and psychodynamic role of cognition in the human psyche. In: S. Arieti (Ed.), *The World Biennial of Psychiatry and Psychotherapy*, Vol. 1. New York: Basic Books, 1970, pp. 3-33.
5. Arieti, S.: *Interpretation of Schizophrenia*, Second ed. (Completely Revised and Expanded). New York: Basic Books, 1974a.

6. ARIETI, S.: The cognitive-volitional school. In: S. Arieti (Ed.), *American Handbook of Psychiatry,* Second ed., Vol. 1. New York: Basic Books, 1974b, pp. 877-903.

7. ARIETI, S.: Affective disorders: Manic-depressive psychosis and psychotic depression: Manifest symptomatology, psychodynamics, sociological factors and psychotherapy. In: S. Arieti (Ed.), *American Handbook of Psychiatry,* Vol. III. New York: Basic Books, 1974c, pp. 449-490.

8. ARIETI, S.: Psychoanalysis of severe depression: Theory and therapy. *J. Amer. Acad. Psychoanal.,* 4:327-345.

9. ARIETI, S. and BEMPORAD, J.: *Severe and Mild Depression. The Psychotherapeutic Approach.* New York: Basic Books (in press).

10. BERTALANFFY, L. VON: General system theory. *Main Currents in Modern Thoughts,* 11:75-83, 1955.

11. BERTALANFFY, L. VON: The model of open system. In *General System Theory,* New York: Braziller, 1968.

12. FESTINGER, L.: *A Theory of Cognitive Dissonance.* Stanford, Calif.: Stanford Univ. Press, 1957.

13. FREUD, S.: An outline of psychoanalysis. In *The Standard Edition of the Complete Psychological Works of Sigmund Freud,* Vol. 23. London: Hogarth Press, 1940; New York: Macmillan, 1964, 141-408. First published as "Abriss der Psychoanalyse."

14. HARTMANN, H., KRIS, E., and LOWENSTEIN, R. M.: Comments on the formation of psychic structure. In *The Psychoanalytic Study of the Child,* Vol. 2. New York: International Universities Press, 1946, pp. 11-38.

15. PAPEZ, J. W.: A proposed mechanism of emotion. *Arch. Neurol. Psychiat.,* 38: 725-743, 1937.

16. RAPAPORT, D.: The structure of psychoanalytic theory. In *Psychological Issues,* Vol. 2, No. 2. New York: International Universities Press, 1960.

Part IV
RELATED FIELDS

26

New Views on the Psychology and Psychopathology of Wit and of the Comic

Published in 1950, this is my first article on creativity. Struck by the observation that psychotics may in all seriousness use expressions which to the normal person appear as real witticisms, I embarked upon a psychological study of wit and of the comic. This study opened for me new avenues which later led me to the formulation of the concept of the tertiary process.

AS FREUD WROTE, wit is worthy of psychological investigation, not only because it is an important element in social life, but also and especially because the study of it reveals material of extreme pertinence to many other problems of the human psyche (1).

In dealing with mental patients I have repeatedly been impressed by the fact, noted by many others, that psychotics may in all seriousness use expressions which to the normal person appear as real witticisms. When I later studied the mechanisms of thought in schizophrenia, I became convinced that this apparently witty way of expression was the result of the application of a special archaic logic which the patient must follow. It then occurred to me that perhaps this primitive logic is applied also in witticisms expressed by normal people and I undertook the research which I am reporting in the present paper. This investigation led me necessarily to the study of the comic, which is closely related to the problem of wit.

Wit has aroused strong interest in not a small number of philosophers, psychologists, psychiatrists, and neurologists. In the monograph referred to, Freud reviews the theories advanced by several authors and shows

367

their inadequacies. Fischer (2) for instance defines wit as "a playful judgment" but does not state what kind of judgment. Paul (3) defines wit as "the ability to combine with surprising quickness many ideas," but does not say how the ideas are combined. Kraepelin (4) thinks that wit is "the voluntary combination or linking of two ideas which in some ways are contrasted with each other, usually through the medium of speech association." He does not seem to take notice of those witticisms where contrast does not enter. Many authors find that wit is based on "sense in nonsense" or in the "succession of confusion and clearness." These last points of view appear to this writer essentially correct but vague in their formulation, inasmuch as no explanation is given of how there could be sense in nonsense or clearness in confusion.

An important contribution which Freud overlooked is that of the great neurologist Hughlings Jackson (5), who in 1887 delivered an address on the Psychology of Joking at the opening of the Medical Society of London. Jackson compared puns to dreams. He found that in both puns and dreams "two very dissimilar mental states pretending to be stereoscopic" are in reality diplopic.

In his monograph published in 1924, Gregory (6) adds a rich bibliography to that of Freud. Gregory himself, after reviewing the literature on wit, comes out with the interesting remark that "wit is a quick, vivid illumination of a truth." Recently Froeschels (7) has published a monograph on "Philosophy in Wit." Although this author is a physician as well as a philosopher, he has dealt with this problem only from a philosophical point of view. He considers witticisms the means by which philosophical truths, congenitally known but not yet expressed, become "ripe for expression."

Koestler has dealt with the problems of wit and of the comic in his book *Insight and Outlook* (8). This author's theories are based on the concept of what he calls "bisociation." Bisociation is "any mental occurrence simultaneously associated with two habitually incompatible contexts." Though it is true that many jokes may be explained by the concept of bisociation, it is also true that bisociation does not always imply an element of comic.

CRITICAL REVIEW OF FREUD'S CONTRIBUTIONS TO THE PROBLEM OF WIT

Of all the contributions to the problem of wit, the one by Freud is the most outstanding. The great master has been the first to penetrate this problem, too. It will be worth-while to review in detail his major findings, because the understanding of wit owes much to his findings and also because I take issue here with some of his findings. Freud became interested in the problem of wit when he noticed that certain dreams resembled jokes, especially when they were interpreted (9). He did not disregard this apparently accidental similarity and studied this problem more and more to discover numerous analogies between witticisms and dreams (1). He studied the various techniques of wit and found them similar to those of the dream-work. He noticed that formation of mixed words or "condensation with substitutive formation" occurs in witticisms as well as in dreams. For instance, in a famous witticism by Heine the word "famillionaire" condenses two meanings, familiar and millionaire. Double meanings or plays on words are found by Freud to be among the preferred techniques in jokes. This is one of his examples: *A physician, leaving the bedside of a wife whose husband accompanied him, exclaimed doubtfully: "I do not like her looks." "I haven't liked her looks for a long time,"* was the quick rejoinder of the husband. The physician, with the word *looks* refers to the patient's condition of health; the husband to his wife's ugliness. According to Freud, other witticisms are based on ambiguity, as in the joke popular during the trial of Dreyfus, *"This girl reminds me of Dreyfus. The army does not believe in her innocence."*

Freud summarizes the technique of wit, which he divides into three groups: techniques of 1) condensation, 2) application of the same material, 3) double meaning. Each of these groups is divided into several subgroups. He admits that the technique is very important in wit, because the wit "invariably disappears when we remove the effect of these techniques in the expressions." For instance, if somebody says: "I was driving tête-à-tête with Mr. X and Mr. X is a stupid ass," this sentence is deprived of the witticism contained in the expression, "I was driving with Mr. X tête-à-bête." Freud rightly thinks that there must be something in common in all these techniques which confers a witty character on the expression, and he makes an attempt to find this common denominator. At first he thinks that this quality consists of the condensation or tendency to economy, as when a single word in the witticism gathers several different or even opposite meanings. He realizes soon however that the nature of wit does not lie in the tendency to economize in expression, because "laconism is not necessarily wit." The intellectual work required in putting together several meanings in order to make a witticism often requires more energy than is saved by the economy of expression.

Freud then takes puns into consideration. Whereas in a play on words both meanings are expressed in the identical word, in the pun only a certain phonetic similarity or structure is necessary. A pun reported by

Brill is quoted as typical. At a party someone spoke disparagingly of a certain drama and said, "It was so poor that the first act had to be rewritten." "And now it is rerotten," added the punster. Freud goes on to examine other forms of wit whose technique cannot be classified under the three groups mentioned. Having in mind the displacement in dreams, that is, the displacement of the focus of attention from the original theme to another, he finds the same phenomenon in jokes, as in the following example: *A needy man borrowed twenty-five dollars from a wealthy acquaintance. The same day he was found by his creditor in a restaurant eating a dish of salmon with mayonnaise. The creditor reproached him, "You borrow money from me and then order salmon with mayonnaise. Is that what you needed the money for?" "I don't understand you,"* responded the debtor. *"When I have no money I can't eat salmon with mayonnaise. When I have money, I mustn't eat it. Well then, when shall I ever eat salmon with mayonnaise?"*

According to Freud, the technique of this joke does not lie in words or play on words, but in the displacement of the psychic accent. The creditor does not blame the debtor for eating salmon on the day he borrowed the money, but reminds him that he has no right to think of such luxuries at all. Freud goes on to illustrate other techniques, for instance, unification or repartee in wit, as in the following joke: *While Duke Karl of Würtemberg was riding horseback, he met a dyer working at his trade. "Can you color my white horse blue?" "Yes, sire," was the rejoinder, "if the animal can stand the boiling."* Freud remarks that the technical factor would have been omitted if the dyer's reply had been, "No sire, I am afraid that the horse could not stand being boiled." Another common technique, according to Freud, is "the representation through the opposite," as in the following example from Heine: *This woman resembles the Venus de Milo in many points. Like her, she is extraordinarily old, has no teeth, and has spots on the yellow surface of her body.* In this case, ugliness is depicted by making it agree with the most beautiful.

It is not necessary to report here all the possible techniques described by Freud. He has described them accurately, but in spite of his attempts he has failed to find what is the common and *essential* characteristic in all of them. His conclusion, undoubtedly correct, is that the same techniques are to be found in dreams. Then he goes on to study the tendencies of wit. He thinks that wit may be harmless when it has no hidden meanings and its pleasurable effect is due only to its technique. On the other hand it may be "tendency-wit" when its content tends to convey something which would not be expressed in a different way. Freud discloses how tendency-wit permits expression of feelings and ideas which otherwise would be repressed, as in hostile and obscene wit. He shows very well how sexual exhibitionism, invective, rebellion against authority, and so on, are made possible by the technique of wit. He then reaches the conclusion, which is one of the most important of his contributions on this subject, that the pleasure in tendency-wit results from the fact that a tendency whose gratification would otherwise remain unfulfilled is actually gratified. But Freud goes further and asserts that a certain psychic expenditure is generally necessary for the retention of a psychic inhibition —that is, for the inhibition of the tendency which cannot be gratified. The joke permits release of the inhibition and sets free some repressing energy. Freud seems to become confused, however, when he asks himself to find the economy of psychic expenditure in what he considers harmless witticisms; that is, in wit without tendency.

After examining other doubtful hypotheses, he expresses the idea that pleasure in some "harmless" witticisms is due to the discovery or recognition of the familiar, where one expects to find something new instead. Recognition of the familiar occurs in witticisms which use unification, similar sounding words, and so on, as technique. Freud adds that the source of pleasure in rhyme, alliteration, refrain, or repetition of similar sounding words in poetry is due to the discovery of the familiar. If it is so, there must be some other fundamental characteristics which make one distinguish the pleasure derived from a poem from the one obtained from a joke.

Freud devotes a whole chapter to wit as a social process and another one to the relation of wit to the comic. They will be referred to later in this paper.

One may conclude that Freud has indeed made remarkable contributions to the understanding of wit, and that the most important of them is the discovery that wit and dreams have many points in common, inasmuch as they use techniques, like condensation and displacement, which belong to the unconscious. Freud has examined the various techniques in jokes, but has failed to find the common formal mechanism which makes a witticism witty. He thinks that the pleasure in some witticisms consists in the gratification of a tendency which otherwise would not be gratified, but does not believe that this occurs in every case.

PALEOLOGIC

This points of view expressed in this paper about wit and the comic cannot be properly understood without some knowledge of opinions expressed in some of my previous works (10). The reader who is acquainted with them will excuse some repetitions which are made here only for the sake of clear understanding.

The exigencies of social life require that at least most of the time man thinks and acts logically. This logic of the human mind, whose laws, first enunciated by Aristotle, are applied more or less automatically by every normal adult, gives us a certain interpretation of reality, which is relatively immutable and rigid: *A* is only *A* and cannot be *B*. Under the stress of strong emotions the human being may find it very unpleasant or even intolerable to accept reality as long as he continues to live and act in accordance with this Aristotelian logic. Some of his wishes and drives cannot be satisfied, no matter how strong they are. The dreamer, the neurotic in his symptoms, and the psychotic abandon this Aristotelian logic and revert to an archaic system of logic called by me paleologic, which is more elastic, more complaisant and which may permit an interpretation of reality in accordance with one's wishes.

Furthermore this type of logic, permitting a highly individualistic or subjective choice of several possibilities, allows that mode of thought which Fromm (11) calls experiential—that is, that mode of thought which makes reality appear as it is emotionally experienced.

Paleologic preceded Aristotelian logic in phylogenetic and ontogenetic development. Its laws may be studied in the mythology and customs of ancient societies, in primitives of today, in normal children, in psychotics, and in dreams. The first of its laws, enunciated by Von Domarus, is the following: "Whereas the normal person accepts identity only upon the basis of identical subjects, the paleologician accepts identity based upon identical predicates." For instance, if a normal person knows that "Socrates is a man; all men are mortal," he will be able to conclude that "Socrates is mortal." This conclusion is justified because the subject of the major premise (all men) contains the subject of the minor premise (Socrates). On the other hand, given the following premises, "The Virgin Mary was virgin; my name is Mary and I am a virgin," a schizophrenic in all seriousness could conclude: "I am the Virgin Mary." The common predicates, the name Mary and the state of being a virgin, led to the identification of the patient with the Virgin Mary. Inasmuch as the paleological type of thinking permits a choice of predicates, out of numerous possible ones, it may lead to deductions which are gratifying for the individual or which correspond to his emotional experiences. For instance, the patient mentioned could think that she was the Virgin Mary as she wished to be, and also as she experienced herself to be, on account of the intense emotional closeness to the Virgin Mary.

The same law of paleologic is applied in dreams. The person or object *A*, having a certain characteristic of *B*, may appear in the dream as being *B* or a composite of *A* and *B*. For instance, the penis may appear symbolically in the dream as a snake, fountain pen, or stick on account of the common elongated shape.

The second principle of paleologic requires familiarity with the concepts of connotation, denotation, and verbalization. For instance, the connotation of the term *table* is its meaning, or the concept "article of furniture with flat horizontal top, set on legs." The connotation is in a certain way the definition of the object and *includes the whole class or category of the object.* The denotation of the term is the object meant— that is, the table as a physical entity. The verbalization of the term is the word as a word—that is, as a verbal representation or symbol of the object table or of the concept table.

The second principle of paleologic states that "whereas the healthy person in a wakened state is mainly concerned with the connotation and denotation of a symbol but is capable of shifting his attention from one to another of the three aspects of a symbol, the person who thinks paleologically is mainly concerned with the denotation and the verbalization, and experiences a total or partial impairment of his ability to connote." Two phenomena are thus implied in this principle: first, the reduction of the connotation power; second, the emphasis on the verbalization.

The reduction of the connotation power is manifested by the fact that the verbal symbols cease to be representative of a group or of a class but only of the specific individual objects under discussion. For instance, the word table is not used as relating to any table, but to a specific table, such as "the wooden table in the kitchen." Figurate or metaphorical language is not possible because it increases the connotation of the word. There is therefore in paleological thinking an extreme literalness in the interpretation of symbols. The proverb "Don't cry over spilt milk" is interpreted by the schizophrenic as "If you spill the milk you should not cry," because "spilt milk" cannot acquire the meaning of unpleasant past events. The language of primitive people, too, discloses a wealth of terms related to specific objects but lack of terms which include groups and categories.

Because of the emphasis on verbalization, the word is not just a symbol in paleological thinking but acquires a greater significance. The attention of the patient is often focused not on the connotation or denotation of the term but on the word as a word. Other paleological processes may take place after the attention has been focused on the verbalization. For instance, a patient who was asked to define the word "Life" tried to define *Life* magazine.

Von Domarus' principle is often applicable after the emphasis has been focused on the verbalization. Thus different objects may be identified because they have names which have a common characteristic—that is, identical or similar (partially identical) phonetic or written symbols. A schizophrenic had the habit of wetting her body with oil. Asked why she would do so, she replied: "The human body is a machine and has to be lubricated." The word *machine*, applied in a figurative sense to the human body, had led to the identification with man-made machines. The verbalization thus may become the identifying predicate.

The third, fourth, and fifth principles of paleologic will not be mentioned here because they are not directly connected with the problem of wit and the comic. The fact has to be emphasized, however, that many other laws of paleologic, or rules derived from the laws which are known, have not yet been differentiated or studied adequately. One of these rules is probably this: "This denial of a statement is the assertion of its contrary." If an object is not black, the person who thinks paleologically may assume that it is white. An obsessive-compulsive patient always walked on the right sidewalk of the street. According to him, walking on the right sidewalk must bring good luck, because he had bad luck (lost his job) one day when he walked on the left side.

Between paleologic and logic many intermediary stages obviously may be traced. One may see them in attempts to explain things plausibly and yet not according to proper logical methods. One may call them, as one usually does, rationalizations or processes pertaining to faulty logic. And we all know how numerous are our rationalizations when emotions have the upper hand.

Up to this point, I have directed the attention of the reader particularly to the fact that these archaic logical processes appear again in dreams and in pathological conditions. They do appear, however, even in special normal instances. An attempt will be made here to demonstrate that wit is an example of archaic logical processes.

PALEOLOGIC IN WIT

I shall take as the first example the witticism which Freud quoted from Heine: "This woman reminds me of the Venus de Milo in many points. Like her she is extraordinarily old, has no teeth and has white spots on the yellow surface of her body." Heine in reality wanted to say that a particular woman was ugly; but to say that to a woman in our society would be tantamount to an act of overt hostility. Heine therefore resorted to a method which would allow him to gratify this hostility but not too overtly. The method he resorted to is indeed a very predictable and bizarre one: he identified the ugly woman with the most beautiful—the Venus de Milo. But how could this identification, logically impossible, be made possible? By abandoning Aristotelian logic and reverting to paleologic. The woman and the statue of Venus are identified because they have some predicates in common, namely, being old, having no teeth, and having white spots on the yellow surface of the body. Freud emphasizes in this joke "the representation through the opposite." I believe that trying to identify a subject with its opposite reinforces the wit in the joke, but that the fundamental factor in this joke is the possibility of the identification when this seems impossible. This identification is made possible by the application of Von Domarus' principle.

To take another example from Freud: The physician leaving the bedside of a woman says to her husband, "I do not like her looks." The husband of the woman adds, "I have not liked her looks for a long time." In this little joke a marital drama is disguised. The husband experiences some feelings of aversion for his wife—feelings that he has to repress until an opportunity presents itself for unpredicted and less prohibited letting-off-steam. The physician uses the word "looks" as a symbol of the concept, "physical appearance, as indicative of a state of health." The husband uses the word "looks" as a symbol of the concept, "physical appearance, as indicative of a state of attractiveness." The two concepts are identified because they have the same verbalization, that is, the same verbal symbol, "looks." The identification here is made possible by the application of the first and second principles of paleologic.

To take another of the above-mentioned Freudian examples: There is the joke which was very common at the time of the trial of Dreyfus, the French Jew unjustly accused of treason by the French Army. "That girl reminds me of Dreyfus. The army does not believe in her innocence." Freud believes that the technique of this joke is mainly that of ambiguity, but it is obvious that the first and second principles of paleologic are here applied. Dreyfus and the girl are identified because they have a common predicate, "innocence not believed in by the army." The predicate is common to both subjects only inasmuch as the same verbalization is applied to two different concepts. In fact, in the case of Dreyfus, innocence means "state of not being guilty of treason"; in the case of the girl it means "lack of sexual experience." Also the word army has a different slant in the two cases. In the case of Dreyfus, it means "general staff," in the case of the girl it means "group of men" with emphasis on their being male. The ambiguity of this joke, emphasized by Freud, is due to the difficulty encountered in making the three or four paleological identifications and certainly adds charm to the joke; but the fundamental factor seems to me to be the possibility of identification.

To take still another example from Freud. "I was driving with him tête-à-bête." The latent meaning obviously is "I was driving tête-à-tête with this stupid ass." The disparaging content of this expression is smoothed and transformed into a joke by the application of paleologic. The concept of tête is identified with the concept of bête because the two French words tête and bête have similar, that is "partially identical," verbalization. All the jokes based on play on words imply the first and second principles of paleologic.

The formal mechanism appears more complicated in other jokes. In the example given by Freud of the man who had borrowed twenty-five dollars and who was found by the creditor in the act of eating salmon with mayonnaise, one finds that when the creditor reproached the debtor and asked him whether that was what he needed the money for, the latter answered, "I don't understand you. When I have no money I can't eat salmon with mayonnaise. When I have money I mustn't eat it. Well then, when shall I ever eat salmon with mayonnaise?" First of all, what is the latent of this joke? Here is the problem of a poor fellow who, being a human being, thinks that he too is entitled occasionally to eat salmon with mayonnaise, in spite of his economic condition. Salmon with mayonnaise was apparently considered a luxury in Europe, even at the time of Freud. The debtor does not take into consideration the fact that, in a capitalistic society, to have borrowed money does not really mean to have money. When he is reproached by the creditor, he has to find an excuse to justify himself. He cannot find an acceptable logical justification and has to resort to paleologic. "If I cannot eat salmon when I have no money, I should be allowed to eat salmon when I have money!" That is, "the denial of a statement is the assertion of its opposite." But according to Freud the technique of this joke results in the displacement of the psychic accent, as mentioned above.

In other jokes the mechanism is even more complicated, consisting of transitional stages from paleologic to logic, or of discarded, and obsolete ways of thinking, as in the following example: *Mother goes for a walk with her little boy. They come to a nudist camp which is sur-*

rounded by a high board fence. The little fellow peeps through a low hole. Mother asks: "What do you see?" Boy: "A lot of people." Mother: "What are they, men or women?" Boy: "I don't know; nobody's got any clothes on." In order to justify logically his ignorance, the child resorts to a childish form of thinking. How do children distinguish, or believe that they distinguish, men from women? Mostly by their garments. People wearing masculine garments are identified with men, and people wearing feminine garments with women. The child could have another source of information, which is the most reliable and which in this case is unexpectedly available: the direct observation of the anatomical characteristics of the nudists. He is not able to resort, however, to this logical method because he does not know of anatomical differences in the two sexes. He is able to justify his ignorance by resorting to his infantile thinking, but by doing so he lets his naïveté come to the surface. Many other factors are involved in this joke, such as the contrast between the surprising availability of the source of information and the non-use of it, and obviously there is a sexual tinge.

The transition from paleologic to logic is almost complete in the following joke. *A woman sues a man by whom she claims she has been raped. The plaintiff and the defendant are in front of the judge. The judge looks at both of them and sees that the woman is very tall and stout; the man very short and thin. With some astonishment he asked the woman, "Is this the man who raped you? How did he do it?" The woman answered, "He pushed me against a wall and he raped me." "But how is it possible?" added the perplexed judge. "You are so tall and he is so short!" "Well," said the woman, "I bent my knees a little bit."* The woman is logical. If she bends her knees, the sexual act is possible. In the attempt to use logic in self-defense, however, she accuses herself, because the bending of the knees would imply her willingness to be a partner in the sexual act and would automatically exclude the act of raping. The logic to which she resorts to defend herself actually accuses her. Though in this case no paleologic is involved, it is still the logical mechanism which is the basis of the joke—a logical mechanism which is used by the woman in self-defense and which on the contrary turns out to be a self-accusation. The woman's logic sustained her contention as to the possibility of the sexual act, but at the same time it excluded her innocence.

In another of the examples quoted from Freud, the mechanism is not too dissimilar from that of the joke just examined. While Duke Karl of Würtemberg was riding horseback, he met a dyer working at his trade.

"Can you color my white horse blue?" "Yes, sire," was the rejoinder, "if the animal can stand the boiling." The reply of the dyer was perfectly logical; but the premise was wrong, because no horse would stand the boiling. The use of a logical deduction inferred from a false premise is resorted to by the dyer in order to outsmart the silly duke, who had implied the false premise.

In some jokes the mechanism consists of comparing two different ways of thinking and of discarding one of them. The thinking of mental patients is often quoted in the jokes which belong to this group, as in the following one: *Mussolini visits an insane asylum and all the patients greet him with the fascist salute. The duce sees a man who does not greet him. In a fit of anger he asked him, "And you, why don't you greet me?" "I am not a patient," replied the man. "I am the attendant."* Why was this joke so popular in Italy and, with the appropriate variations, in Germany and other fascist countries? The latent, though obvious, meaning of the joke is, "Only insane people should greet Mussolini." The anti-fascist attendant had to defend his behavior by rejecting the opposite behavior of the patients, inasmuch as they were insane.

Somehow the opposite occurs in the following joke. *A deluded patient visits a psychiatrist. "Doctor, Doctor, help me!" he says. "Look, I am full of bugs," and tries to brush off from his clothes the imaginary parasites. "Be careful," replies the pyschiatrist, quickly recoiling, "don't brush them on me."* The story is witty because the psychiatrist accepts the patient's way of thinking, whereas he is expected to reject it. The other way of thinking, which would lead the psychiatrist to behave logically, is omitted but is implied. The meaning of the joke is obviously this: "Psychiatrists are not supermen; they may be fooled too."

Even more complicated is the alleged acceptance of a psychotic way of thinking in order to prove something. Referring to the fact that during the recent presidential campaign Governor Dewey seemed to go to each city where Truman had been shortly before, the President said in one of his witty speeches, "I went into consultation with the White House physician and I told him that I kept having the feeling that wherever I went there was somebody following behind me. The White House physician told me not to worry. He said, 'You keep right on your way. There's one place where that fellow's not going to follow you and that's into the White House'" (12). Truman identifies himself with a deluded patient, because of the common characteristic of deluded patients—the feeling that somebody is following them. The doctor reassures the patient: the follower will not come into the White House.

From all these examples it is apparent that a joke is in a certain way a means of proving something, sustaining an allegation or a desire. The sustaining of the story is made possible by the adoption of special intellectual mechanisms. At times these mechanisms consist of archaic processes called paleologic, at other times of transitional methods from paleologic to logic, at other times of logical processes with false premises, or of logical ways of thinking, different from those generally accepted. In special cases the technique consists in comparing two different ways of thinking and in the rejection of one of them.

The importance of the intellectual part of the joke cannot be overlooked, because it is *exclusively* upon it that the joke is based from a *formal* point of view.

GRATIFICATIONS OF TENDENCIES IN WIT

Even more important, however, is the content of the joke, that something which has to be proved, those tendencies and emotions which seek gratification. The formal mechanisms which have been described represent wit-work, which, like dream-work, transforms the content of the joke into one which is more acceptable. Whereas the dream is only for the dreamer and is to be accepted only by the unconscious of the dreamer, the joke has to be accepted *socially* and has to be understood by others. This social characteristic of the joke prevents complicated wit-work or an intense distortion such as occurs in dreams. Both the repression and the gratification achieved in the joke are not so marked as in dreams. The gratification is due to the fact that oral expression of the forbidden becomes permissible, and with this oral expression a certain excitement and release of emotions is obtained. What are the tendencies whose gratification is sought by means of witticisms? They are several. One of the most common is sexual in nature. Frank admission of sexual drives, as well as of sexual exposure and consummation, is made possible in telling a joke. That sexual jokes are extremely numerous is understandable because of the repression to which sexual drives are subjected in our society. However, since the repression in the joke is very weak, sexual jokes too are forbidden in numerous milieus and, of course, all of them cannot be published. Homosexual jokes are relatively rare because the repression in the joke is indeed too feeble to compensate for the ostracism to which this form of sexuality is subjected. It is possible that in the future, because of the changing concepts of our sexual code, sexual jokes will become at first more numerous even in conservative environments, and then will decrease considerably in number, because sexuality will not be strongly inhibited and there will be less necessity to find gratification by this method. As far as the technique is concerned, sexual jokes do not differ from others. Often they resort to very primitive paleological laws, as in the following example taken from Freud. *A wealthy but elderly gentleman showed his devotion to a young actress by many lavish gifts. Being a respectable girl, she tried to discourage his attentions by telling him that her heart was already given to another man. "I never aspired as high as that," was his polite answer.* The technique of this joke consists of the paleological identification of two concepts, because they have the same verbalization in the word "high." The gentleman used the word in an anatomical sense and not in a figurative sense as he pretends. The latent meaning of the joke is obviously this: "Let's do away with this false sentimentality. My attentions are caused only by my physical desire for you."

A second group of jokes, perhaps even larger than the group with sexual content, consists of what may be called hostile jokes. In these jokes the tendency is toward the expression of anger, enmity, disparagement, and denigration. It is not a surprise to find so many hostile jokes, since civilization requires repression of hostility as much as of sexuality. The target of hostility in the joke is attacked not directly, but through wit-work. The reader will remember the witticism about the husband who manifests his feeling toward his wife by agreeing with the physician about her looks. Heine's joke about the Venus de Milo and the "tête-à-bête" joke have a similar tendency. Jokes expressing rebellion against socially-recognized authority may be included under this category. The new crop of jokes about psychiatrists, which has appeared recently in the American press, expresses the resentment about the prominent position that psychiatry has acquired as a social science. "Psychiatrists may be fooled too," imply all these jokes. One of them has already been reported in this paper. The joke about the Duke of Würtemberg who wants to embarrass the dyer also expresses resentment against authority. The dyer actually outsmarts the duke and tells him in a latent way: "You are a duke and I am one of your poor subjects, whom you want to confuse and mock; but in reality you are more stupid than I am." When Germany and Italy were under fascist domination, jokes manifesting resentment against the dictators and their stooges were very numerous in those countries. The reader remembers the joke about Mussolini visiting an insane asylum. But even in our democratic way of living repressed hostility is a matter of everyday life, both within the family and in society at large. In many situations the joke has become an actual act of hostility, ranging through a gamut of variegated tonalities, from bland teasing to vitriolic contumely. The schizoid personality, which is particularly sensitized to environmental hostility, is often said to have no sense of humor. This is because the schizoid, alert as he is to external antagonism, is not deceived by wit-work and recognizes the hostile element in wit.

It may not be out of place to mention that those parents and teachers who have always frowned upon any form of physical punishment have instead often applied punishment by the use of witticism or by emphasis on the comical aspect of situations. Confucius himself is said to have used humorous reproof as an educational method about 2500 years ago. In spite of our respect for Confucius, it must be stated that the effects of this method are at times even more paralyzing and disturbing than other types of punishment, as disclosed by patients under intensive psychotherapy.

Hostility due to prejudices may also be ventilated through jokes, as revealed by the following example. *A Jewish gardener answered an advertisement for a job in a nunnery. The Mother Superior told him that since he was Jewish she'd have to give him a week of trial service. At the end of the week the Mother Superior came up to the gardener and said, "Well, you have done pretty good, but there are several habits I want you to lose. I don't mind so much your lighting cigarettes from the holy candles, or washing your hands in the holy water, but, for God's sake, stop calling me 'Mother Shapiro.' "* This joke, apparently innocent and harmless, may have an anti-Semitic touch. What is its latent meaning? It is the same accusation made time and again that Jews do not want to lose their Jewish habits and traditions, even when these are sharply contrasting with those of the gentile society in which they live. The gardener should be very grateful to the Mother Superior. Though he is Jewish, he has found employment in a Catholic cloister, a place where it is hardly conceivable that a Jew would be hired. He should feel a sense of obligation and try to conform as much as possible. What does he do instead? He lights his cigarettes from the holy candles and washes his hands in the holy water. These habits are overlooked by the Mother Superior because they disclose only his poor judgment. What the Mother Superior cannot tolerate is her being called "Mother Shapiro." Shapiro is a common Jewish name, and the gardener, who is used to pronouncing it, confuses it paleologically with "Superior." Even in the cloister which has been so generous to him, he remains a typical Jew.

In a third important, though not quite so numerous, group of jokes, the tendency which wants to be expressed is the assertion of one's rights or the frank admission of human frailty as a truth which has to be accepted and defended. This tendency, though justified, has to be repressed generally on account of the pattern of living which civilization imposes upon us. Typical of this group is the above-mentioned joke of the man who was caught by the creditor in the act of eating salmon with mayonnaise. The debtor had to resort to wit-work in order to assert his human right and defend his wish to eat salmon with mayonnaise once in a while. To him this desire had the validity of a truth. Several jokes, especially those belonging to this group, assert what may be considered "natural truths." In a certain way they are reminiscent of those dreams, which as Fromm (11) teaches, do not express the fulfillment of irrational and immoral wishes but the fulfillment of some of our good impulses which, for social reasons, have to be repressed. They also show that, at least in some cases, the assertion of Gregory (6) that "wit is a quick, vivid illumination of a truth" is correct. Also the assertion of Froeschels (7), mentioned in the introductory paragraph—that witticisms are means by which philosophical truths congenitally known but not yet expressed become "ripe for expression"—appears now much more plausible.

A fourth group which is quite common consists of jokes which tend to repress, because unrealistic, the tendency of the inadequate man to cover his own inadequacy. This tendency, like the others, is not really fulfilled in the joke, which therefore in a certain way becomes a hostile joke. Nevertheless, since it is especially the covering of one's inadequacy which is emphasized in these jokes, I think they deserve to be classified in a special group. There is an example in Koestler. *"Mr. Dupont, an elderly notary, has for years suffered from the annoying habits of his clerk Jules. Returning home unexpectedly from a journey he finds Jules in bed with his wife. Mr. Dupont surveys the scene with a mournful eye and says, 'That's enough Jules! Once more and you're fired'"* (8).

According to one way of thinking, the notary's action is logical. The clerk is warned. If he makes the same mistake again, he will be fired. But according to another way of thinking, more acceptable to our society, Mr. Dupont should have been more energetic and found an immediate and more drastic punishment for Jules. The faithfulness of one's wife is connected with one's honor in our society, and one is expected to defend it with all his power. But Mr. Dupont is an inadequate man, too weak to defend his honor by drastic action, and what he really wishes is just to find a method to keep peace and save appearances. He resorts to a method which is logical according to a certain way of thinking: warning the clerk.

These four tendencies are, in my opinion, the principal ones but probably there are many more. Often more than one of these tendencies are combined in the same joke; at times even all four. An example is found, for instance, in the joke of the tall woman who sues the short man on the charge of rape. In this joke, there is certainly a sexual exposure, which satisfies the sexual tendency. There is also hostility for women, for the joke illustrates very well what many men think of such charges made by women —that sexual intercourse with conscious adult females is not possible without her consent, or without a certain degree of acquiescence. From the point of view of the man there is assertion of his own right; he is unfairly accused of having raped the woman. Finally, the joke shows how the woman attempts to cover up her own inadequacy or the inadequacy of her story.

The study of the repressed tendencies in jokes is useful in considering the repressing activities of the psyche in general. Every generalization is liable to lead to error; however, if one were to attribute to the psyche in general what has been noted in this study of jokes, it would appear that the sexual instinct is only one of the tendencies which are repressed. Hostility, self-assertion, and covering up of one's inadequacies seem to play important roles too. Of course these tendencies do not appear repressed or distorted in jokes as they would appear in dreams or in the unconscious; one may say that in wit only a futile attempt to repress is made. The tendency to cover up one's inadequacy, which is expressed in many jokes, is perhaps comparable to those so-called defenses of the ego which appear in every analysis.

SPECIAL CASES OF WIT AND RELATED FORMS OF EXPRESSION

This presentation would be far from complete if certain special types of witticism and kindred expressions were not considered, for instance, the witticisms usually called puns. The reader will remember one about the play which had to be rewritten and was "rerotten." Another example may be taken from another speech of President Truman's, delivered during a political campaign. Alluding to the fact that the Gallup and other private polls, which predicted the victory of his opponent, discouraged Democrats from going to vote on election day, he called them "sleeping polls" (13). He obviously meant that they acted as sleeping *pills*. Other examples, mentioned by Freud, are the Latin *"Amantes-Amentes"* (Lovers-Lunatics) and the Italian *"Traduttore-Traditore"* (Translator-Traitor). All these examples are witty, and yet they decrease, in the order they are presented here, in comic content. What meanings do these expressions really convey? The play is both rewritten and "rerotten"; the polls are in a certain way (sleeping) pills; the lovers (amantes) act foolish and therefore are like lunatics (amentes); the translator (traduttore) does not convey the real meaning of the original text, and he is therefore a traitor (traditore). It is obvious that in these examples the latent meaning is sustained not only by the paleological identification; in other words there is no contrast between the logical and the paleological stream of thought. The paleological identification is used either to add something to the logical meaning or to give additional support to it. These witticisms are not like that about the woman who was identified with the Venus de Milo. Such identification was only possible from an exclusively paleological point of view. In the case of the play which was rewritten and "rerotten" the meaning of the expression is still mainly sustained by paleological identification, and therefore there is still a considerable amount of wit. In fact the punster was more interested in conveying the notion that the play was "rerotten" than the notion that it was rewritten. But the more the logical meaning is accepted and the less is the need for paleological sustenance, as in the cases mentioned, then the less witty is the expression. The expression, however, acquires emphasis and strength. When the logical thought is entirely accepted, there is very little, if any, witty effect. The paleological identification mainly reinforces the expression and confers on it greater effectiveness. Modern commercial advertisements often use this paleological reinforcement. The puns or proverbs, in which the paleological meaning mainly reinforces the logical one, may be compared to those rare dreams whose manifest content coincides with the latent. A beautiful example of paleological reinforcement is found in Benjamin Franklin's historical statement "If we don't hang together, we'll hang separately." This sentence has great vigor and effect because it is both logically and paleologically correct. It has very little comical effect because the meaning is not sustained by paleologic alone. Franklin says: "We must hang anyway: let's hang together, rather than to hang separately"; but "to hang together" means to remain united, and "to hang separately" means to be executed on the gallows. This expression is particularly efficient for its unusual technique; the similar verbalization of two opposite concepts is used to emphasize one of the two concepts—namely, the impelling need to hang together.

To take another example which has been used throughout the centuries as an example of persuasive efficaciousness: In the Gospels of St. Luke, St. Mark, and St. Matthew it is written that people who wanted to confuse Jesus asked him whether it was proper to pay taxes to Caesar.

Jesus requested that the money be shown to him and then asked whose image was on the coin. They replied "Caesar's." Jesus then said, "Render therefore to Caesar the things that are Caesar's." The Gospels say that the people were astonished at such an unexpected answer, just as an increasing number of people have been throughout the centuries. But in reality there was no Aristotelian logic in what Jesus said. He had to resort to paleologic in order to sustain his point. The image on the coin was *of* Caesar only inasmuch as it represented Caesar, not because it *belonged* to Caesar. Why, then, does the story not appear humorous, in spite of its paleological foundation? This expression reinforced the already accepted fact that taxes had to be paid, in spite of the unfairness of it. It was not on the validity of Jesus' sentence that people paid taxes. The unfair tribute to Caesar had to be paid; and Jesus tried to placate the discontent of the people by showing, through a play on words, that it was right to do so.

ACCESSORY FACTORS

The emphasis given in this paper to the use of a different logic or different way of thinking in the formal technique of witticisms should not induce one to think that this is the only factor involved. There are many other mechanisms, which were first recognized by Freud. Whereas Freud thought that these factors constituted the basis of witticism, I think that they are merely accessory mechanisms which are not necessary in themselves but confer additional charm to the joke. The necessary factor in the joke remains the necessity to demonstrate something by resorting to an unusual way of thinking. For instance, what Freud calls *ambiguity* is interpreted here as the suspense and effort necessary to make the paleological identification. *Displacement* of the psychologic accent is based on the fact that often the paleological identification needs a predicate or characteristic which is a secondary one or adventitious or loosely associated to the original meaning. *Representation through the opposite* also confers charm and beauty on the joke; for example, the joke of the ugly woman who was identified with the symbol of beauty, the Venus de Milo; and the child who could not recognize the sex of people because they were naked. In these cases representation through the opposite increases the element of surprise, but the intellectual element—demonstration of something, for instance, beauty or justification of one's naïveté—is the fundamental factor. In many jokes these secondary characteristics are purposely devised and at times exaggerated in order to increase the suspense or the element of surprise. For instance in the following joke, there is an *apparent* thesis—namely, to prove how you are born either a pessimist or an optimist.

There were twins, about seven years of age. One had been born a pessimist, the other an optimist. Came Christmas and their father gave the pessimist a nice little automatic plane that, once wound, would do all sorts of tricks; and he filled the optimist's shoe with some horse manure. On Christmas morning an uncle came to visit, and asked the pessimist: "Well, how did Santa treat you?" "Terrible," was the answer, "I got a little plane that will do everything by itself—no fun for me, nothing to do." "And you?" asked the uncle of the optimist, "How was Santa with you?" "Couldn't have been nicer," said the little boy, "he brought me a little live pony; only, before I woke, unfortunately the pony ran away . . .!"

The emphasis on the opposite attitudes of the twins, confers charm on this joke. However, most of the content of this joke is technically unnecessary. The really witty part consists not in the attitude of the pessimist —mention of which may be even completely eliminated—but in the attitude of the optimist—that is, in the optimist's interpretation of the presence of manure as proof that he had received a pony as a gift. At a latent level this joke is a very pessimistic one, inasmuch as it shows how unfounded is the optimism of one of the twins. The witticism is due to the attempt of the optimistic twin to cover his own inadequacy.

Another characteristic mentioned by Freud—condensation—is a very important accessory factor. The more condensed the latent meaning, the more significant is the joke—a phenomenon found also in dreams. This condensation is due to the paleological identifications or compositions which were mentioned before. Condensation occurs also in the emotional content. For instance, in the joke about the tall woman and the short man at least four different tendencies and emotional drives are condensed.

WITTY EXPRESSING OF MENTAL AND NEUROLOGICAL PATIENTS

The present research started with the study of witty expressions in mental patients. This topic deserves to be examined in detail. I have already quoted from one of my previous works (10) the case of the schizophrenic who used to wet her body with oil because the human body was a machine and had to be lubricated. This example is typical of the apparent witticisms of schizophrenics. These witticisms are generally due to paleological identifications and to extreme literalness, which is the result of the reduction of the connotation power and of the emphasis on the verbalization. One of Levin's (14) patients thought that she was in a colored ward. Asked why she thought so, she replied, "Because I was brought here by Miss Brown" (the nurse who had accompanied her to the hospital). One of Bychowski's (15) patients, asked where her husband was, replied: "On our wedding picture." Patients make these remarks in all seriousness. The way of thinking to which the ordinary person occasionally regresses when he wants to be witty is a usual way of thinking for these patients. One should note that these apparent witticisms are present not only in schizophrenics—they are often found in other psychotic conditions. In nonschizophrenic psychoses, however, they are based on less primitive forms of thinking. When I was still a medical student, I visited the psychiatric department of the medical school, where the instructor showed me a patient who was suffering from the expansive type of general paresis. The patient boasted that he was extremely healthy, strong, enormously rich, and able to do anything he wanted. Without any tact, I asked him, "If you are in such a wonderful condition, why are you here?" "I am surprised at you," replied the patient. "Don't you know the latest news? I have been appointed director of this hospital." This may be considered a real witticism, although expressed seriously by the patient. In fact there is an attempt to explain something logically and to cover one's inadequacy. Only patients and doctors are in the hospital. Since the patient denied being a patient he had to be a doctor and of course the chief doctor.

Many expressions of mental patients are really witty because they attempt to cover the inadequacy which is due to the symptoms of the illness. These expressions are found predominantly but not exclusively in organic syndromes. In Korsakoff psychosis, senile psychosis, and cerebral arteriosclerosis we find often confabulations and expressions of a witty nature. If the patient is asked what is the date, he may reply, "I don't know; I don't read the paper." To the question, "How long have you been in the hospital?" the patient may answer, "What difference does it make?" In an apparently rational way he tries to cover his shortcomings. I have the impression that the symptom described in patients with frontal lobe tumors (called moria or with the German word "Witzelsucht") entails often the same mechanism. Such a mechanism, I feel sure, was involved in a case of this kind which I had occasion to study in detail (11). The patient was irritated at the discovery of her shortcomings and tried to cover her inadequacy with apparently witty expressions. In other cases described in the literature, the patients appear comical because of the extreme literalness of their interpretations and the general inappropriateness of their behavior. However, these patients are not willingly facetious as the textbooks say. Often they do not even know that they are facetious, but appear that way to the listener only. The same thing could be said of some epileptics in twilight states and of some mental defectives. Recently several authors, most of them writing in German, have described the symptomatology of the cerebral type of Buerger's disease. It seems that when Buerger's disease involves the brain, the patient manifests a peculiar sensation or, rather, perception of the comic (Komisches Gefühl). "It is as if the patient would think it is funny to find himself, suddenly and for a period of brief duration, unable to function intellectually as usual" (17). I have had no experience with cases of this kind and refer the reader to these original works (18).

In manics and hypomanics one finds productions which range from real witticisms to clever expressions revealing uninhibited thoughts. The following is an example. The residents of a State hospital were obliged by the chief of the service to follow a prepared outline for psychiatric examination and to do in each case a long and painstaking examination of the sensorium, even in functional cases where it was not only unnecessary but often irritating and traumatic. One of these residents was examining a hypomanic female patient, and, following the book, asked her to "name five oceans." The patient replied, "Who the hell cares for five oceans? I care for my five children." This clever and in a certain way witty reply does not represent a paleological identification, but a process intermediate between identification and association, which is often found in manics. The link, of course, is the number five, her children coincidentally being as many as the oceans. What is the latent meaning of her reply? Perhaps I may undo the laborious work of condensation and find the numerous meanings which are implied in her expression. She might be saying: "What a fool you are! You ask me these questions as if I would be here to have my education or my intelligence examined. I know I am not too well educated, but that does not matter. It is not on account of my poor education that I left my five children and came here. You better hurry and stop losing time with these silly questions. My five children need me and are anxiously waiting for me. That's my real concern at this time."

One might summarize what has been said so far by stating that the witty expressions found in schizophrenics generally consist of the application of primitive paleological mechanisms. They are not real witticisms, because there is no contrast between latent and manifest meaning, *from the point of view of the patient*. In organic psychotics witty expressions are, in a certain way, real witticisms because by means of them the patient tries to cover up his inadequacies or the symptoms of his illness. Manic patients use witty expressions whose mechanisms range from paleological to associational ways of thinking. In all these cases, however, the patient is never aware of the comical aspect of his productions.

This question of appearing facetious brings up an important problem. Very often the schizophrenic uses very primitive paleological mechanisms in order to demonstrate his point of view. At times he appears facetious to the normal listener; but often he does not appear facetious. From the foregoing, it would seem that he should appear witty each time he uses paleologic. Why is it not so? This problem is most important—so important that if no solution is found, this whole theory would have to be revised.

The explanation of this problem forces me to a consideration of the comic, of which wit is only a subcategory.

THE COMIC

The study of the nature of the comic has been undertaken by many philosophers and psychologists. Aristotle, Plato, Kant, Spencer, Freud, and many other great thinkers have tried in various ways to delve into the intricate mechanism of this purely human phenomenon. No prehuman species, as far as it is known, conceive things as comical. Koestler in a very effective way writes that "on the level of biological evolution where laughter arises, an element of frivolity seems to creep into an essentially humorless universe" (8).

In this paper, I cannot attempt to summarize even the most important theories about the comic. It would require so much space that only a monograph on the subject could do it justice. The reader is referred to the works of Greig (19) which contain an extensive bibliography. One may state, however, that although many people have tackled this problem, it is still far from being solved. Each author believes he has found the essential quality of that to which people respond with laughter, a smile, or a humorous attitude. However, when one probes the validity of each proposed theory, he sees that that theory seems correct for some particular aspect of the comic but completely wrong for others. The common denominator or stimulus to which one reacts as perceiver of the comic has not yet been found.

An observation which I made many years ago led me recently to the formulation of a theory which I am going to present here for the first time. I noticed that when Italians for the first time in their life hear or read something in the Spanish language, they start to laugh or smile— that is, they react as perceivers of a comical stimulus. Now is there anything comical in the beautiful Spanish language, which Charles V, the polyglottal emperor, called the language of the angels? Of course not. There must be therefore something in the situation which makes the Italian react this way to the Spanish language. An Italian who listens to Spanish for the first time recognizes that he is listening to a foreign language with different grammar and different vocabulary. And yet the two languages, in spite of the differences, are so similar that an Italian is often able to understand the meaning of what is said. In other words, an Italian often understands the meaning not because he has studied Spanish, but because he knows Italian. He is prepared to respond to Spanish but he often finds himself responding to Italian—the Italian which appears in the Spanish—and he experiences a comical sensation.

This observation led me to formulate the following hypothesis: *A subject is a perceiver of a comical stimulus when he is set to react to A and then finds himself reacting to B, on account of a confusion between the identity and the similarity of A and B.* *

In order to see whether this theory is valid in other comical situations, I shall begin with the most comical instance, the mistaken identity of persons. Let us take for example Shakespeare's "The Comedy of Errors," which is perhaps the most comical work of the great dramatist. What happens in this play? Two brothers, unknown to each other, are identical twins, and are continuously confused with each other, even by their wives. To increase the confusion they have the same name, one being referred to as Antipholus of Ephesus and the other as Antipholus of Syracuse. Each Antipholus has a servant who is an identical twin of his brother's servant. Each servant is called Dromio. The situation is

---

* The non-philosophically minded reader may think that in my views on paleological thinking and on the comic too much importance is attributed to the concepts of identity and similarity. But it is exclusively on the ability to compare and to identify that logical thought is based. James wrote: "Logic has been defined as the 'substitution of similar,' and in general one may say that the perception of likeness and unlikeness generates the whole of 'rational' or 'necessary' truth" (W. James, *Some Problems of Philosophy;* New York, Longmans, Green & Co., 1911). Jackson wrote (5) : "The process of all thought is 'stereotypic' or 'diplopic,' being the tracing of relations of resemblance and difference."

According to the law, which logicians generally call Leibniz's law, "x is identical to y if x has every property that y has and y has every property that x has." Von Domarus' law, which the paleologician follows, can be reformulated in the following way: "x is identical to y if x has at least one property that y has and y has at least one property that x has."

My theory about the comical may then be reformulated in the following way: "A subject is a perceiver of a comical stimulus when he realizes that he is identifying x with z not in accordance with Leibniz's law but in accordance with Von Domarus' law."

extremely comical and causes the audience to roar with laughter, because when one thinks he is reacting to the presence of Antipholus of Ephesus he is instead reacting to Antipholus of Syracuse, and vice versa. When the audience thinks it is in the presence of one servant, it is in the presence of the other servant. The wife of one of the twins allows certain intimate expressions to a man whom she thinks is her husband, but this man does not even know her. This comedy of Shakespeare's is a very close imitation of the comedy of Menaechmi by the Latin Plautus (254-184 B.C.). Plautus in his turn imitated the Greek Menander (343-291 B.C.).

The error or misidentification of person is from ancient times one of the most powerful stimuli of the comical. The simplest form of mistaken identity of A for B occurs in the case of two persons who look very much alike—as with identical twins. Even today in plays, movies, and vaudeville shows, twins appear frequently as a source of the comic. The comical element is maintained if the two persons are identified not only because they look alike, but, for instance, because they have a predicate in common, as when A has the same name or dress as B, or is located geographically in a place where B is supposed to be.

The audience tends to laugh when a character C, in a theatrical performance, is set to react to A and instead reacts to B, thinking that B is A. The audience does not accept C's apparent paleological identification of A and B; therefore, the spectators laugh. Moreover, the spectators themselves are set to react to A but find themselves reacting to B; they become aware of the mistaken identity and laugh. The performer C, however, allegedly does not know that the person whom he thinks is A really is B; so he cannot laugh. He continues to identify paleologically—somewhat like the schizophrenic. It is because the audience cannot accept the paleological identification. that it continues to laugh.

I would now like to examine what happens in other comical situations. The intensity of the comic persists but is diminished when A and B are in the same person. For instance, in plays and masquerades there is a tenuous comical elements because we know that the person who acts or is dressed like A is not A but B. In the horse pantomime we laugh because we are set to react to a horse and instead find ourselves reacting to two men functioning as the legs of the horse. In the caricature we look at a picture of a person anatomically distorted, and yet recognizable. We recognize the similarity in the dissimilar. The caricature uses exaggeration of traits to make a B of an A, but in spite of the deformation we recognize A and laugh. Images seen in distorting mirrors produce the same effect. We react comically also to a photographic picture which has not turned out well. Generally we react comically to the inadequate but only when the inadequate has unconsciously deceived us in the paleological identification. For instance, a child who uses big words like a grown-up makes us smile because at first we react to him as to a man and then we realize that he is not a man. In a certain way, however, we feel that there is a man in him; this feeling is furthermore reinforced because we know that a child is potentially a grown-up. We are deceived until we focus our attention on the fact that he is a child.

Now I want to examine again what happens in the perception of wit, which in my opinion is one of the highest types of the comic. *One is a perceiver of a witty stimulus when he is set to react to logic and then realizes that instead he is reacting to paleologic or to other forms of thinking.*

I have tried to show in the foregoing how important is the intellectual process in wit. The listener is temporarily deceived because unconsciously somehow he apprehends the intellectual process of the joke as logical. Almost immediately, however, he realizes that it is not logical at all, and he laughs. The listener discovers that he is not reacting to A but to B—not to logic, but to paleologic or to faulty logic. Logic, faulty logic, and a paleologic are very similar, and may deceive us as do identical twins. It is just a temporary deception, however. As soon as we become aware of it, we laugh. If we know that we are going to listen to a joke, we prepare ourselves to be temporarily deceived. Wit, therefore, distinguishes itself from the comic in general inasmuch as the confusion between A and B takes place in the realm of logic. It is true that some jokes are not only witty but also comical in a more general sense. This is due to the fact that often the confusion necessarily involves not only logic and paleologic but some specific elements of the joke.

Now it is possible to understand why every paleological expression of the schizophrenic is not laughable. The language of the schizophrenic is often so remote from reality that no similarity or possibility of confusion with logic is left. Only when such confusion is possible are his expressions both paleological and witty.

COMIC AND WIT AS INTERPERSONAL AND CULTURAL MANIFESTATIONS

The interpersonal aspect of the comic and of wit were also studied by Freud. He made an important observation in comparing the comic and wit: Whereas in the comical situation only two persons are necessary—the observer and the object in which the observer finds something comical—in wit generally an interplay of three persons occurs—the person who tells the joke, the hero in the joke, and a third person who is the listener. It is true that a person may enjoy reading a joke with nobody present, but in the typical situation a third person is expected to be present. In my opinion Freud has not explained adequately why this third person is, if not necessary, at least important in the wit situation and not in the comical. I think that the reason for this phenomenon has to be found in the nature of wit itself. In wit an attempt is made to demonstrate something by resorting to some kind of intellectual process. This something— that is, the theme of the joke—has to be demonstrated to a somebody who is generally represented by the third person. When the third person explodes in laughter, he shows that for a moment he has been deceived by the logic of the joke and that he has been able to correct himself.

In my discussion on the gratifications of tendencies achieved through wit, the importance of this form of expression as an interpersonal agent could not be overlooked. It is obvious that witticisms are used by people to convey to each other not only pleasure and laughter but, in a subtle way, intimate truths, resentment, and hostility, or, from a general point of view, to express feelings and ideas that culture forbids. Thus wit becomes a cultural manifestation. It would be interesting to study the types of wit occurring in cultures different from ours. My limited knowledge of anthropology does not allow me to state whether such a study has ever been made. My guess is that probably sexual jokes may be absent or completely different in cultures which have sexual codes different from ours. On the other hand, since any organized society, no matter how primitive, necessitates repression of hostility among the members of the same group, it is probable that jokes with hostile tendencies are present in every society.

Studies of the comic in the various subgroups of the Western society have been done. Eysenck (7) stated that "the agreement found between different nationals is far more striking than are the differences." But undoubtedly differences exist not in the fundamental principles but in accessory characteristics, such as the timing of the joke, and in the preference for certain contents. Local historical factors play an important role. For instance, when Germany and Italy were under fascist rule, an enormous number of jokes were created which expressed hostility against the tyrannies. Literary traditions influence culture. Thus, the fact that in England, the United States, and other English-speaking countries, a joke is interpolated as comic relief in a serious situation—such as in a lecture, political speech, diplomatic discussion, and so on—probably originated with Shakespeare. Ignoring Aristotle's principles about the classic drama, the great Elizabethan mixed comic scenes in the tragic context and, as it was said, mingled kings with clowns. Neither the French Corneille and Racine nor the Italian Alfieri would dare to do so. The result is that even today in Anglo-Saxon countries the interpolation of a comic element in the middle of a serious situation is not only permissible but also appreciated, whereas in a French or Italian environment it may be considered completely out of place and incongruous to do so. In German-speaking countries the tradition is intermediate between the Anglo-Saxons and the Latin countries.

Another important point in the study of wit as a cultural manifestation is the use of it as expression of social prejudices. The common use of Jewish jokes as manifestation of anti-Semitism has already been mentioned. This problem is complicated by the fact that Jews themselves seem to create anti-Jewish jokes. How is this to be explained? Freud himself attempted to give an explanation. He thought that Jewish jokes made up by non-Jews are nearly all brutal, whereas Jewish jokes originating with Jews are sincere admittance of one's real shortcomings. Freud then adds, "I do not know whether one often finds a people that makes merry so unreservedly over its own shortcomings." This explanation of Freud seems to me unsatisfactory. Granted that Jewish jokes originated by non-Jews are more offensive than those originated with Jews, the fact remains that even the latter may be offensive. Jews know that even mild jokes dealing with dirtiness and thriftiness may be used by anti-Semites as a disparaging weapon.

I have the feeling that this habit of the Jews is paradoxically an unconscious defense against anti-Semitism. Aware as they have been in the course of centuries of the great hostility by which they were surrounded, the Jews have tried to make the gentiles discharge their hostility by means of these not too harmful jokes. It is better to be accused of stinginess and dirtiness than of ritual murder. It is better to be laughed at than to be massacred. Freud is right in being surprised at this tendency of the Jews. The peculiarity of this tendency is due to the peculiarity of the history of the Jewish people.

Something similar to this, though on a much lesser scale, I have noted among Italians in New York City. In some sections of New York City, where there is a prejudice against Italians, I have seen vaudeville shows, performed by Italians, in which Italian characteristics like the excessive eating of spaghetti and the poor pronunciation of English were made fun of. Again, it is better to be accused of eating too much spaghetti than of being gangsters. Similar jokes about Italians would horrify an audience in Italy. If my impression is correct, Jewish jokes should be or should quickly become very unpopular in the new state of Israel. Just as a patient may accuse himself in order to placate his cruel superego, so social groups under environmental stress may resort to the neurotic social defense of creating self-accusatory jokes.

CONCLUDING REMARKS

I hope that this presentation has at least revealed how complicated are the phenomena of wit and of the comic. Human emotions, repressed with Freudian mechanisms, and formal intellectual processes—ranging from the stern logic of Aristotle to that of Marie Antoinette, who thought people could eat cake if they had no bread, or even to that of the schizophrenic who confuses identity with similarity—may meet in the most casual witticism to confer on it artistic creativeness in what would be a trivial occurrence, an element of truth in the midst of absurdity, a great deal of doubt and a touch of belief, explosive laughter and hidden tears. But what may be even more important is the attempted demonstration of the fact that certain phenomena, such as the comic and wit, which seem irrational or not logically understandable and therefore seem to pertain to the realm of philosophy, are in reality psychological issues.

What is not understandable logically is not necessarily transcendental, but may pertain to archaic psychological mechanisms, some of which in the history of the human race have been diverted from their original goals.

REFERENCES

1. FREUD, S.: Wit and its relation to the unconscious. In *The Basic Writings of Sigmund Freud*. New York: Modern Library, 1938. All the quotations from this book are reproduced with the permission of Routledge and Kegan Paul, Ltd., London, holders of the copyright.
2. FISCHER, K.: Quoted by Freud. Reference footnote 1.
3. PAUL, J.: Quoted by Freud. Reference footnote 1.
4. KRAEPELIN, E.: Quoted by Freud. Reference footnote 1.
5. JACKSON, J. H.: An address on the psychology of joking, *British Medical Journal,* Oct. 22, 1887. Reprinted in *Selected Writings of John Hughlings Jackson*, Vol. 2. London: Hodder and Stroughton, 1932, p. 359.
6. GREGORY, J. C.: *The Nature of Laughter*. London: Kegan Paul, Trench, Trubner & Co. Ltd., 1924.
7. FROESCHELS, E.: *Philosophy of Wit*. New York: Philosophical Library, 1948.
8. KOESTLER, A.: *Insight and Outlook*. New York: The Macmillan Company, 1949.
9. FREUD, S.: *General Introduction to Psychoanalysis*. New York: Garden City Publishing Co., 1949.
10. ARIETI, S.: Special logic of schizophrenic and other types of autistic thought. *Psychiatry*, 11:325-338, 1948.

11. Unpublished lectures given in a course on theory and practice of dream interpretation, 1948, at the William Alanson White Institute of Psychiatry in New York City.
12. Speech delivered in New York City, Oct. 28, 1948.
13. Speech delivered in Cleveland, Oct. 26, 1948.
14. LEVIN, M.: On the causation of mental symptoms. *J. Mental Sci.* 82:1-127, 1936.
15. BYCHOWSKI, G.: Physiology of schizophrenic thinking. *J. N. and M. Disease*, 98: 368-386, 1943.
16. ARIETI, S.: Frontal lobe tumor expanding into the ventricle: Clinicopathologic Report. *Psychiatric Quart.*, 17:227-240, 1943.
17. CARRERA, E.: Sintomatologia psichica del 'Buerger cerebrale.' *Rivista Patologia Nervosa e Mentale*, 69:475-480, 1948.
18. For complete bibliography on the cerebral type of Buerger disease. See E. Carrara, "Sul 'Buerger' cerebrale." *Rivista Patologia Nervosa e Mentale*, 69:13-43, 1948.
19. GREIG, J. Y. T.: *The Psychology of Laughter and Comedy*. London: Allen & Unwin, 1923.

27

The Rise of Creativity: From Primary to Tertiary Process

This paper, written 14 years after the previous one, continued the work presented there and advances the concept of the tertiary process.

I

AN ATTEMPT will be made in this paper to show how some studies of the primary process may lead to a broader understanding of the creative process.

Many years ago, while studying schizophrenic thought, I became convinced that this type of thinking, which I called paleologic, followed an immature form of cognitive organization, which could be included in Freud's concept of the primary process. While Freud (8) and his followers (11) were mainly interested in studying the primary process as a carrier of unconscious motivation and as a consumer of psychic energy, I became particularly involved with the study of the organization of this type of thinking (3).

By the term "creative process," I mean, to borrow an expression used in a different context by von Bertalanffy (14), the process by which man tries to transcend the usual psychological formula Stimulus-Response. Although there is a fundamental difference between the infrahuman animal which has a limited number of responses and the symbol-making human being (9), we must admit that man too tends to respond in fixed ways. Whether his response occurs immediately after the stimulus or whether it follows a complicated set of symbols and of choices, man tends to react in accordance with a repertory of responses provided by his usual psychological faculties or by ways which have become the common style of his culture. If his responses are mediated by cognitive processes, those generally follow what Freud called the secondary process, which corresponds to what logicians call Aristotelian logic or our ordinary logical thinking.

The creative process allows man to liberate himself from the fetters of these secondary process responses. But creativity is not simply originality and freedom. It is more than that: it also imposes restrictions. First of all, although it uses methods other than the secondary process, it must not be in disagreement with the secondary process. Otherwise the result would be bizarre, not creative. Secondly, it must attain an additional aim: a desirable enlargement of human experience—either aesthetic pleasure, as in art, or usefulness, understanding and predictability, as in science. Thirdly, the creative process tends to fulfill a longing or a search for a new object or for a state of experience or of existence which is not easily found or easily attainable. Especially in aesthetic creativity, the work often represents not only the new object but this longing, this indefinite search, this sustained and yet never completed effort, with either a conscious or unconscious motivation.

One of the main ways in which the creative process operates is by using the primary process. The primary process which seemed relegated to pathology or to the unconscious, re-emerges instead as an innovating power.

The relations between the primary process and the creative process are many. I shall focus my presentation on one of these relations, identification based upon similarity. For the sake of clarity and continuity, I shall summarize some concepts already presented in my writings on schizophrenia (1, 3, 4, 5).

The seriously ill schizophrenic, although living in a state of utter confusion, tries to recapture some understanding and to give organization to his fragmented universe. This organization is to a large extent reached by connecting things which have similar parts in common. Many patients force themselves to see similarities everywhere. In their relentless search for similarities they see strange coincidences, that is, similar elements occurring in two or more instances at the same time or at brief intervals. By considering these similarities as identities they attempt to find some clarity in the confusion of the world, a solution for the big jigsaw puzzle.

A red-haired young woman in a post partum schizophrenic psychosis developed an infection in one of her fingers. The terminal phalanx was swollen and red. She told me several times, "This finger is me." Pointing to it she said, "This is my red red and rotten head." She did not mean that her finger was a symbolic representation of herself, but in a way incomprehensible to us, really herself or an actual duplicate of herself. Another patient believed that the two men she loved in her life were actually the same person, although one lived in Mexico City and the other in New York. In fact both of them played the guitar and both of them loved her. Another example that I often quote is that of a patient who thought she was the Virgin Mary. Asked why, she replied, "I am a virgin; I am the Virgin Mary."

Many patients at this stage of regression indulge in an orgy of identifications. The patient tries to find glimpses of regularities in the midst of the confusion in which he lives. He tends to register identical segments of experience and to build up systems of regularity upon them. Not only does he experience an increased immediate grasping of similarity but he responds to such similarities as if they were identities. If we want a logical formulation for this disorder we could say, with Von Domarus, that, "Whereas the normal person accepts identity only upon the basis of identical subjects the schizophrenic, when he thinks in a typical schizophrenic way, accepts identity based on identical predicates" (15). In other words, in the primary process type of organization, similarity becomes identity. In Aristotelian logic, only like subjects are identified. The subjects are fixed; therefore, only a limited number of deductions are possible. In paleologic thinking the predicates lead to the identification. Since the predicates of the same subject are numerous, the deduction reached by this type of thinking is not easy to predict. The choice of the predicate which will lead to the identification is psychodynamically determined by conscious or unconscious motivational trends.

This cognitive organization of the primary process is susceptible of different interpretations which actually refer to the same phenomena. We may, for instance, state that the primary process organizes classes or categories which differ from those of secondary process thinking. In secondary process thinking a class is a collection of objects to which a concept applies. For instance, Washington, Adams, Jefferson, etc., form a class of objects to which the concept "President of the United States" applies. In paleologic or primary process thinking a class is a collection of objects which have a predicate or part in common (for instance, the state of being virgin), and which, therefore, become identical or equivalent. The formulation of a primary class is often an unconscious mechanism. Whereas the members of a secondary process class are recognized as being similar (and it is actually on their similarity that their classification is based), the members of a primary class are freely interchanged; for instance, the patient becomes the Virgin Mary.

Another characteristic of the paleologic organization is the change in the significance of words. They lose part of their connotation; they may not refer to a class any more, but the verbalization, that is, the word, as a phonetic entity, independently of its meaning acquires prominence. Other primary process mechanisms may take place after attention has been focused on verbalization. In many expressions of patients who think paleologically two or more objects or concepts are identified because they can be represented by the same word. The verbal symbol thus becomes the identifying predicate. This leads to what seems to be plays on words. For instance, a patient who was asked to define the word "life" started to define *Life* magazine. An Italian patient, whose name was Stella, thought she was a fallen star. Another patient thought she was black like the night. Her name was Laila, which means night in Hebrew.

II

Freud developed his concepts about the primary process first in his studies on dreams, and later he applied them to his studies of psychoneurotic symptoms. He opened a direct path toward the understanding of the creative process with his book on the psychology of wit. Freud (7) became interested in the problem of wit when he noticed that certain dreams resembled jokes, especially when they were interpreted. He did not disregard this apparently accidental similarity and on studying this problem discovered numerous analogies between wit and dreams. In wit as in dreams, Freud focused his attention on the unconscious motivation of the joke—a very important point indeed. However, he made a rather hasty analysis of the formal mechanisms of the joke.

Let us examine some examples of jokes, quoted by Freud. One of them is a famous witticism of the poet Heine, who in talking about a lady, said, "This woman is like the Venus de Milo in many ways. Like her, she is extremely old, has no teeth, and has spots on the yellow surface of her body." Freud believed that the technique of this joke consists of "representation through the opposite." Ugliness is made to agree with the most beautiful. I believe that trying to identify a subject with its opposite reinforces the effect of the joke, but that the fundamental factor in this joke is the possibility of identifying two apparently unidentifiable subjects. Heine in reality wanted to say of a particular woman that she was ugly. The artistic method he resorted to, to carry this meaning, was indeed unpredictable and bizarre; he identified the ugly woman with the most beautiful—the Venus de Milo. How could this logically impossible identification be made? By abandoning Aristotelian logic and reverting to the paleologic of the primary process, like the logic of the schizophrenic. The woman and the statue of Venus are identical because they have some predicates or parts in common, namely being old, having no teeth, and having spots on the yellow surface of their bodies.

To take another example from Freud, a joke which was very common at the time of the trial of Dreyfus, the French Jew unjustly accused of treason by the French Army. "That girl reminds me of Dreyfus. The army does not believe in her innocence." Freud believed that the technique of this joke is mainly that of ambiguity, but it is obvious that here again an improbable identification is made. Dreyfus and the girl are identified because they have a common predicate, "innocence not believed in by the army." The predicate is common to both subjects only as the same verbalization is applied to two different concepts. In fact, in the case of Dreyfus, innocence means "state of not being guilty of treason"; in the case of the girl it means "lack of sexual experience." Also the word "army" has a different slant in the two cases. In the case of Dreyfus, it means "general staff"; in the case of the girl it means "group of men," with emphasis on their being male. We see thus how identity based only upon a similarity of a part or a predicate is an important formal component of jokes. However, as I have discussed in much greater detail elsewhere (2), the cognitive mechanisms of witticisms are more complicated in some cases. Let us examine another joke, this time not from Freud.

> A woman sues a man by whom she claims she has been raped. The plaintiff and the defendant are in front of the judge. The judge looks at both of them and sees that the woman is tall and stout, the man short and thin. With some astonishment he asks the woman, "Is this the man who raped you? How did he do it?"
>
> The woman answers, "He pushed me against a wall and raped me."
>
> "How it it possible?" adds the perplexed judge. "You are so tall and he is so short!"
>
> "Well," says the woman, "I bent my knees a little bit."

The woman is logical. If she bends her knees, the sexual act is possible. In the attempt to use logic in self-defense, however, she accuses herself, because the bending of the knees implies her willingness to be a partner and automatically excludes the act of rape. Though in this case no paleologic is involved, it is still the logical mechanism which is the basis of the joke—a logical mechanism which is used by the woman in self-defense and which, on the contrary, turns out to be a self-accusation.

This example shows that in some jokes faulty cognitive mechanisms, which technically belong to the secondary process, are used instead of primary process mechanisms. These faulty mechanisms consist at times of correct logical processes which are based on false premises; at other times of logical ways of thinking which implicitly invalidate the allegation made or prove only an inconsequential issue. These faulty mechanisms are used not only in jokes, but also in rationalizations of normal as well as psychoneurotic and psychotic persons, who want to defend an allegation, a hostile attitude or a desire (6).

I must be clearer on a specific point in order to avoid conveying a wrong impression. It has not been suggested here that the witty characeristic of the joke is due simply to the use of primary process paleologic or to faulty logic. More than that is necessary. Let us examine again the Dreyfus joke and let us assume that the girl who was identified with Dreyfus was Jewish. If a person had said, "This girl has something in common with Dreyfus; she is Jewish," this would have been a logically correct statement but platitudinous. It would have been a statement made with the application of a secondary mechanism. Let us assume that a schizophrenic patient had said, "This girl is Dreyfus; she is Jewish." This would be a paleologic primary process identification because of a common predicate (being Jewish). This statement would be delusional but not witty.

Thus, it is not the use of primary process paleologic or of faulty logic which confers the witty characer to the joke. In my opinion, *one perceives a stimulus as witty when he is set to react to logic and then realizes that he is instead reacting to paleologic or to faulty logic.*

The listener is temporarily deceived because he first apprehends the intellectual process of the joke as logical. A fraction of a second later, however, he realizes that the intellectual process is not logical at all, and he laughs. The listener discovers that he is not reacting to logic but either to paleologic or to faulty logic. Logic, faulty logic, and paleologic may be very similar and, when they are associated as they are in the joke, may deceive us as do identical twins. It is just a fleeting deception, however. As soon as we become aware of it, we laugh. If we know that we are going to listen to a joke, we prepare ourselves to be temporarily deceived.

In the creation of a joke, the creative process is thus based on the following facts: (1) Primary process mechanisms, or cognitive mechanisms which are usually discarded because of faults, become available to the creative person. (2) Out of those primary process and/or faulty cognitive mechanisms which have become available, the creative person is able to select those which give the fleeting impression of being valid secondary process mechanisms. The witty or comic response on the part of the listener occurs when there is recognition of logic-paleologic discordance.* The listener recognizes that what seemed a logical process is instead a primary or paleologic process, and he laughs. The creative process of wit consists in putting together the primary and secondary process mechanisms and automatically comparing them. It is the comparison which reveals the discordance and provokes laughter.

It is possible now to understand why most paleologic expressions of the schizophrenic are bizarre but not witty. The language of the schizophrenic is often so remote from reality that no similarity or possibility of confusion with logic is left. Only when such confusion is possible for the listener are expressions witty. Occasionally they are; as a matter of fact, I owe to some witty expressions of schizophrenic patients the origins of my interest in the psychology of creativity. For instance, a patient, whom I examined many years ago, had the habit of wetting her body with oil. Asked why she would do so, she replied; "The human body is a machine and has to be lubricated." The word "machine," applied in a figurative sense to the human body, had led to the identification with man-made machines.

The creative process, as we have described it, is not involved in what this patient said. She did not know that what she was saying was witty. She meant literally what she said. Her delusional remark is witty only for us. In this case we, not the patient, create the joke, because we recognize her illogicality in her apparent logicality.

It is from the appropriate matching of a secondary process mechanism with a primary process mechanism that a product of creativity emerges, that a primitive or faulty form of cognition is transformed into an innovation. I propose to use the expression "tertiary process" for this special combination of primary and secondary process mechanisms. In the different fields of creativity there are specific ways in which the secondary process is matched with the primary process so that innovation emerges.

---

* If faulty logic is used instead of paleologic, then there will be a logic-faulty logic discordance. In the following discussion, we shall take into consideration only logic versus paleologic and secondary process versus primary, because these seem the most typical and most frequent combinations in creativity. However, the same notions could be repeated for logic versus paleologic and secondary versus faulty secondary process.

We have seen that in wit the specific way consists of pairing similar logical and paleological mechanisms and in recognizing the logic-paleologic discordance. We shall now consider the specific modalities which are used in the arts and sciences.

III

In such products of creativity as puns, proverbs, parables, and even in some commercial advertisements, expressions are used in which there is no logic-paleologic discordance but the contrary, namely paleologic reinforcement. Here paleologic actually strengthens logic. The result is not humor but great verbal effectiveness.

These expressions may be compared to those rare dreams whose manifest content coincides with the latent, or to those neurotic manifestations which coincide with reality demands. A beautiful example of paleologic reinforcement is found in Benjamin Franklin's historical statement, "We must all hang together, or assuredly we shall all hang separately." This sentence has great vigor and effect because it follows both logic and paleologic. It has practically no comical effect because the meaning is not sustained by paleologic alone. Franklin wanted to convey the message, "We must remain united," but he did not use this ordinary phrase. He said instead something like this, "We must hang anyway; let's hang together rather than hanging separately"; but to "hang together" means to remain united, and "hanging separately" means to be executed on the gallows. In a fleeting preconscious moment all the meanings of the words "to hang" are identified. When they are recognized as being different, the artistic effect is experienced.

To take another example which has been considered with veneration throughout the centuries: In the Gospels it is written that people who wanted to confuse Jesus asked him whether it was proper to pay taxes to Caesar. Jesus requested that money be shown to him and then asked whose image was on the coin. They replied "Caesar's." Jesus then said, "Render therefore unto Caesar the things that are Caesar's, and to God the things that are God's." The Gospels say that the people were astonished at such an unexpected answer, just as an increasing number of people have been throughout the centuries.

Jesus' answer is enigmatic and has been interpreted in many ways. And yet we immediately perceive its great vigor and we sense that it conveys a great meaning. Why is it so? It is difficult to examine Jesus' sentence from an exclusively formal, strictly literal and concrete point of view, because as soon as we hear it we become inundated by its various and deep abstract meanings.* Nevertheless, it seems that if we make an effort we can recognize in this sentence a concrete and literal basis, as we do in parables in general. The image on the coin was Caesar's only as it represented the likeness of Caesar, not because it belonged to Caesar. In other words, only the image was Caesar's, not the ownership of the coin. Therefore, if we take this sentence in an extremely literal, concrete sense, Jesus would be wrong, having based his statement only on a play on words, on the fact that the expression "Caesar's" would paleologically acquire the meaning "being property of Caesar." The coin then would have to be given back (rendered) to Caesar, its rightful owner. But taxes would have to be paid even if the coins did not show the image of Caesar, and as a matter of fact some Roman coins did not show Caesar's image or name.

Why then does the story not appear humorous, in spite of having a partially paleologic foundation? The expression reinforced the important message that Jesus wanted to convey to the people: that money *did* belong to Caesar, not in a literal but metaphorical sense. Monies were material things and belonged more to Caesar and to the materialistic world of Rome than to the spiritual world of Jerusalem. Jesus' followers should not be concerned with such things but only with "things which are God's and must be rendered to God." Jesus was trying to placate the discontent of the people by showing, in an unusual, unpredictable way, that it was right to pay the unfair tribute to Caesar. With his words he did not show a pro-Roman attitude, nor did he come out against payment of taxes. This would have been a rebellious position. At the same time, in a new and highly artistic way, he supported the old religious Hebrew tradition which stressed the antithesis between God and Moloch. Moloch is a contemptuous word for king, a king being interested in temporal, earthly values only. In this parable, Caesar is Moloch.

We can see in this example the fusion or contemporaneous occurrence of several levels of meaning. Had Jesus resorted just to a play on words, his remarks would have been witty but not epoch-making. Had he tried to placate discontented taxpayers, his intent would have been a noble one but not a revelation. Jesus wanted to reveal what for him was the highest truth. This revelation was made not through a scientific demonstration

---

* An additional difficulty is due to the fact that in the King James version of the Bible, which imitates the Latin Vulgate translation, the word "render" is used. The verb "to render" in English has predominantly the meaning "to give," whereas in Latin, French, Italian the equivalent words used in this passage *reddere, rendre, rendere* mean to give back, to return, to make restitution of anything borrowed to its rightful owner.

but through paleologic reinforcement. Paleologic reinforcement is the opposite of logic-paleologic discordance. It does not pertain to the cosmic, but to the general realm of art, and occasionally of science, as demonstrated below.

IV

The poet too is looking for a similarity which will reinforce his theme. This occurs in that creative process called the metaphor. Aristotle wrote, "The greatest thing by far is to be a master of metaphor; it is the one thing that cannot be learnt from others; and it is also a sign of genius, since a good metaphor implies an intuitive perception of the similarity in the dissimilar." (*Poetics*, xxii).

Poetry, of course, is not based exclusively on metaphor, but metaphorical language is one of its fundamental components. Let us take as an example Blake's beautiful poem "The Sick Rose":

> O Rose, thou are sick!
> The invisible worm
> That flies in the night,
> In the howling storm,
>
> Has found out thy bed
> Of crimson joy;
> And his dark secret love
> Does thy life destroy.

Ostensibly the poem is about a beautiful flower which has been invaded and is being destroyed by an ugly worm. But there are many more levels of metaphorical meaning. What comes easily to mind is that the rose stands for a beautiful woman and that worm stands for a fatal illness which soon will destroy her. Such comparisons between flowers and women, and worms and illnesses, do not occur only in poetry but also in dreams and in schizophrenic ideation.

We have seen how in psychopathologic conditions and in dreams common predicates lead to metamorphosis, that is, to identifications of what seem to normal or waking people dissimilar subjects. In poetry there is no *metamorphosis* but *metaphor*. The poet knows that the rose is not a woman, but he feels the woman is like a rose.

In order to compare the sick flower to the sick woman the poet has accessibility to the formation of a primary class, as we have described at the beginning of this paper. As we have mentioned, a primary class consists of equivalent or interchangeable members. Now, is a primary class involved in the making of a poetic metaphor? Yes and no.

The poet does not *actually* substitute the sick rose for the sick woman. The sick rose is not the sick woman; but in the sick rose he sees the sick woman. In schizophrenia the interchangeability or displacement is complete instead of partial: for instance, in the example in which the patient becomes the Virgin Mary. In the schizophrenic the primary class of virgin women was an unconscious class.

In poetry the dipslacement, for instance, from the woman to the rose, is conscious. The poet wants to react to the sick woman as he would to a sick rose. Whereas in psychopathologic conditions and in dreams the displacement is from the real object to the symbolic, in poetry it is from the symbolic object (the rose) to the real (the woman). The difference is deeper than that. Let us take Blake's poem again. As we have already mentioned, the rose does not *replace* the woman (as the Virgin Mary replaces the patient, who is no longer the patient but who has undergone the delusional metamorphosis of becoming the Virgin Mary). In the poem we see the woman *in* the rose. The woman and the rose are fused; but it is not that bizarre fusion that we see in schizophrenic drawings and delusions. The woman and the rose, though fused, retain their individuality. The retention of their individuality permits a comparison, yet does not lead to identification. How is this possible? It is possible because by putting the sick rose and the sick woman together, we become at least partially *conscious* of a class: the class of "beautiful life destroyed by illness." As a matter of fact, it is enough for the human cognitive faculties to be aware of only two members of a class to become aware of the whole class.

But is this class primary or secondary? Both, and in a certain way, neither. In the act of being created, the class is primary. Finding common predicates among different subjects and identifying by virtue of these processes tends to remain primary: the rose and the woman tend to interchange or to remain together, but as the concept of the class "beautiful life destroyed by illness" emerges, their fusion does not become, so to say, consummated. They remain distinct. However, the level of secondary class is not reached completely in the poem, or does not remain independent from the primary process origin. The poet does not deal on a cognitive level with "beauty destroyed by illness." Only the student of art may translate the poem into a secondary level content. The poem itself oscillates between a primary level and a secondary level which is inferred. Here is thus an important difference between art and psychopathology: *Whereas in the psychopathologic use of the primary process there is no consciousness of abstraction* (as a matter of fact the power of abstraction is impaired and has to find concrete channels), *in art the use of the primary process does not eliminate the abstract. On the contrary, it is through the medium of the primary process that the abstract concept emerges.*

A physician would not compare a woman to a rose in order to clarify the outcome of a fatal illness or in order to lead to the formation of a new class. Why does a poet need a rose invaded by a worm to tell us that fatal sickness in a beautiful woman is a horrible thing? Why does he need to resort to his unusual accessibility to primary classes?

The poet discovers that things abound with similarities. New similarities take on new meanings, because each recognized similarity is a concept and implies the formation of a new class. The formation of new classes or categories is one of the main ways of expanding knowledge, which the aesthetic fields have in common with science, as we shall see below.

Let us remember what happens in jokes: the joke is based on the eventual recognition that logic and paleologic are not identical but only similar. The recognition of the logic-paleologic discordance leads to the comic reaction. In some puns and parables there is more agreement than disagreement between the logic and the paleologic. In poetry, there is agreement between paleologic and logic. Paleologic actually reinforces logic.

Art indeed is founded to a great extent on *paleologic reinforcement.* At the same time that the work of art elicits the abstract concept, it sustains itself upon the paleologic reinforcement, or identification with a concrete example. There is almost a perfect welding of the abstract concept with the concrete example: of the replaced object with its metaphor. The concrete object of the metaphor is not only a symbol, it is a participant in producing the effect. In paleologic mechanisms, as used by the schizophrenic, the object which is replaced or symbolized fades away (at least from consciousness) or is replaced by its symbol. For instance in our example the virgin patient disappears and is replaced by the Virgin Mary. In dreams, too, what is symbolized is no longer present. For instance, in a dream a gorilla may stand for one's father. The image of the father is completely absent and only psychoanalytic work can recapture it. In art the replaced object fades also, but not entirely. It fades away only in its concrete essence; its presence is felt in its absence. For instance, the woman is not mentioned in Blake's poem, but her presence is felt. She indeed exists in the artistic assumption. At the same time that she is eliminated by the art work she is there as a rose. Symbolism and reality hold hands.

There are other factors to be considered in the study of the metaphor.

In a brief poetic passage we may find only one metaphor, but in highly artistic works more than one metaphor is combined. Let us re-examine Blake's poem. We have seen that the rose stands for a beautiful woman who is sick and that we are, so to say, invited to pity the fate of this woman. In some respects this is actually a recurring theme in literature. It is enough to think of an ailing woman, named after the flowers she liked so much, *la dame aux camelias* of the French literature. We can also think of many heroines in Italian operas. In La Bohème, Mimi is not a sick flower but a sick maker of artificial flowers. Her beauty is compared to the crimson beauty of dawn and of the sunset. Something vaguely associated to this image is also found in Dante. In the first of the dreams reported in his early book *La Vita Nuova,* he describes how Beatrice appeared to him, in the arms of a male figure, Eros or Love (13). Beatrice is partially covered by a red cloth. The whole scene takes place in a cloud, red as fire. Dante knows that Beatrice is going to die because of something Love has made her eat.

In Blake's poem, however, many other metaphorical meanings are suggested. As in Dante's dream, the invader is a male (*his* dark secret love). The bed of crimson joy conveys the image of femininity and sexuality, from the point of view of a male (crimson are the cheek, lips, and perhaps the vagina of the woman). The rose becomes more female, the worm more male. Accessory predicates which lead to more identifications increase the artistic value, just as they do in jokes.

But there is much more in the poem. The invisible worm that flies in the night, in the howling storm, which with his secret love invades the bed of crimson joy and destroys life, may suggest evil producing sexuality, a sadistic passion, a "dark" love, not something appropriate for crimson joy.

At this level of understanding the poem would represent a drama between two people, woman and man, the battle of the sexes. But the poem can be interpreted at a much more abstract level, representing beauty and evil which must but cannot coexist in the same universe, as evil often ends up by destroying beauty. The worm may represent the seed of spiritual decay. And yet the worm may even appear not so evil in its evil, because it is capable of loving and it is only its love which leads to destruction.

We could find other levels of meanings. The rose and the woman appear like sisters, in the sense in which Francis of Assisi saw brotherhood and sisterhood in the disparate existences of the universe. The new class or "family," to which the rose and the woman belong, reasserts the universal encounter with life, love, sorrow, decay, and death. We enter thus into an indefinite realm of symbolism, for the classes of symbolized objects accrue by a sequence of paleologic analogies which are like more and more windows, more and more doors, which open into unguessed aspects of reality, into unpredicted worlds. In the great work of art we can seek and find more and more analogic expansions. Thus, though the new object has been found, the longing and the search continue. The finiteness of the new object contrasts with the indeterminacy of the search. And yet the search itself becomes part of the newly created work, of the new unity, an aesthetic entity which in its totality appears for the first time in the universe. This is occasionally referred to as the unfinished statement of the work of art.

We are ready to appreciate new aesthetic unities. All of us respond to phonetically beautiful words and to their rhythm; we also pity beautiful women who become sick and die; we are all concerned with evil that destroys beauty; we are also receptive to the sensuous beauty of flowers and have some distaste for earthy worms. Everything was ready for the fitting of all these elements together, but somebody had to make them click. Blake did this by blending harmoniously primary and secondary processes as in a symphony, never heard before, of unsuspected predicates. The synthesis Blake achieved can be easily communicated and shared. The originality of the new unity contrasts with the response to such a unity, which is almost a general one.

Can then a poetic fusion of primary and secondary processes be compared to a discovery? In a certain way, yes; but only to a special type. An aesthetic discovery may not make us know things that we did not know before. However, it creates a new affective experience.

Schizophrenic language and dreams, too, have different meanings and different levels of cognition. However, in psychopathological conditions these different meanings are discordant; furthermore, often they do not coexist but replace one another. That is, the dreamer and the talking schizophrenic are only aware of what they see in the dream or of what they say at a manifest level. They need the therapist to recapture all or many of the meanings. If there is a unity, it is in the atmospheric feelings or in a sort of primitive affective gestalt. Although the schizophrenic experience is also a new experience, it is actually a reduction to a concrete level, a restriction, not an enlargement, unless some new understanding or the recapturing of the abstract meaning is obtained through recovery or therapy.

At times the artist has a capacity for imagery almost to the extent that the dreamer has or that capacity for "orgies of identification" which the schizophrenic has. He is able, however, to use them in unpredictable syntheses, which become works of art. For instance, Victor Hugo in his poems compares the stars, in multiple, and, to the average person, inconceivable ways: to diamonds, other jewels, golden clouds, golden pebbles, lamps, lighted temples, flowers of eternal summer, silvery lilies, eyes of the night, vague eyes of the twilight, embers of the sky, holes in a huge ceiling, bees which fly in the sky, drops of Adam's blood, and even to the colored spots on the tail of the peacock.

v

I have re-examined the classic work on creativity by the great French mathematician Poincaré, who described accurately the moments of creative illumination that he experienced (10). In the morning, following a sleepless night spent working on a mathematical problem without finding the wanted results, he entered a bus. At the moment he put his foot on the step, the idea came to him, apparently without any conscious effort, that the transformations he had used to define the Fuchsian functions were identical with those of non-Euclidian geometry. This sudden illumination was a breakthrough leading to great expansion in the field of mathematics.

Poincaré described his subjective experiences extremely well, but he did not stress the fact that his creative insight consisted of seeing an *identity* between two previously reputed dissimilar transformations; the Fuchsian and the non-Euclidian. In the previous night, and for fourteen days prior to that night, Poincaré had accumulated facts. But accumulation of data is not yet creativity. Many people are able to accumulate facts. The creative leap occurs when observed facts are correlated, that is, when by perceiving a heretofore unsuspected identity, a conjunctive path or a new order is discovered.

We could multiply endlessly the instances where great discoveries were made by the act of perceiving an identity among two or more things which had seemed dissimilar or unrelated. Newton observed an apple falling from a tree and saw a common quality in the apple attracted by the earth and the motions of heavenly bodies. Newton perceived the similarity between two forces, that which caused an apple to fall to the earth and that which retains the moon in its orbit. He validated this insight by comparing the rate of falling bodies on the earth with the rate at which the moon deviated from the straight line which it would have followed had the earth not existed.

Darwin saw a similarity between Malthus's theories and the life of the jungle, and this association led him to conceive his theory of evolution. Freud saw similarities between dreams and jokes, and this observation opened the path to the study of the creative process.

Of course, the observation of similarity is not enough. For instance, the transformations used by Poincaré and those of non-Euclidian geometry are not in every respect identical. An apple is very dissimilar in size, origin and chemical structure from the moon, and yet Newton saw a similarity. In what way are the moon and the apple similar? What does their partial identity consist of? Of being members of a class of bodies subjected to gravitation. Thus, at the same time that Newton saw the similarity between the apple and the moon, *a new class was formed* to which an indefinite number of members could be added. The new object for which he was searching and which he found was a class.

The discovery of this class revealed a new piece of the order of the universe, because each member of the class came to be recognized as having similar properties. Is this new class a primary class, as we have described it at the beginning of this paper? Obviously not. It differs on many counts:

First, when Newton perceived the identical element he did not respond to the stimulus but to the class. Had he been a regressed schizophrenic, after seeing a similarity between the moon and the apple he could have paleologically identified the moon with the apple and could have thought that the moon could be eaten like an apple, or sucked like the maternal breast, as Renée, a by now famous schizophrenic patient reported by Sechehaye, did during a stage of her illness (12).

Second, Newton's creativity consisted in seeing a common property in the moon and the apple, and in not identifying them but in seeing them as members of a new class. An increased ability to see similarities, which is a property of the primary process, is here connected with a concept and the tertiary process emerges. The secondary class loses all its original connections with the primary process. Here too, however, although the new class is very well defined, the search is not ended. The understanding of the Newtonian system is a prerequisite to the eventual opening of the Einsteinian world of classes.

VI

We could, at this point, as a sort of summary, state that in wit an ostensibly secondary class is recognized as primary. In poetic metaphor a primary and a secondary class reinforce one another; in science what originated as a primary class proves to be a secondary class.

If now, in ensemble, we look at the three basic processes, primary, secondary and tertiary, we may conclude that an important common characteristic of them resides in the ability to differentiate similarities from manifold experience.

Similarity indicates that there is some kind of recurrence and, therefore, regularity in the universe. It is from these segments of regularity that the human mind plunges into the understanding of the cosmos. In psychopathology, normality, and creativity, the ability to register similarity is the common guiding principle—a tremulous and lonely light with which to break the secret of the universal night! It is on the varying responses to similarity that the ultimate rise or the ultimate fall of man depends. We can represent these variations by resorting to the imagery of a sentence: for the primary process all that glitters is gold. It will be the labor of the secondary process to discover that all that glitters is not gold. The tertiary process will do at least one of two things: either it will bestow the glittering of the gold to other substances to beautify them artistically or it will create a new class of glittering objects.

I might even apply these selfsame criteria to my own presentation. Have I myself been caught in the very problem with which I was groping? I have found a common characteristic in the three processes. How am I to interpret my findings? What can I do with them? Is this a delusional identification of mine, like that of the patient I mentioned at the beginning of the paper? Is it a primary process identification? Or could it be that an artistic striving, dormant since my adolescence, has rekindled in me a flair for aesthetic metaphors?

The consideration of these alternatives deals with a problem to be heeded by whosoever dares to advance new views.

REFERENCES

1. ARIETI, S.: Special logic of schizophrenic and other types of autistic thought. *Psychiat.*, 11:325, 1948.
2. ARIETI, S.: New views on the psychology and psychopathology of wit and of the comic. *Psychiat.*, 13:43, 1950.
3. ARIETI, S.: *Interpretation of Schizophrenia.* New York: Brunner, 1955.
4. ARIETI, S.: The microgeny of thought and perception. *Arch. Gen. Psychiat.*, 6:454, 1962.
5. ARIETI, S.: Studies of thought processes in contemporary psychiatry. *Amer. J. of Psychiat.*, 120:58, 1963.
6. ARIETI, S.: The schizophrenic patient in office treatment. *Psychoth. Schiz.* Karger: Basel, 1965.
7. FREUD, S.: Wit and its relation to the unconscious. In *The Basic Writings of Sigmund Freud.* New York: Modern Library, 1938.
8. FREUD, S.: *The Interpretation of Dreams.* New York: Basic Books, 1960.

9. LANGER, S. H.: *Philosophy in a New Key*. Cambridge, Mass.: Harvard University Press, 1942.
10. POINCARÉ, H.: Mathematical creation. In *The Foundation of Science*. Lancaster: The Science Press, 1946.
11. RAPAPORT, D.: Toward a theory of thinking. In: D. Rapaport (Ed.), *Organization and Pathology of Thought*. New York: Columbia University Press, 1951.
12. SECHEHAYE, M. A.: *Symbolic Realization*. New York: International Universities Press, 1951.
13. SPIEGEL, R.: *Dante's Dreams in La Vita Nuova* (Unpublished manuscript).
14. VON BERTALANFFY, L.: The mind-body problem: A new view. *Psychosom. Med.*, 24:29, 1964.
15. VON DOMARUS, E.: The specific laws of logic in schizophrenia. In J. S. Kasanin (Ed.), *Language and Thought in Schizophrenia: Collected Papers*. Berkeley: University of California Press, 1964.

28

Anti-Psychoanalytic Cultural Forces in the Development of Western Civilization

This paper, published in 1952, represents one of my early attempts to correlate socio-cultural forces with the development of psychiatry and psychoanalysis. It searches for answers to two questions: Why did a Freud appear on the world stage at the end of the nineteenth century? Why did dynamic psychiatry originate in this period and not before or later?

WHY DID FREUD appear on the world stage at the end of the nineteenth century? Why did dynamic psychiatry originate in this period and not before or later?

An historian or a sociologist could attempt to solve this problem by the usual method; that is, by investigating what chains of events or what previous discoveries were necessary for the development of psychoanalysis. This method is best illustrated by examples from the field of mathematics and physics, where it is impossible, for instance, to conceive an Einstein without a previous Newton, a Newton without a Galileo, a Galileo without a Copernicus, and so on, backward to Euclid, Archimedes and Pythagoras.

However the situation of dynamic psychiatry is different from that of physics, or any other science, including every other branch of medicine. In other words, there is no series of previous necessary discoveries which made a Freud possible only at the end of the nineteenth century, and not, let us say, in the fifteenth or twelfth century, or even before the Christian Era.

I suspect that many readers may doubt the validity of this statement. They might think that there would be no psychoanalysis without hypnosis and its application to psychiatry by the French school. Others might feel that a Charcot was necessary to orient Freud toward the psychoneu-roses. Still others might think that it is impossible to conceive of a Freud without a previous Darwin, because Freud's thinking was so greatly influenced by Darwin's evolutionary and genetic concepts.

As to hypnosis, it is true that it was, for the first time in Western his-tory, officially accepted as a therapeutic method by the French medical schools of the nineteenth century, especially on account of the teaching of Mesmer, Braid and Bernheim. Actually, hypnosis has been practiced since ancient times. It is well known not only that the Babylonian sooth-sayers and the Hebrew physicians practiced hypnosis repeatedly, but that in Europe, too, throughout the Middle Ages, alchemists were concerned with it and officially accepted it in the scientific world of those times. Therefore, what is really strange is not that Freud and Breuer were able to observe that forgotten memories reappear under hypnosis, but that nobody else before them ever paid serious attention to these rescued memories.

As to Charcot, he undoubtedly influenced Freud's thinking and career like many others did; but it is one thing to influence a man's thinking and another to have the kind of effect without which no further growth is possible. Few people nowadays attribute to Charcot such a decisive influence for the development of psychoanalysis.

Darwin's influence on Freud has to be considered more seriously. Horney, too, has discussed this influence in her book, *New Ways in Psychoanalysis* (1). Freud believed that stages of development are repeti-tions of phylogenetic stages, and such belief has influenced his theories of fixation and regression of the libido. However, these theories, conceived probably under Darwin's influence, are not fundamental in psychoanal-ysis. Horney, in her school of thought, conceives and practices a psycho-analysis deprived of these Darwinian influences. Furthermore, similar ideas, similar comparisons about phylogenetic and ontogenetic develop-ments had been formulated previously, but did not evolve into anything comparable to psychoanalysis. The philosopher Giambattista Vico (2), in the seventeenth century, compared primitive people to children, and studied myths and mores in a way which has great resemblance to the analytic method. Though his writings became part of the background of every philosopher, they did not hasten the development of psychoanalysis. In his writings Freud shows no evidence of having been influenced by Vico, either directly or through some other indirect source.

In my opinion it is not true that psychoanalysis could have been born only at the end of the nineteenth century and not before, because the state of knowledge and science prior to that period would have made it impossible. As a matter of fact, I think that a suitable time for the development of psychoanalysis—much more suitable than the end of the nineteenth century—was that period in Greek history which immediately preceded the great Periclean era. At that time, of course, no neuropathology, genetics or biochemistry were known; but these and many more technical sciences may be easily dispensed with in psychoanalysis. What was available, however, was a general interest in the irrational impulses of man, in his uninhibited emotions, and a concern for the individuality of man's thinking. Heraclitus, who lived between the sixth and the fifth century B.C., expounded the idea that people do not live according to reason, but as though they have an understanding of their own. According to Zilboorg (3), he "implied the need of thorough individualization in psychology."

Empedocles, who lived during the fifth century B.C., stressed the importance of emotions in man's behavior and thought. With an insight reminiscent of Freud, he described the role that the two fundamental emotions, love and hate, play in the problems of living.

Hippocrates, the father of medicines, lived already at the beginning of the classic period of Greek history, but he was one of the first great men of this period and was not yet entirely influenced by the prevailing thoughts of his era. Though he was predominantly what today we would call an internist, he was very much interested in the diseases of the mind. He gave an excellent description of psychoneuroses which far surpasses the definitions of generations of physicians after him. Hippocrates also expressed the belief that emotional conditions may cause physiological and even anatomical changes, thus conceiving the fundamental principle of what twenty-five centuries later was to be called psychosomatic medicine.

But many other important things were going on in Greece at the time, prior to the era of Pericles. The old sacerdotal medicine was still very popular. Although that type of medicine was mostly magical and animistic, it contained many valid psychological elements.

At the same time, the so-called Eleusian and Orphic mysteries were very popular. When a person had some kind of psychologic problems, he would visit these holy places and, while in a state of ecstasy or trance caused by alcohol or by hypnotic procedures, he would feel completely disinhibited and give vent to his emotions. Often these people would attain a twilight or dreamlike state and utter apparently nonsensical words.

In the classic Greek literature examples are reported of these obscure expressions, at times similar to the schizophrenic word-salad, which the priests tried to interpret, often with keen psychoanalytic insight. Dreams were interpreted in the same way and continued to be interpreted in Greece by a few who continued the old tradition even much later. Freud himself, in his introductory lectures on psychoanalysis (4), reports a dream which Alexander had while he was laying siege to the city of Tyre. The dream-interpreter, Aristandros, gave an interpretation of the dream which Freud calls "undoubtedly the right one."

It would seem then that in this period of Greek history, many elements existed which may be considered pre-psychoanalytic or even fully psychoanalytic. It is not too far-fetched, therefore, to envisage the possibility that an intellectual of those days, influenced by all these factors, could have conceived something similar to psychoanalysis.

Actually this era lasted a short time only—too short a time to give that possibility a fair chance to materialize. Adverse trends soon started to operate with such force that the foundation of anything resembling psychoanalysis was definitely not only not encouraged, but actually prevented for twenty-five centuries.

I have made an attempt to study three of these antipsychoanalytic cultural forces, but many more similar forces undoubtedly existed which I have not been able to differentiate.*

The first of these three cultural forces was the increasing supremacy in the Western World of the objective, rational thinking prevalent in Greece.

We have seen that in the sixth and at the beginning of the fifth centuries, B.C. people in Greece were aware of strong emotional and irrational forces which operated in the human psyche. Physicians under these cultural influences, but mostly under the influence of the Dionysian

---

* The term "antipsychoanalytic," which is here used is not correct, and it is used only because I could not find a better one.

These cultural forces are antipyschoanalytic in the same sense that in psychoanalysis the process of repression or of resistance is antipsychoanalytic; that is, in the sense that they prevent other psychological material from gaining access to the center of consciousness. Thus in a certain way these forces are psychological and psychoanalytic.

From this presentation one may obtain the impression that I consider the cultural forces operating in Western civilization as having only an inhibitory, repressing effect. Nothing is farther from the truth. It happens that in this particular presentation I have taken into consideration only this particular aspect. When I use the term "Western civilization" I include in it the Greek and the Jewish cultures. According to some historians this is not correct. However, it will be clearly seen that for the purpose of this paper it is convenient to accept this broadening of the concept of Western civilization.

religion, were still paying heed to these factors. But then what happened? The great philosopher, *Plato,* appeared on the scene. Why he appeared, and who his precursors were, cannot be discussed here. One must admit, however, that it is with him that psychology took a step backward, the first in a long series of setbacks. Since, as Alfred North Whitehead wrote, all Western philosophy from Plato's time on is a series of footnotes to Plato's writings, we may realize the importance of this first step.

First of all, Plato preached that the soul consists of two parts, the rational and the irrational. The irrational soul is the source of the emotions, is mortal, resides in our chest, heart and diaphragm, and belongs to a much lower level than the rational soul. The interest of Plato, therefore, and of those who fell under his influence, became focused only on the rational soul. But Plato's influence went far beyond that. On account of his theories about the nature of Ideas, the interest of the whole Western civilization was centered on—and limited to—what is considered the universal and not the particular. For instance, in the case of horses, according to Plato, it is not important to study this horse or that for its individual qualities like color, strength, speed; what is really important is to study the "horseness" in horses; that is, what is common to horses, what corresponds to the abstract idea of the horse, which, in his opinion, is the perfect, and "pre-existing" reality of the horse.

Now it is obvious that this conception is in essence very antipsychological. Contact is lost with the individual. The individual—be it a horse or a man—is examined in terms of what he has in common with others, in what is objective, not subjective.

Thus Plato, who in reality is a mystic and a poet, paradoxically becomes an ultrarationalist and an antipsychologist. The situation becomes much worse with the appearance on the scene, of Plato's great pupil, *Aristotle.*

As a founder of the new science of logic, Aristotle emphasized the rational to an unprecedented degree. By his system of logic he demonstrated how the mind works when it works well and how one is to avoid irrational thoughts. In addition, he, too, emphasized the universal, not the particular. An individual thing or man belongs to a category, and the category is more important than the individual. The "here and now" is not important—important is only what holds true "everywhere and always." Thus the fleeting contact with the fleeting experiences of the world, which is so important in dynamic psychology, was ignored.

This is an example of how Aristotle reasons (5). History, he says, tells us that the enormously rich king, Croesus, fell and, also, that the enormously rich king, Polycrates, fell. But is history in a position to conclude that rich kings are bound to fall? Of course not. Therefore, history is not a science—it is a mere aggregate of perceptions and facts. No universal judgments may be drawn from it.

Aristotle would probably have said the same thing about the clinical histories of our patients under analysis. Of what universal value would be such histories, each different from the other?

It is from Aristotle's time on that physicians focused their attention on what is common to certain types of patients, with the purposes of identifying and classifying them. This tendency has continued in psychiatry down to our times, having had its best representative in *Kraepelin*. The whole Western civilization has been conquered by these Aristotelian ideas. Ever since, only what is lasting, universal, applicable to all cases of a given category has attracted the main interest of the student. The momentary sensuous perception of change has not only been overlooked, but actually suppressed and, finally, to a large extent repressed.

This tendency, this love for the universal, was due to a need to clarify the world, which otherwise appeared in a chaotic, constantly changeable, perceptual flux.

After the fourth century, B.C. all Greek life, including religion, became influenced by this rationalist conception. The cults of Dionysius and Orpheus, and the practice of the mysteries decreased, and were to a great extent replaced by the cult of Athena, the goddess of wisdom, who was born not from a womb of a goddess but from the head of Zeus.

Although the teachings of the great Greek philosophers acquired increasing importance in Greece, and later in the whole Western world, it would be incorrect to think that their influence was the only important one in Greece. Even among the great writers we find examples like the historian, Herodotus, and the three big dramatists, Aeschylus, Sophocles and Euripides, who did not seem to have the same mental attitude. However, these undercurrents always remained secondary. The main stream of Greek civilization remained concerned with this problem of the universal and the rational, transmitting this concern to the Western world to such an extent that Western people came to think much more like Greeks than the Greeks themselves.

The Romans, and later the Catholic Church, transmitted this manner of rational objective thinking to the whole Western world. In the Middle Ages this Greek conception of the world was almost universally accepted. The scholastics, the philosophers of that period, kept themselves busy trying to reconcile this way of thinking with the tenets of the Catholic Church. Scholasticism created little new knowledge, but tried unceasingly to make more and more orderly and intelligible this otherwise confusing world of perceptions. Its great exponent, *Thomas Aquinas,* is perhaps the greatest formal thinker of all times. He trusts reason entirely and reason only. He tries to explain by the use of Aristotelian logic what appears in the world as a disorderly, fragmentary collection of perceptions and sensations.

Mumford (6) calls the work of Aquinas "an immense textile factory with a thousand looms, each bringing forth a uniform product." The Catholic Church adopted the teachings of Aquinas as her own, so that they were diffused and assimilated by the whole Western world.

In the Middle Ages too, as in ancient Greece, there was a cultural undercurrent which was not rational at all. As a matter of fact, if we consider the problem statistically, we may think that the irrationalities of the Middle Ages by far overcame the rationalism of its philosophers. That is the Middle Ages as it is known to the masses: an era full of superstition and fantasy, an era in which people saw themselves haunted by demons, ghosts, and witches.

These fantasies and myths, however, were permitted and accepted only as long as they did not interfere with the dogmas of the Catholic Church. They gradually diminished in number and at the time of the Renaissance they played a relatively small cultural role, although they have never entirely disappeared. At any rate, it is not this mythical, superstitious atmosphere that the Middle Ages predominantly transmitted to subsequent eras—what the Middle Ages successfully transmitted from the ancient to the modern world was, in spite of appearances to the contrary, Greek rationalism. This rationalism had its greatest triumph later when men started to think that the universe works the same way as the human mind is supposed to work: that is, by the objective, logical, mathematical method.

Descartes is one of the greatest figures in this development. His ideal of the perfect science was geometry, and he tried to mold his philosophy according to a geometrical pattern. Descartes stressed the distinction between what he called clear, distinct ideas from what in our mind is confused, vague, doubtful, fantasy-like, and he based his whole system of philosophy on these ideas. According to him, all things that we conceive very clearly and very distinctly are true. We cannot find a better example of an anti-psychoanalytic attitude. Psychoanalysis, in fact, is the science of the marginal thoughts, of the ideas and feelings which are not clear and distinct, but confused, doubtful, and fantasy-like.

Vico, the philosopher mentioned as one of the precursors of psychoanalysis, fought Descartes' ideas vigorously. However, Descartes' doctrines prevailed in Western civilization, and he really became the founder of the modern geometrical world.

Eventually, everything was interpreted according to mathematical and geometrical laws. Even God changes. He is less of a person and becomes the great architect of the universe. Newton included everything in that grandiose conception called the Newtonian World Machine—something similar to what Aquinas had done on a purely intellectual, abstract level.

As soon as this mechanical geometrical quality of the mind was applied on a large scale to the production of machines, the machine era started. The machine is a reproduction or imitation of part of our mind. (Cf. Cybernetics.)

With the triumph of science and of the industrial revolution, man tried to imitate the machine, which is only part of himself; by doing so, he reduced his possibilities, he tried to suppress other parts of his personality which did not fit into the comparison.

At this point, I would like to recapitulate the foregoing. I have attempted to demonstrate that in the fifth century B.C., immediately before the periclean era, social and cultural factors were at work in Greece, which were very favorable to the advent of psychoanalysis. However, with the beginning of the great Greek era, a rationalist philosophy started which diverted the interest of the people from the irrational, the specific and the subjective. This rational thinking was transmitted and maintained first by the Romans, and then by the Catholic Church; later it was applied to the scientific world in general and received its greatest application in the era of the machines. This rational objective thinking, by diverting the attention of Western man from the irrational, the specific and the subjective, delayed the birth of psychoanalysis for twenty-five centuries.

This objective, rational thinking would probably in itself have been enough to prevent dynamic psychiatry for twenty-five centuries; however, in certain periods of Western history, and especially in the Middle Ages, it lost some of its strength and might have failed to prevent the study of the irrational had it not been reinforced by other cultural factors which had the same preventive effect.

The second of these factors is what I call the suppression of the sensory and of the emotional. This factor has many connections with the first one, but should not be confused with it; as a matter of fact, it is of even more ancient origin. It has been recently stated that the seventeenth century belief in the rational control of the emotions had in the nineteeth century become the habit of repressing the emotions (7). That is true. However, this would not have been possible—at least not to such a large extent—if the habit of repressing the sensory and the emotional had not been formed much earlier in history. As a matter of fact, if one wants to examine the beginning of this tendency in Western civilization, one has to take early Jewish culture into consideration.

If we go back thirty-five centuries, we find the tiny Jewish nation embedded between two great civilizations of that era—the Egyptian and the Mesopotamian.

For reasons which cannot be fully explained, a fundamental idea distinguished the Jewish from the surrounding cultures. That idea is: Nature is not God. Whereas the Egyptians and the Mesopotamians considered the gods in nature, nature itself representing the gods, or the divine being immanent in nature, the Jews regarded nature only as a product of God, therefore inferior and subservient to God.

This idea is extremely important; here its probable connections with the establishment of the patriarchial society can be mentioned only in passing. Mother Earth and all the other female divinities, which were connected with Nature, were abolished by the Jews. Femininity, which was also associated with Nature, lost importance. God is male; Nature, female, is only his product. God is eternal; Nature had a beginning, when it was created by God. The patriarchate is thus officially recognized in the Jewish theocratic system. At the beginning of the Genesis, Eve is made an obedient follower of Adam. The legend implies, however, that it was not so before the intervention of God.

God is different from Nature, is abstract and completely disembodied; God cannot even be represented by a concrete image. Men have bodies, which are not very important because they are part of Nature. Here we see the beginning of that dichotomy between mind and body which has to play such an important role in Western civilization.

The Jews considered the body and the sensual inferior to the abstract; however, they did not actually despise the body or the natural aspect of life. The goal of the Jewish religion is, as a matter of fact, sanctification of life. The body is not despised, inasmuch as it is necessary for life. This tendency to consider the abstract life more important, however, and the sensual and physical secondary has continued to prevail among the Jews.

Among the Jews, too, as among the Greeks, opposite undercurrents existed; for instance, in the hassidic movement, which gave a prominent role to the sensuous, the emotional, the irrational and the mystical. The predominant rabbinical schools, however, throughout the centuries, emphasized the abstract, the incorporeal, like the content of the Book, the Law, etc.

I have already mentioned that in Greece Plato considered emotions and sensations on a lower plane, in comparison to the rational aspect of the mind. Sensations and emotions, like pain, thirst, hunger, anger, fear, love, are relegated to the second-rate, irrational soul.

Paul of Tarsus who, from an historical point of view, is the founder of Christianity, combined these Jewish and Greek cultural forces and expanded them. The purpose of Christian religion is no longer santification of life, but salvation of the soul. The body is conceived as something which imprisons the soul; therefore, it has to be considered as nothing but a hindrance. Carnal urges have to be suppressed.

All emotions which may originate in the body, should also be suppressed. Only love is permitted and esteemed; but it is a love removed from any sexual connotation.

Jerome, one of the most important Church fathers writes, "Regard everything as poison which bears within it the seed of sexual pleasure." It is impossible to discuss the importance of the Church as a cultural force which represses the sexual part of life. Certainly, its influence has been immense. It is true that the majority of cultures have some kind of sexual taboos, but they put emphasis on the general avoidance of sexual gratification per se. For instance, one may see this different attitude even in the attitude toward masturbation. The Greeks did not see anything wrong in masturbation provided the golden mean was respected: not too much indulgence. The Jews condemned male masturbation, as it is described in the biblical episode of Onan, because it produces a waste of the seeds of life. (How can life be sanctified if its seeds are wasted?) The Catholic Church considers masturbation a mortal sin because it brings about carnal pleasure.

This early Christian approach to life did not attempt to repress only sexual pleasure, but all pleasant sensations and emotions. Only a rigid, monastic, ascetic life was advocated with its special kind of love. One wonders whether the failure of love to expand on earth as had been hoped, was partially due to this forced separation from many other vital forces.

During the Renaissance, this attitude toward emotions and the sensuous relaxed somewhat. But the tremendous repression that prevailed in the early part of the Middle Ages was too strong to disappear despite the new Renaissance spirit.

This repression, on the other hand, was reinforced by the advent of the scientific era. I have mentioned how the prevailing objective, rational thinking, by tending to consider the universal rather than the particular, made people lose some contact with sensations and emotions. This loss of contact increased when men started to measure or to interpret everything mathematically. Quality ceased to be quality in the minds of many; it became quantity. Sensations became numbers. The weather, which had appeared to the ancients as something bizarre, irrational, unpredictable, the result of Zeus' whims, is now seen by the meteorologist as something rational and predictable, explainable in terms of isobars and pressure systems. The meteorologist, however, does not hear the wind blowing, does not perceive the cold of the winter, is not afraid of the thunder. In other words, he has lost direct contact with the phenomenon itself.

This abstract attitude is again very unsuitable for psychoanalytic research. It is, therefore, surprising that Freud should have appeared in the midst of this era; unless we consider him a reaction to the prevailing cultural climate. Furthermore, this antipsychological attitude of Western civilization has continued even after Freud and has invaded the field of psychology itself. The school of behaviorism, which advocates the elimination of the subjective experience and attempts to interpret the phenomena in mathematical terms, is in a certain measure an antipsychological school.

We come now to the third force which, for many centuries, has diverted the attention of students from psychoanalytic research. This cultural force is the concern with moral evaluation. The magnitude of this problem permits only a fragmentary and superficial discussion.

In interpreting psychological phenomena, Western man has always been preoccupied with the question of right and wrong, of good and evil. When a phenomenon is examined from this point of view, the wish of the individual or the psychological motivation is not what matters most. This ethical preoccupation is, to a certain extent, present in every society. However, in Western civilization it has acquired a specific importance and it has become confused with the religious attitude.

In ancient Greece morality did not coalesce with religion. As a matter of fact, the Greeks were much more ethical than their religion was. For instance, they practiced monogamy and could not reconcile themselves to the idea that Zeus, with his "dirty" tricks, was allowed to rape goddesses and poor women. More than any other ancient people the Jews were concerned with ethical problems. With the legend of Adam and

Eve, they attributed awareness of the ethical problem to the first couple that existed on earth. Adam and Eve ate the forbidden fruit and acquired knowledge of the good and the evil. The Jews, having accepted the idea that they were the chosen people, had to live up to God's expectations by acting morally. By acting morally, they could recapture the lost paradise in the messianic era. This paradise, however, is a terrestrial paradise; it belongs to this world. With Christianity the paradise ceases to belong to this world; it belongs to the world of eternity. With Christianity, therefore, the moral evaluation of a deed acquires tremendous importance. For instance, if any deed is examined in the light of objective, rational thinking, it appears merely as the effect of a previous cause, a temporary link in an interminable chain of causes and effects. But if a deed is examined from a moral point of view, in Middle-Age theological terms, its moral significance becomes eternal. A deed is good or bad for eternity, and the person who has committed it will be eternally responsible for it.

In the Middle Ages, therefore, the moral evaluation of a deed was much more important than the emotional motivation of the deed, or its rational interpretation. Life was examined not as it was, but as it should be. *Augustine* is the most typical representative of this concept of life. From his writings it appears obvious that he was obsessed by a sense of sin. His goal was to make this world a city of God, a place free of sin— but this was an almost impossible task, because he saw sin all over. He committed a sin when, as a child, he stole some pears from a neighbor's tree; and even in his late years he besought God to forgive him for this sin. He thought that the newborn baby may experience sinful pleasure at the mother's breast.

Augustine's ideas spread to the whole Christian world. This obsession about sin dominated the early Middle Ages; everything was examined from a judgmental point of view. This judgmental tendency which culminated in the Middle Ages, continued in the Western world, and plays a predominant role even today. It is true that in the Renaissance people tried to shake off this moralistic attitude, but they did not succeed fully. One of the best examples of these half-successful compromises can be seen in Dante's *Divine Comedy*. Dante also examines people in general from the point of view of whether they deserve hell, purgatory or paradise. However, he does this very reluctantly. He has to put in hell people he really admires; for instance, Frances of Rimini, a gracious lady, too frail to resist a powerful love to which she succumbs. Dante is not Augustine. He is a Christian and has to put Frances in hell because she sinned;

but when he visits her in hell he has no contempt for her but admiration and pity. He is overwhelmed by sympathy and is not ashamed to admit that he fainted while he was listening to her story.

Though people in general, like Dante, have tried to shake off this judgmental attitude, they have never quite succeeded. At times this attitude decreases a little, as at the beginning of the seventeenth century, or it increases, as during the Victorian Era. The fact remains, however, that it has diverted people from studying the psychological, nonjudgmental motivation of phenomena.

We have seen that these three forces—the prevalence of rational thinking, the tendency to suppress emotions and sensations, and the tendency to evaluate life morally—have in the course of the centuries, diverted the attention from the study of dynamic psychology.

Freud had to fight against these very forces and to overcome them not only in the society at large, but also in the single patient. It is not coincidental, but part of the same phenomenon, that the three forces mentioned operate not only in society, but in the single individual as well. They are part of his resistance and his defenses.

When a patient starts his analysis, he has to start to pay more attention to what appeared to him irrational, what he had a tendency to repress. He often appears afraid of revealing the irrational, just as the Western world was afraid after Plato's time. The patient also has the tendency to use exclusively objective, rational thinking, and to talk in general terms. Many patients, at the beginning of analysis, are reluctant to bring up the specific, the objective, the "here and now." Their tendency is to generalize, to ask the analyst, "but don't all people feel or act in this way?" In other words, they want to lose their individuality and put themselves into a category. By doing so, they may lose contact with the perceptual and emotional experience. In the course of time, they must eliminate this tendency and become more subjective, more specific, in order to proceed favorably in analytic treatment. At the same time, they must become more aware of their sensations and of their emotions. That emotional insight which, to a great extent, was lost twenty-five centuries ago, has now to be recaptured.

At the same time, the patient's focus of attention is shifted from the judgmental point of view to that of his inner genuine feelings. He learns to see the world not from a point of view of what is right and wrong, of the "should's" and "should-not's", but from the point of what his feelings really are, once they are divested of this authoritarian ethic.

Freud recognized these forces; in his system they inhabit the superego which, to use his own words, is the representative of parental authority and of the cultural past. There is no doubt that Freud understood the importance of the cultural past in our ethical, punitive attitude. However, I am doubtful whether he completely understood the importance of the cultural past in repressing irrational thinking and emotions. Generally, the attitude of orthodox analysts has been the opposite of the one taken here. They feel that in the culture man represses the same tendencies that he represses in himself.

Before finishing this presentation, another important point must be mentioned.

If it is not the lack of previous, necessary knowledge, but only the impact of these cultural forces which prevented the development of dynamic psychiatry, how is it that the birth of psychoanalysis finally did take place? What in our culture made psychoanalysis possible? Was there a relaxing of these forces or an antithetic reaction to these forces which were becoming too powerful? Was the new romantic movement, with its emphasis on the individual, enough of an inspiration for psychoanalysis, enough to overcome the traditional rationalistic tendencies?

It is not possible, in my opinion, to answer these questions at the present time. I feel, however, that this problem may be solved, if we consider the advent of psychoanalysis not as an isolated phenomenon, but in connection with other more or less contemporary developments, which are apparently unrelated.

One of them is the development of existential philosophy. Its founder, *Kierkegaard,* died in 1855, one year before the birth of Freud. Existential philosophy is fundamentally a rejection of the Greek and of most of Western philosophy. It is a purely psychological philosophy, as it advocates examining every phenomenon from a psychological, subjective point of view.

According to existentialism, reason is not so powerful; categories lose importance. Objective knowledge is a classification of beings put into more and more general categories. The larger these categories are, the more worthless they become. Abstract philosophical systems are an interference, a curtain between the philosopher and the thing. The problem of death is not important. The important thing is that *I* die. It is not important to seek *the* truth, a universal abstract detached truth. What is important is to seek *my* truth. Even from these brief remarks, it is possible to see the connections with psychoanalytic practice and doctrine.

Another interesting development occurred in 1895, the same year in which Freud and Breuer published their famous book on hysteria, which marked the beginning of the psychoanalytic era. In 1895, in Paris, *Paul Cézanne* had the first one-man show of modern paintings, the first exhibition of modern painting in the world. The *Journal des Artistes* called the exhibition "an apparition of atrocious nightmares." People were shocked as they were at Freud's interpretation of dreams. Cézanne was called a primitive and in a certain way he was; that is, he did not observe the Greek laws of esthetic. To find something similar one had to go back to a time prior to the Greek era, or to countries which were not touched by Greek civilization. Aristotle said, "Art is imitation." With Cézanne art was no longer imitation; it became predominantly an expression of the artist's feelings.

At approximately the same time that Cézanne worked in Paris, the same expressionistic trend was independently followed by *Van Gogh* in Holland, by *Munch* in Norway, and by many others.

Later even mathematics seems to have been affected by this anti-intellectual trend. Intuitional mathematics was the result.*

It is a debatable question why these new anti-intellectual developments should appear at the same time, relatively speaking. The cultural climate, of course, is responsible; but how and why it is responsible, remains to be determined.

REFERENCES

1. Horney, K.: *New Ways in Psychoanalysis.* New York: W. W. Norton & Co.
2. Vico, G.: *Principi di Una Scienza Nuova.* Naples, 1725.
3. Zilboorg, G.: *A History of Medical Psychology.* New York: W. W. Norton & Co., 1941.
4. Freud, S.: *A General Introduction to Psychoanalysis.* New York: Garden City Publishing Co., Inc.
5. Quoted by R. G. Collingwood in *The Idea of History.* Oxford: Oxford University Press, 1946.
6. Mumford, L.: *The Condition of Men.* New York: Harcourt, Brace and Co., 1944.
7. May, R.: *The Meaning of Anxiety.* New York: Ronald Press Company, 1950.
8. Arieti, S.: Special logic of schizophrenic and other types of autistic thought. *Psychiatry,* 105:325-338, 1948.
9. ———: Primitive intellectual mechanisms in psychopathological conditions. *Am. J. Psychotherapy,* 4-15, 1950.
10. ———, Autistic thought, its formal mechanisms and its relationship to schizophrenia. *J. Nerv. & Ment. Dis.,* 3:288-303, 1950.

---

* Intuitional mathematics denies the absolute validity of the aristotelian principle of the excluded middle (that is, that every proposition is either true or false). In dreams, too, and other psychological functions this aristotelian principle is not respected. (Arieti, 8, 9, 10)

29

The Double Methodology in the
Study of Personality and
Its Disorders

This theoretical paper asserts the difficulty inherent in the studies of the personality and its disorders. We must use not one, but two methodologies or philosophical trends which are difficult to reconcile with each other.

THE PURPOSE of this presentation is to demonstrate how a double methodology is adopted in the study of personality and its disorders, how the duality of this methodology is not recognized by many, and how for many others such a problem does not even exist, because they follow exclusively one of the two possible methods.

This dilemma does not concern only psychiatry and psychology but many other disciplines. In fields related to our own, perhaps only the anthropologists have made an accurate study of this problem (3, 8, 9).

I shall start with some very brief and general historical data which, although certainly well known to the audience, I must mention in order to lead to the main thesis of this paper.

Each body of transmitted knowledge is at the beginning a collection of data, a description of facts. Phenomena are observed, described and accepted for what they are without attempts being made to go beyond their appearance. Such readiness to accept things as they are is due, first, to the fact that the pioneers in any field have so much work to do in collecting data that they cannot do anything else, secondly, to the fact that they have not yet developed the means to go beyond apparent facts. Psychiatry, too, has gone through this collective and descriptive stage represented by the pre-Kraepelin era and, to a large extent, by Kraepelin himself.

It is already at this point, when an attempt is made to go beyond the descriptive stage, that a double line of approach, a double possible methodology presents itself. I shall follow here the neokantian approach of Dilthey (5) and Windelband (14) and point out that already at this stage any field of knowledge may proceed in two directions which may be called the *scientific* or *nomothetic* and the *idiographic* method.

Maybe a brief definition of the two methods is appropriate at this point. The scientific or nomothetic approach studies phenomena in order to abstract the laws which rule these phenomena. The knowledge of these laws is considered necessary to enable the student to interpret, to predict, and eventually to alter the course of the phenomena, if it is desirable to do so. This approach is more concerned with quantities than with qualities, more with categories than with the individual. The idiographic or historical approach deals more with qualities than quantities, with specific entities and with the sequence of events more than with laws and classes.

Being a physician, raised in a positivistic, biologic fashion, Kraepelin, like most of his contemporary colleagues, found it natural to orient himself toward the scientific method. The next step in the scientific method, after collection of data, is *classification* or taxonomy. Kraepelin did this job remarkably well. His classification of mental diseases has remained essentially the same to this day.

But science does not stop at the stage of classification. Even the stage of classification is to be considered a very primitive one. The pursuit of the scientific method requires the search of laws ruling the phenomena which have been described and classified. It requires the discovery of the causes of the phenomena, the finding of a construct within which the phenomena are placed in a state of necessary integration, so that each part may be subsumed from the rest of the construct. For instance, in chemistry, after the first stages of description and classification of the elements, laws or constructs were discovered, like Mendeleev's periodical table which permitted to interpret and to predict, at least partially, the properties of the elements.

The pursuit of this method in psychiatry has, as a whole, been extremely unsatisfactory. The pursuers of the scientific method first tried to find organic interpretations of mental disorders, mostly in the biochemical and histologic fields. Some results, like those obtained for such conditions as general paresis and Alzheimer's disease, must be considered very modest when viewed in relation to the whole field of psychiatry. The same modesty must be seen in relation to the organic types of treatment which, although achieving at times dramatic results, must be adjudged symptomatic.

Researchers could have followed the scientific method at a psychologic level and some of them attempted to do so, although not with great success. Watson's behavioristic approach which, at first, seemed to lead to great achievements, was eventually recognized as very limited. In its attempt to reduce everything to quantitative data, it omitted entirely the study of the most important aspects of the psyche, such as, consciousness and subjective experience.

Freud actually revolutionized the methodology in psychiatry and psychology. Unlike his predecessors and contemporaries, he was not so much concerned with how things are, but much more with how things come to be what they are. Freud was very much interested not only in finding the previous cause of an event, but also the purpose of the event. He did not follow only "mechanical causality" but also "teleologic causality." What the philosophers call teleologic causality became for the psychologist *motivation*. Phenomena like symptoms, dreams, defenses are seen as having a purpose, a goal, a certain direction which is part of the general directedness of life. Freud also gave emphasis in his approach to the subjectivity of the experience rather than to the objectivity. Other authors, like Sullivan, Fromm and Horney, have accepted and modified his methodology. But by revolutionizing the methodology, by accepting teleologic causality, by being interested primarily in development, by relying on the subjective experience, Freud actually abandoned the scientific method.

What Freud and the Neofreudians did was to apply the historical method to psychology and to call it psychodynamic. If we consider the following definition of history, given by the historian Bernheim (2) "History is the knowledge of the development of human beings in their activities as social beings," we understand immediately how this definition could also be applied to dynamic psychology and psychotherapy.

The dynamic therapist, like the historian, never treats an event as an isolated happening in time; he views every event as a result and as a cause of change. In this he does not differ from the scientist who sees in every event a ring in the endless chain of causes and effects. But whereas the scientist places the event into a category of similar events and tries to explain the event by attributing to it the properties which the whole category has, the psychodynamic therapist and the historian focus on the differences, on whatever is unique in the event.

But the uniqueness is generally connected with motivation, that vital characteristic which cannot be fully explained by mechanical causality. If Anthony is madly in love with Cleopatra and thus alters the whole course of Roman history, and perhaps of Western civilization, the unpredictability of the motivation and of the consequences has to be explained only in terms of the idiographic historical method and not of the nomothetic scientific.

As an offspring of the historical or psychodynamic method in psychiatry, one may consider another method of which we see early trends in Freud himself, in Jung, Fromm, and especially Horney. This is the characterologic method, which attempts to explain synthetically the inner life of the individual as an expression of a particular type of personality. More important than the temporal sequence here are the functional aspects of the traits and symptoms, all to be subsumed under a particular type of general functioning, or of personality. For instance, in the Freudian context, the tendency to hoard is the expression of the anal character. The drive toward recognized success is, from Fromm, the expression of the marketing personality; the tendency to be submissive and self-effacing is, for Horney, the expression of a "moving-toward-people" personality. Mixed and therefore conflictual personalities are described by all these authors.

As the sociologist Mannheim (10) has emphasized, the characterologic method should not be confused with the classificatory or taxonomic. It does not put just a label on a person in order to classify it; it tries to go much further. It actually tries to explain the motivation, the whole behavior of the individual in terms of a global and enduring pattern, the personality, which gives a special stamp to every behavior manifestation of the individual.

This method corresponds in sociology and history to those methods which see every manifestation of peoples as related to a special type of society or culture, as manifestation of their *Weltanschauung*. In sociology, especially Mannheim, with his sociology of knowledge, has emphasized this point. In history, it corresponds to the interpreting of certain happenings as expressions of the prevailing, feudal, authoritarian, democratic system, etc.

There is no doubt that we owe a great deal to the introduction of the historical method into the field of psychiatry. With the (very important) partial exception of Sullivan, to whose complicated position we shall come back later in this paper, we must say that the psychoanalytic profession has accepted the historical-idiographic method. The longitudinal character of the study, the temporal sequence, the detail, the motivation, the global outlook, the emphasis on the uniqueness, on the autonomy of the individual, are all characteristics which pertain to the psychoanalytic procedure.

But now, let us ask ourselves: Granted that these characteristics are very important and that their study is absolutely necessary, can we say that the only important method in psychology and psychiatry is the historical-idiographic one? Can we say that this method includes everything which is important to know about the human psyche?

To answer this question we must participate in the animated controversy between the advocators of the idiographic-historical method and the advocators of the nomothetic-scientific method. In what follows I shall try

First: to present the arguments in favor and against the two approaches, trying to maintain as much impartiality as I am capable of;

Second: to present the position on this matter of the two major teachers of the William Alanson White Institute, namely Fromm and Sullivan;

Third: to present some personal points of view, resulting especially from studies on schizophrenia.

The advocators of the scientific-nomothetic method feel that although it is true that psychoanalytic matters are important in their particularity, it is also true that nothing is completely known under the aspect of particularity. For instance, if John Smith is a man, I know many things about Smith, which will occur and which cannot occur to him, because John Smith is not only John Smith but also a man. I know, for instance, that sometime he is going to die, that he will never be affected by distemper because distemper is a disease which affects only dogs, etc., etc. The scientific method transposes to John Smith the characteristics of the category to which he belongs and, in this way, our knowledge of him is very much increased. The advocators of the all inclusive idiographic-psychodynamic method retort that whatever we learn from the scientific-nomothetic method is really not of historical, psychodynamic significance; it may refer to men only inasmuch as men are also things, but not to the humanity of man. This extreme position is taken by some historians. For instance, the well-known Spanish historian Ortega y Gasset (11) goes to the extreme of saying "that man has no nature; what he has is . . . history."

Another controversy between the scientific nomothetic and the historical-idiographic methods refers to the actual procedure of observation. The scientist feels that if this procedure is to have validity both the observer and the object under observation should not change and, especially the object, should be in a state of isolation from disturbing variables. But in the psychotherapeutic situation, there is no isolation and both the patient and the therapist are in a process of change. As far as the patient is concerned, the change is actually what we want. As far as the therapist is concerned, we all know that the therapist is not only an observer, but a participant, who changes on account of the countertransference.

To this criticism the advocators of the psychodynamic-idiographic method reply that it is actually this change, or rather changing, that is studied by the psychodynamic method. Whereas the scientific method crystallizes moments of time and studies them in a static cross-section situation, which actually does not exist but is abstracted in an artificial way, the idiographic-historical-dynamic method attempts to recapture the perennial change, the movement which is the essence of life. People and things always act upon one another; there is no state of isolation, of pure experimental condition, of pure culture, etc. . . . Even in the scientific procedure this is never achieved.

The critics of the psychodynamic method point out also some other limitations. The most important is that this method permits only the determination of degrees of probabilities but not of absolute certainty. For instance, if we know everything that is possible to know about the childhood and later life of a patient, we may make the statement that *probably* this patient, later in life, will develop schizophrenia or a homosexual pattern of behavior. We may say "probably" but not "certainly," with that certainty with which an astronomer, let us say, may predict an eclipse at such and such a time.

The historian also deals with probability and not certainty, when after studying the past and present conditions of a country, he predicts, let us say, a war or a revolution.

At most, the historian and the psychodynamic psychologist are able to determine the recurrence of certain patterns, like certain cycles of history which tend to repeat and certain patterns of behavior which tend to recur. But this recurrence is indicative only of a *relative empirical regularity*, not of universal laws, like for instance the law of gravity.

To this criticism the advocators of the psychodynamic method reply in two different ways, which are almost self-contradictory. One way consists in accepting the limitations of the idiographic-historical-psychodynamic method. All right, they say, let us accept these limitations of the historical method. In spite of these limitations, this method opens horizons which are psychodynamically very significant. The scientific method, too, has limitations. The scientific method produces a decomposition of the phenomena, which is artificial, a dissection which is the negation of life, a crystallization of the isolated elements. In the scientific procedure, we amputate the whole, by removing the accessory or concomitant parts, and never apprehend things as wholes and never see them in their totality. In its rigidity the scientific method follows certain dogmas which cannot be applied to the idiographic-psychodynamic method; it studies such problems as the following: *If* an event happens, *then* another event happens. In other words, it studies invariable associations. But in dynamic or historical matters, there are no invariable associations. Science tends to abstract from wholes only those properties which may be measured or to which can be attributed certain properties that numbers have. Only these measurable properties, that is, properties which may be translated into quantitative data, are studied by science which, therefore, has a limited scope.

But, even more than that, the extremist supporters of the idiographic-psychodynamic method feel that the scientific method tends to reduce the role of the therapist and of the historian to that of a technician. In a scientific world, it is only the discoverer and the inventor who are creative. All the others are technicians who repeat in a routine manner what the creative persons have introduced. In the historical, psychodynamic method, no procedure could be repeated in a routine manner. Every therapist and every historian is a creator.

As I mentioned before, there are, however, some people who defend the psychodynamic and historical method in a completely different way. These people state that the limitations of the psychodynamic-historical method are due only to the fact that we do not know all the variables. Were we to know all the facts, we could be able to predict how the patient is going to turn out, just as an historian would be able to predict a war with absolute certainty if he would know all the facts which were involved in the decision of waging a war, from the economy and military power of the enemy to the philosophic outlook of the rulers and the convictions of each individual citizen. But it is impossible to know all the facts. Such knowledge would require computations of millions or rather billions of variables which act upon one another. The solution of such mathematical problems is not possible, in spite of cybernetics and computing machines. Instead of trying to find the algebraic sum of all the innumerable factors, the psychodynamic therapist and the historian select a few facts as representatives of quantitatively undeterminable conditions. For instance, certain incidents which have occurred in the childhood of a patient are taken as representative of the whole childhood, or of certain periods of the childhood.

In other words, people who emphasize the fact that we do not know all the variables, deny that the psychodynamic method is an historical one, and affirm that it is scientific. Freud himself thought that this method was scientific and would have resented a statement to the contrary. Like all the scientists, he was induced to formulate laws, similar to the laws formulated in mathematics and physics. For instance, he and his orthodox followers considered as valid as a law the statement that every psychoneurosis was derived from an unsolved Oedipus complex. Actually, this is a generalization but by no means a law. Freud should have said that in his Viennese culture, at the turn of the century, many neuroses were caused by what he called an unsolved Oedipus complex.

The staunch supporters of the idiographic method attack this reasoning. They feel that in the understanding of psychodynamic mechanisms it is not the mathematical knowledge of all the variables, which counts, but a certain emotional intuitiveness which also many artists, writers, and uneducated people possess. These staunch supporters of the idiographic method, direct their criticism to the founders of psychoanalytic schools, too, when they feel that these founders have abandoned the pure historical method. The critics state that psychoanalysts have vainly attempted to build general theories of personality and neuroses which would include all the facts. These analysts are comparable to some historians, like Spengler and Toynbee, who have tried to explain events as manifestations of underlying structures.

The builders of psychiatric and historical systems see in their creation an architecture which sustains all the things which they are investigating. The critics see in them a skeleton without flesh. The builders see in their system an enduring pattern and an interrelation of apparently unrelated things; the critics see in them an esthetic illusion. According to the latter, big theories are artifacts. They have a certain beauty and therefore satisfy the esthetic sense which searches for repetition, for cycles and symmetry in a world which is instead under the continuous urge of creative and unpredictable drives. As Spengler's, Toynbee's and other builders' systems are destined to crumble, in a similar way Freud's theory of personality, with its division in id, ego, and superego will collapse. The systems built by Jung, Horney, Sullivan, etc., will also

collapse. In a realm of knowledge which is not scientific all the archi-
tectures will fall, only the individuality of the human being will emerge
in the context of the human community. In other words, to use existentialist terminology, there is no essence but only existence.

Now, that we have given an account of this controversy from a general
point of view, we shall examine in particular the thinking of the
William Alanson White School on this subject. What is Fromm's position? Fromm's position seems to me clear, unequivocal. He has enhanced
completely the idiographic-historical method and has paid little attention
to the scientific-nomothetic. If we study his writing carefully, we see that
he has consistently taken this attitude. His fervor and zeal in his position
make him integrate into his psychodynamic teachings a great deal of
material coming from other predominantly idiographic subjects, like
history and sociology. His emphasis on the uniqueness, on the individuality, his characterologic trends, are all features pertaining to the idiographic method. His approach to psychologic problems is predominantly
idiographic. Let's take for instance his study of dreams. Fromm (6) maintains that what we should aim at is not an *interpretation* of dreams, as
Freud did, but an *understanding* of dreams. This word "understanding"
rather than "interpretation" reveals his whole allegiance to the idiographic method.

Plato, too, thought that the two highest forms of knowledge are understanding and interpretative reason. Understanding is the intuition of the
single particular: interpretative reason, instead, according to Plato, is
what put things into interrelated systems. Thus Fromm feels that the
language of dreams and myths has to be understood in its own right, not
interpreted, that is not related to or translated into another language.

Fromm's characterological trends, also are part, as we have mentioned,
of his striving for unity, and are idiographic. His existentialist leanings
have to be interpreted in the same way.

It is much more difficult to determine the position of Sullivan. A man
who speaks of selective inattention, of security operations, of parataxic
distortions, is certainly psychodynamically, teleologically and idiographi-
cally oriented. However, Sullivan did not entirely accept this historical-
idiographic position. One thing bothered him, and indeed is one thing
which has bothered all the thinkers since the dawn of our Western
civilization. This is the problem of the individual, of the particular.
Sullivan seems not to accept the existence of individuality; he, therefore,
rejects an extreme idiographic position, like that of Fromm and Horney,
and wants to remain in a scientific frame of reference. To what extent

he rejects the concept of individuality, is difficult to ascertain. At times, he seems to mean that, since we are all in a system of interrelated and interpersonal forces, there is really no isolated entity or individuality; we are all participating in a large interrelated whole. Now, if this is all he means, this concept would be acceptable even to idiographic thinkers. But it seems that he means more than that; that he actually does not believe in the uniqueness of the participants in the interrelated whole, or in the uniqueness of the whole, or in the uniqueness of the whole personality. In fact, although Sullivan speaks of enduring patterns of response, he does not seem to believe in the concept of total personality. He writes (13), "For all I know every human being has as many personalities as he has interpersonal relations." In the same article he speaks of the viewpoint of personal individuality as "an inescapable illusion." Thus Sullivan, like Freud, although advocating the historical-idiographic method, does not reject the scientific method. Like Freud, however, he remains somewhat obscure on this point, inasmuch as he cannot integrate the two methods.

Thus, as far as Fromm and Sullivan are concerned, we find ourselves in this situation: in Fromm's orientation we find consistency and clarification but, at the same time, simplification. We have to give up almost entirely one of these two methods. In Sullivan we find an acceptance of both methods, but not a complete integration of them. It could be that, had untimely death not interrupted his work, Sullivan would have made great advancements toward this integration.

Since the beginning of the psychoanalytic era, great achievements have occurred in the field of idiographic psychodynamics. The orthodox Freudian school as well as the schools of Adler, Horney, Fromm and Sullivan himself, have enlarged the understanding of personality by following chiefly the idiographic method. The recent trends, which tend to incorporate existentialism and Zen-Buddhism, two extremist idiographic schools of thought, seem to tend more and more toward the idiographic method.

My own point of view in this matter has been influenced by anthropologists. Kroeber (8) states that anthropology is both science and history, and I feel that a similar attitude must be taken for psychiatry, psychoanalysis and all the social sciences. Now, since there is no doubt that the idiographic method has won so many sweeping victories in psychoanalysis, a person who wants to maintain the point of view that both methods are important must concentrate on the defense of the nomothetic-scientific method which has been so badly neglected. This, of course, does not mean that the writer attempts to minimize the idiographic method, but that he suggests an adoption of both of them.

We have already seen that the scientific method has failed in psychiatry because it has resorted chiefly to histology and biochemistry and has attempted to bypass the psychologic level, except for the pseudopsychology of behaviorism. But it is on a psychologic level that the scientific method must assert itself. In some psychoanalytic groups this need has already been felt for some time and pertinent studies have been made. In orthodox Freudian circles these investigations have been grouped under the label of "ego psychology." In other words, these investigators have tried to force their findings within the framework of the libido theory. This seems to me a difficult task. I have found it more useful to adopt some conceptions of other authors, like Piaget, Cassirer and Susanne Langer, than those of the Freudian ego-psychologists, and have consequently come to consider every psychologic phenomenon, like everything else in nature, under two different aspects: form and content (1).

Whereas the content is studied best by the idiographic-historical-psychodynamic method, the form is studied better by the nomothetic-scientific-epistemological method. At present, in my opinion, it is in the study of the forms that the scientific-nomothetic-epistemologic method must reassert itself.

Let's take an example. A schizophrenic woman hears an hallucinatory voice which tells her repeatedly, "You are a prostitute." If we try to interpret this phenomenon with the psychodynamic-historical-idiographic method, we shall learn many things which are of the greatest therapeutic importance. First of all, we shall examine this phenomenon not in isolation but in relation to the whole life and whole personality of the patient. This study will tell us that before becoming overtly psychotic this person was self-effacing and self-accusatory. The voice is a symbolic reproduction of the voice of the significant adult who repeatedly injured the self-esteem of the patient. Before the psychotic outbreak, this voice of the significant adult was introjected and experienced as a feeling of inadequacy and guilt. Now it is projected again into the external world. By being projected, this feeling of worthlessness and guilt is not experienced any longer as coming from the self, but from the symbolic persecutor. There is thus a defense, an attempt, although a vain one, to raise again the self-regard. An experience occurs which is a little more tolerable than what the patient underwent before. All this is very important and therapeutically valid. But is this interpretation all inclusive? Obviously not. For instance, it does not explain the fact that similar feelings of inadequacy and guilt which remain as such in the average person do not acquire this form. In the neurotic they may appear as compulsions or phobias. In the depressed patient they may assume the form of suicidal depression or of manic denial.

The answer that our patient was subjected to more violent traumata than the neurotic or that she had a specific constitutional vulnerability are not complete answers. As a matter of fact, I am sure that many of us are willing to accept both these explanations. We know from their life history that schizophrenics, as a rule, have been subjected to more violent traumata than neurotics, and, at our stage of knowledge, we cannot deny nor affirm a constitutional vulnerability. But this does not explain the essence of the hallucination. In other words, the psychodynamic-idiographic method will explain the psychic conflict but will not explain the form which the psychic conflict will assume. But it is the form that distinguishes the schizophrenic condition from others.

Now, what does the scientific study of the psychologic form "hallucination" tell us? Undoubtedly, not all that we would like to know; but a few important things which may open new avenues of research and may enrich our psychodynamic understanding. *First*, it tells us that a particular mental content which is susceptible to being studied psychodynamically, has assumed the form of perception. A high conceptual construct, a large constellation of thoughts and feelings, in our case predominantly of guilt and self-effacement, has assumed the form of a simple perception, a real perception, not a faked one. In fact, electroencephalographic studies of experimentally induced visual hallucinations have demonstrated the same changes as when normal visual perceptions occur (4). Possibly, future researchers will demonstrate similar alterations for auditory hallucinations.

Second, the voice seems to the patient to come from the external world, in spite of absence of a real auditory stimulus. How is this to be explained? This point which seems so difficult to understand is, on the other hand, easy, if we see it under the category of the phenomenon of perception. As a matter of fact, not only in hallucinations but in every perception, there is a projection to the external world. For instance, in front of me I see a group of people. The visual perception of a group of people will occur in my cerebral cortex, in proximity of the calcarine fissure. At the same time, however, that my cortex perceives this visual image, the image of the group of people is by my nervous system projected to the external world. Now, why and how the perceiving baby learns to project his first experiences is not to be discussed here. The important thing is not that the hallucinatory voice is projected externally, since this projection is implied in the category of perception. What is important is the fact that an abstract complex has been perceptualized.

Third, how could it be that such a large abstract complex, like the one about disparagement, self-effacement and guilt, with which thousands and thousands of feelings and thoughts could be associated, has been reduced to a simple auditory perception, to the little sentence, "You are a prostitute"?

Here we must explain very briefly a fundamental concept. In the biologic scale we find that expansion of form goes together with expansion of content. From the simple level of unconditioned reflexes to the level of the high symbolic processes of the human being we find a crescendo in both form and content. Now, in psychopathology, especially as a result of the disintegrating effect of anxiety, we find the following characteristics: both forms and contents tend to assume less advanced types, for instance, infantile and immature aspects. But in conditions of more severe psychopathology, as in schizophrenia, not only both content and form tend to assume simple types, but also there is a discrepancy between form and content, in the sense that the form acquires a much more elementary type than the content. For instance, we have seen that in our patient who hallucinates the complex of guilt and self-effacement has taken the type of a symbolic reproduction of an infantile expression, as far as the content is concerned, but has assumed a much more elementary type, as far as the form is concerned: a highly abstract concept and complex has become a simple auditory perception.

This discrepancy is seen very well in schizophrenia. In other conditions we see less discrepancy between the regression of form and content. For instance, in phobic reactions the complicated and, to a certain extent, abstract phenomenon of anxiety becomes transformed in the simple mechanism of fear. Feelings of inadequacy and fears of interpersonal relations, like doubts about being loved, may become transformed into a concrete fear, like fear of horses. In other cases, anxiety about ability to love and to be loved becomes transformed into the simpler fear of sex. Children who cannot get love and affection from their parents and do not know what they want, say that they want toys. Neurotic parents also give food and toys for something else they cannot give. In these reductions of forms and contents we see a mechanism which is the opposite of the one described by Freud. In these cases, it is not the infantile strivings which on account of their own strength reemerge violently with their original forms and contents, but it is the inability to live at a high level of interpersonal, symbolic relationships, which brings about a retreat to lower forms and contents. Similar things could be repeated for many unclassifiable patients, in whom, because of their inability to live in accordance with their potentiality, it occurs what seems a trivialization of life, or an emergence of "faulty habits," as Adolph Meyer would say.

But let us go back to our schizophrenic patient, the woman who hallucinates. What happens when the complex of disparagement, self-effacement and guilt is reduced to the sentence, "You are a prostitute"? Since, of course, at the level of perception, no abstract concepts are possible, a visual or auditory image must concretize the concept. Here the same thing occurs which occurs in dreams and in fine art. A perceptual fragment of the large context is what is experienced. The voice, "You are a prostitute" is a part of the experiential history of the patient, of the large context of scolding and self-effacement.

The unity of this context is thus broken. But here something of stupendous significance happens. Although the unity is broken, this little fragment, this infinitesimal part, will stand for the whole context. Thus the unity which was destroyed is immediately restored; it re-emerges symbolically because the little part is emotionally equivalent to the whole. The voice, "You are a prostitute" will stand for the whole life, for the whole tragedy of the patient. And from this point we could go into the fascinating field of symbolism, but time does not permit this.

From what I have said, I hope I have been able to express how important I think is the study of forms or formal mechanisms. The term "formal" is unappealing to many, inasmuch as it seems to indicate something static, conventional. But it is not really so. The study of forms leads us to the very vital, ever-surprising, ever-changing world of transformations. As I have indicated, many analysts are studying these problems today. Among these studies Schachtel's (12) works on amnesia are of the greatest importance. Schachtel, although not rejecting the Freudian idiographic-dynamic point of view that we forget because we do not wish to remember, adds a new scientific-nomothetic approach. We do not remember our infantile experiences, because we do not have any longer the same forms, or as he says, the same schemata. In the Horney school, Harold Kelman (7) has recently devoted a great deal of work to the study of forms.

I want to conclude this paper with the anticipation of a criticism. Some of you may feel that this division in form and content, science and history, is a repetition or a surrogate of Descarte's division in body and soul, or one of the many derivatives of the Cartesian impact on our Western civilization. Perhaps it is; I am not sure. I admit that unity rather than duality appeals to the esthetic sense of man. Actually, the opponents of duality have nothing to offer. They reach unity just by dropping one of the two parts or denying its existence. I hope, too, that one day such synthesis will be reached, at least at a philosophic level. But at the present time a duality must be maintained at a psychologic level. It is in maintaining such a double approach that I see one of the main difficulties of the psychologist, psychiatrist and psychoanalyst today.

REFERENCES

1. ARIETI, S.: *Interpretation of Schizophrenia*. New York: Robert Brunner, 1955.
2. BERNHEIM, E.: *Lehrbuch der historischen Methode*, Leipzig, 1889. Quoted in M. Mandelbaum, *The Problem of Historical Knowledge*. New York: Liveright, 1938.
3. BIDNEY, D.: *Theoretical Anthropology*. New York: Columbia University Press, 1953.
4. CHWEITZER, A., GEBLEWICZ, E., and LIBERSON, W.: Action of mescaline on the alpha waves. *Compt. Rend. Soc. Biol.*, Vol. 124, 1206, 1937.
5. DILTHEY, W.: *Gesammelte Schriften*. Berlin: Leipzig, 1923.
6. FROMM, E.: *The Forgotten Language*. New York: Rinehart, 1951.
7. KELMAN, H.: The symbolizing process. *Am. J. Psychoan.*, 16:145, 1956.
8. KROEBER, A.: History and science in anthropology. *American Anthropologist*, 37:539, 1935.
9. KROEBER, A.: *Anthropology*. New York: Harcourt, Brace, 1948.
10. MANNHEIM, K.: *Essays on the Sociology of Knowledge*. New York: Oxford, 1952.
11. ORTEGA Y GASSET, J.: History as a system. In *Philosophy and History, Essays Presented to Ernst Cassirer*. New York: Oxford, 1936.
12. SCHACHTEL, E.: On memory and childhood amnesia. *Psychiatry*, 10:1, 1947.
13. SULLIVAN, H.: The illusion of personal individuality. *Psychiatry*, 13:317, 1950.
14. WINDELBAND, W.: *Geschichte und Naturwissenschaft*. Strassburg, 1904.

30

The Origin and Effect of Power

This study of volition, started long ago and inspired by re-search on catatonic schizophrenia, led me to the study of power, a force which thwarts the will. This chapter advances some ideas, to be expanded in the book The Will To Be Human.

DEFINITIONS

LIKE MANY OTHER CULTURAL FIELDS affecting society today, psychoanalysis is in the midst of a major crisis. More and more we recognize that in spite of its profound explorations of the human psyche, psychoanalysis has ignored, or inadequately studied or wrongly subsumed under too broad or too rigid categories, factors which are of vital importance in the development and function of the personality. One of them is power; and the American Academy of Psychoanalysis has to be congratulated for having devoted this meeting to this significant subject.

As a point of clarification, I want to indicate that in the paper I am presenting the word power is not used in all its possible connotations. It connotes not a function or ability of the person—such as the capacity to paint, to sing, to breathe, or to climb a mountain—but a force, mostly in a negative sense, which derives from the actions of others and which is experienced by the individual as thwarting, deflecting, inhibiting, or arresting one's will, one's freedom, or one's capacity for growth and expansion in accordance with the rhythm of one's personality.

The concept of power in a psychological-psychoanalytic frame of reference is thus connected with the problem of will—another concept which has been badly neglected in psychoanalysis and which only now reappears for reconsideration, especially in the works of Leslie Farber (8), Rollo May (12), Leon Salzman (15), and myself (3, 7). Will, as capacity to make choices and to implement the choices, is the culmination of all psychic functions. This capacity may be hindered by internal

445

forces, such as neurotic and psychotic complexes, or by external, that is social, forces.

These forces are experienced as power, starting from the end of the first year of life and continuing for the whole lifetime of the individual. Theoretically, they do not need to be experienced. If what Erik Erikson, Martin Buber, and other authors have included in the concept of trust, or basic trust, existed in a complete form, such forces would not be experienced. A state of relatedness and communion would exist among people, which would promote the growth and flourishing of the personality, and on account of which the joyful fleeting moment would leave a wake of trust that the next moment is going to be the same. The good mother is the representative of this world of trust.

But, unfortunately, this is rarely the case. Even when the individual was exposed to good motherhood the complexities of human existence make him gradually aware that he must mistrust. He experiences in various degrees people as hostile powers. At times this experience is very mild and may promote constructive vigilance, but most of the time it is better defined as fear, which may be mild, as in most cases, or very pronounced. The child must learn to deal with this external power, with which he must co-exist. He may learn to placate this power: to become a compliant, subservient, pleasing personality. Karen Horney (11) would call this type of personality "moving toward people." But in a language which is more effective today we may call it an Uncle Tom type of personality.

The child may instead learn to fight back, in his turn, to intimidate the power. Karen Horney would say that he moves against people. The case, however, could be that since childhood the person has felt that he had more chance to preserve his own integrity by fighting and arguing than by pleasing, obliging, or submitting. The child may learn to deal with the hostile power by removing himself from it, either by physical distance or by emotional detachment. He may become an aloof, withdrawn person.

These enduring patterns of response, which come to constitute important parts of the personality, actually grow out of fear for the other, when the other is seen as a power possessing various degrees of enmity. When the resulting way of living is not too affected, the person may still be considered normal or mildly neurotic. When the individual exaggerates these tendencies, he may develop a paranoid attitude toward the world, which he sees as a conspiracy of many inimical powers or a single, huge, omnipresent, all-engulfing threat.

The matter is obviously more complicated than I have so far outlined. We know that the external power is incorporated or introjected, so that the individual may have to obey or placate an inner dictate, a should, a superego or conscience, according to whatever terminology we prefer. In another publication (7), I have called this internalized power endocratic, because it dominates from inside, in contradistinction to external power. This internalization is actually a necessity. Social life, with its numerous and complicated possibilities of behavior, would not be possible without such endocratic power.

But as analysts we have to ask ourselves whether this inimical power which the individual experiences from early life is fiction or reality. Is it just a fantasy of the unconscious or of the id of the patient?

THE DYNAMICS OF POWER

We shall consider now the special characteristics and origin of power which tends to influence, deflect, subjugate, or use the will of other people.

The ethological theories of aggression, like those of Konrad Lorenz (12) or the classic psychoanalytic theories of Thanatos seem to explain only a small part of this complicated human phenomenon. The ethological theories focus on adaptational aspects of the problem; i.e., the human being, like the subhuman animals in the jungle, is endowed with aggressive mechanisms with which to fight other animals, secure food, maintain territorial rights, compete sexually, and defend the progeny. It is true that the capacity for aggression is very important for the preservation of animal species. Evolution has preserved this capacity with many selective mechanisms. One of them is to make aggression pleasant for the aggressor. Aggression is not as pleasant or as important as sexuality, but it has nevertheless a major role biologically and psychologically. Although these biological facts are undeniable they cannot explain the full range of human hostility. The neurophysiological functions of rage and physical aggression become in man only part of larger mechanisms. In many elaborated forms of human hostility they may not enter at all in these elementary manifestations.

Freud did not derive his theory of death instinct and aggression from the biological sciences. In formulating the theories of the two instincts he was influenced predominantly by cultural factors: in the case of Eros, by the sexual repression of the Victorian era; as to Thanatos, by what was occurring in Europe during the First World War. In the case of Eros Freud saw suppression, as related to repression, resistance, transference, symbolism, sublimation, displacement, and so on. Here Freud was great. With regard to Thanatos he did not see suppression-repression but, on the contrary, expression and acting out as they were possible in the First World War. Freud here was not so great. He did not work out very well the origin or vicissitudes of aggression and the death instinct. He could not determine the somatic zones responsible for them or their phases of development, as he did for sexuality.

Neither Freud nor the ethologists could give us adequate theories, because at a certain point in the life of man or in the history of the human race new factors emerge that change completely the aim and potentiality of aggression. To view some of man's complex psychological processes purely as behavioral manifestations of instinctual aggression or of neurophysiological mechanisms is part of a reductionistic approach; it is another example of genetic fallacy. The complex functions that range from rage to hostility have at least five aims, often combined: first, self-defense, or elimination of fear; second, hurting others; third, depriving others; fourth, revenging; fifth, dominating others. This paper deals only with this fifth function, which when it is manifested with aggression, bypasses the other four aims. Power is the result: the capacity to manipulate, control, deflect, exploit, crush the will of others. The aim is to dominate irrespective of whether domination, or the means to achieve it, hurts or not. Power affects every interpersonal relation and disturbs it to such a point that a state of communion between two or more people is no longer possible. When two people are together an unequal distribution of power, that is, unequal ability to exert one's will, tends to develop, unless strong measures are taken to maintain the equilibrium. The result will be that one person will be dominant and the other submissive. This need to dominate may disturb the relation between parent and child, husband and wife, teacher and pupil, employer and employee, and so on. A relation which is meant to be based on love, affection, learning, or cooperation becomes corrupted by power seeking—most of the time implemented not just by conscious but also, and in many cases predominantly, by unconscious maneuvers. Generally society sanctions the more common unequal distributions of power, which may thus remain unchallenged for thousands of years, or until liberation movements occur.

Unequal distribution of power first gives origin to a hierarchy, then to control, finally to potential or actual subjugation. I repeat that the aim of power is not necessarily to hurt, but to dominate. Nevertheless the dominated person is hurt. In many cases the experience of being hurt is conscious; in many other cases it is unconscious and the psyche suffers without being aware of the suffering. The person's autonomy and individuality are attacked; the individual becomes an Uncle Tom, an extremely subservient person, a compulsive, a queer, a psychopath, a paranoid, and so on. When the dominated person seems to accept being dominated, he does so in order to avoid stronger fears and anxiety or because he cannot conceive other ways of experiencing life. I can only allude here to the unequal distribution of power in such large groups of people as some social classes or entire countries.

The need for power has characteristics of its own, not found in primitive biological needs such as hunger, thirst, sleep, and sex. These biological needs that we have in common with other animal species are indeed powerful, but also self-limiting. A man cannot eat more than a certain amount of food and cannot have sexual relations with more than a certain number of women. Even very large harems, as they exist in some countries, are built to signify prestige and wealth, more than sexual prowess. Contrary to sexual ability the need for power is potentially endless and boundless. Some people as Alexander the Great and Napoleon in the early period of their political life could have had all the wealth and sexual exploits they wanted, yet they continued to seek more and more power. Even the meaning of money has to be reinterpreted in relation to power. If money is a means to obtain food and sex, it cannot go beyond physiological satisfaction. But money can buy status, prestige, and power.

Marx's theory about the economic interpretation of history is susceptible of revision. It is true that the nineteenth-century bourgeoisie wanted an economic position in which it could prosper and exploit the masses. The whole theory, however, could be understood in terms of the dynamics of power. In a capitalistic society in which birth privileges are not important and the aristocracy plays a minimal role, the most common way to increase power is by accruing capital. If we cannot be aristocrats, we can become plutocrats. Marx's ideology can conceive a classless society as far as economy is concerned, but certainly the system by which the ideology is supposed to be actualized does not lead to equal distribution of power. In Russia there is an elite of the powerful, and a mass of the powerless.

What theories have psychoanalysis and related sciences advanced about the origin of power? Adler has offered very meaningful hypotheses (1, 2). The child starts to feel inferior in the world of adults, and later he learns that "to be human means to feel inferior." This explanation is plausible but leaves unanswered many questions. Why does the individual continue to feel inferior when he grows up? Why does everybody feel inferior, even kings and presidents? And why is inferiority compensated for by domination of others?

Although the inferiority feeling becomes manifest as a feeling of helplessness in the child, it is actually grounded on and perpetuated by intrinsic properties of the human psyche (4). It is based on the fact that a discrepancy exists between the way man sees himself and the way his symbolic processes make him visualize what he could be. Man is always short of what he can conjecture; he can always conceive a situation better than the one he is in. This discrepancy is caused by the power of his symbolic processes, actually by a much larger or inclusive philosophy of life which he comes to build in his contacts with other human beings. I have become increasingly (4, 6) aware that cognitive processes, such complicated structures as so-called philosophies of life, or what the sociologist Gouldner (10) calls domain assumptions, are responsible for many constructive as well as destructive motivations. These domain assumptions operate most of the time at an unconscious level or at the periphery of consciousness. Psychiatrists and psychoanalysts should expand on the work of sociologists by revealing more of these assumptions and elucidating their ramifications. A great deal of human behavior, generally believed to be motivated by primitive instinctual drives, is motivated instead by unconscious presuppositions which are part of elaborate cognitive structures. At the same time these high-level cognitive motivations may reinforce more primitive ones and overdetermine man's behavior.

What are the philosophies of life or domain assumptions which urge people to dominate others? At a certain time in his phylogenetic or ontogenetic development, man transcends his biological nature and becomes aware of a basic irreconcilable dichotomy: he conceives a theoretical or ideal state of perfectibility, and yet he is very imperfect, and in relation to the ideal, inferior. When he sees himself less than what he would like to be, he believes others too are dissatisfied with him. He faces a theoretical infinity of space, time, things, and ideas, which he can in a vague sense visualize but not master. On the other hand, he becomes aware of his finitude. He knows he is going to die, and that the range of experiences he is going to have is limited. He cannot be better than he is capable of being and he cannot enjoy more than a certain amount of food and sex.

But being able to conceive the infinite, the immortal, the greater and greater, he cannot accept his littleness. If frustration were not such a weak and misused word, he could say that he feels frustrated about his own nature and desperately searches for ways to overcome his condition. At a certain period in history some religions have made him conceive compensations in another life, after death. However, these conceptions of immortality were conceived not earlier than 3500 years ago. Earlier in human history the only way to obtain an apparent expansion of the prerogatives of life was to invade the life of others. Since then, this method has remained the prevailing one. My life will be less limited if I take your freedom, if I make you work for me, if I make you submit to me. Thus instead of accepting his limitations and helping himself and his fellowmen within the realm of these limitations, man developed domain assumptions which made him believe that he could bypass his finitude and live more by making others less alive.

These assumptions ramified and built up networks of rationalizations. If someone's life was limited it was only because the others impinged upon him, restricted his potentialities, and infringed his will. If he succeeds in ruling others he will expand and live intensely; he will have the pleasure of exerting an unbounded will; he will increase his ego and decrease his superego. The conception of superman, which reached full consciousness and distinct formulation in the philosophy of Nietzsche, has existed in related forms since prehistoric times in the psyche of the masses of men as an unconscious domain assumption. Because of it the individual tends to confuse the concept of freedom and of individual autonomy with the irrational illusion of infinity, and by doing so he diminishes the freedom of others.

I must stress once more that most of the time these conceptions are not in the mind of men in a state of consciousness or full consciousness. Contrary to the early theories of classic psychoanalysis, it is not just the primitive which is repressed or kept at a preconscious level. Whatever is not acceptable to the self tends to be repressed or to be kept at the periphery of consciousness, whether it comes from primitive, ordinary, or unusually high levels of the psyche. Again I must stress that the mentioned interpretation does not rule out more primitive motivations for dominating others, such as the need to hurt, to deprive, to revenge, or to remove fear and anxiety. The unconscious aim to overcome the human limitation may become the ally of the pleasure principle and of what some authors call id motivation.

When man became the only entity to discover the predicament of his finitude in the midst of the infinite he could, theoretically at least, react in three possible ways:

1. He could accept his finitude with the proviso that by following the endless symbolic processes which are at his disposal he could continue to grow as long as he lived.

2. He could recognize that his fellow human beings shared the predicament of his finitude and try to help them by fostering justice, equality, and individual growth.

3. In a futile attempt to overcome or decrease his finitude he could try to overpower others and make others even more limited.

History shows in an indisputable manner that with rare exceptions man has selected the third possibility as the acceptable domain assumption. Obviously it was the easiest and most gratifying; it was the one which permitted man to be aggressive in a deflected way; it was the one by which he felt he could get quick admiration and approval from others. However, the tendency toward this choice was certainly reinforced by the fear of the other. If you do not dominate the other, the other will dominate you. Thus we go back to the problem of presence or absence of basic trust. We enter a circular process in which it is impossible at the stage of our knowledge to distinguish the initial from the subsequent steps.

At a sociopolitical level the accumulators of power are few, and the subjugated are many. Thus man always lived in fear of being overpowered. This fear has existed from prehistory to present times. Politics is to a large extent the art and science of acquiring power, preserving power, and defeating the opponent's power. But as we very well know, power is also very important in private life within the family. The threat of being overpowered that the little child experiences, as Alfred Adler was the first to describe, is perpetuated in the life of the adult, at a sociopolitical as well as at a family level.

After this reflection the temptation comes again to consider the paranoid and paranoiac patient as a real prophet or proclaimer of the truth. Some authors have accepted this interpretation. In this regard we must remember that people have been able to adapt to the most cruel situations, such as slavery and Nazi concentration camps, without becoming psychotic. Again we may reaffirm that the psychotic is not a prophet, but is one of the first and most severely injured victims. The fact that other factors, including biological, are necessary to make him become the first and total victim is immaterial in the present context. The fact remains that by being so sensitive and so vulnerable he may counteract the callousness that our healthy capacity for adjustment and adaptation has brought about.

As already noted, the most common roles of unequal distinction of power become sanctioned and crystallized by society. The person who wants to achieve autonomy must thus be liberated from inner restrictions and emancipated from some external ties. The greatest episodes of emancipation have so far been left to the unpredictable games of history. It seems that the time is ripe for psychiatrists and psychoanalysts to make in new ways modest contributions to this vast subject. By adding their knowledge of personality to certain social trends, which are quickly developing in our times, they may help the individual acquire a healthy autonomy in a complicated context of collective interdependence.

POWER IN THE THERAPEUTIC SITUATION

Not enough attention has been paid to the topic of power in the transference situation, especially with psychotic patients in psychoanalytic therapy. Obviously the analyst and the patient are not on an equal footing. The patient sees the analyst in a position of power: not just power as a function to illuminate, to interpret, to help, but actually as a controlling power of which the patient is afraid. Perhaps this is unavoidable at the beginning of therapy, as the patient transfers to the analyst the feelings he once had for the parent. At the end of therapy, when the transference is solved—somebody could argue—the patient will no longer experience the analyst in this way. However, this seems to be rarely the case, unless a different therapeutic attitude has been adopted. Even at an advanced stage of treatment the psychotic or formerly psychotic patient tends to see the analyst not as a peer, or a person he respects, but as a person he must obey. Even when many other transferential problems of parental origin have been solved, the problem of personal power remains. In my opinion, as long as the power problem exists no basic trust is established, and a prepsychotic or psychotic potentiality remains.

Perhaps I shall make my position clearer if I say that at an earlier stage in my development I was much impressed by a sentence that the French psychoanalyst Racamier (15) used in defining Frieda Fromm-Reichmann's position in the treatment of the psychotic. Racamier wrote that contrary to John Rosen and Marguerite Sechehaye, who in their treatment entered the world of psychosis, Frieda Fromm-Reichmann assumed and retained the role of ambassador of reality and did not pretend to accept the delusions of the patient. On the contrary, she relied on the part of the patient which was adult and mature in order to guide him back to the world of reality of which she was the ambassador.

In my opinion the analyst must have a double and therefore difficult role: he must be a companion of the patient in his journey in the world of unreality, and at the same time he must remain in the realm of reality. But I do not think that the term ambassador of reality defines this second role, or Fromm-Reichmann's attitude. Fromm-Reichmann had no rose gardens to promise in this world of reality. It is only when the patient feels that the analyst is not an ambassador, but a peer in this imperfect reality, a person who shares the human predicament without succumbing, that he will not necessarily see human beings as hostile powers. Only then will an atmosphere of basic trust and relatedness develop. The analyst is not a representative of any country, society, religion, parents, establishment, and so on; he is just there, involved with the patient whom he considers an equal in his human worth and in his potentiality to will.

In this position of equality it is essential that countertransference be equal in importance and intensity to the transference. To define a therapeutic relation with the psychotic as a working alliance is indication of a misalliance. "Alliance" smacks of militarism. "Working" seems to imply that the analyst and the patient work together as the employer and the employee. Moreover the analytic situation is not for the psychotic only work or mainly work, but also a place, like home is for a small child, where he can grow even without working, or by working very little. The work will increase the more the therapist and patient become peers and share even the negative aspects of the environment.

POWER IN PSYCHIATRIC AND PSYCHOANALYTIC INSTITUTIONS

In spite of excellent training, teaching, research activity, and therapy, psychiatrists and psychoanalysts are not immune to power maneuver, but are as susceptible to it as are other people. And why should they be different? Don't analysts dream like other people or have personal problems like other people? Here are some of the observations:

In many psychiatric hospitals the director acts like a king who rules over the life not only of patients but also of the medical and paramedical staff. The medical staff is generally divided into at least two groups or parties, both of which try in a subtle way to become the one preferred by the director, in order to have special privileges or to have their own policies accepted. One is reminded of the situations described by Theodore Lidz in the family: family schism and family skew. If one party loses, its members live for one thing: the hope that the director will die or retire. It is pathetic to see how submissive and obsequious to the director some members of the staff become in order to be in his good graces. The director is always right, never contradicted. In the hospital with which I was once associated, residents were warned against dating nurses, although they were allowed to date female psychologists, social workers, and occupational therapists.

Faculty appointments in medical schools, especially as chiefs of departments, follow the games of power. In a European country, where the medical schools are controlled by the state, when a vacancy to a chairmanship occurs, all the other chairmen of departments of psychiatry of the country have a meeting during which they choose three candidates. Obviously they are supposed to choose the best or the most qualified. This is seldom the case; instead, power coalitions are formed. Each chairman tries to nominate his assistant or pupil, since (a) the pupil is likely to maintain friendship with his former chief and therefore form with him the nucleus of a new power coalition, (b) the pupil will continue to spread the ideas of the teacher and perpetuate his prestige and power, and (c) because the pupil did the research or writings for papers published under the name of the chairman, the latter must show his gratitude. Inasmuch as it is not possible to nominate more than three persons, coalitions among the chairmen and secret alliances are formed. When a coalition becomes powerful enough it will be able to nominate one candidate, pupil of a chairman, with the understanding that, later on, candidates who are pupils of the other members of the coalition will also be nominated. Finally, the three candidates are selected. The battle does not end there, since the senate of the medical school will have to select one among the three suggested by the commission of chairmen. Strong pressures start to be exerted again by political parties, the church, the members of the cabinet of the government, and so on. The one of the three who is able to collect the greatest political support will finally be chosen: rarely the best.

In the United States there are no pressures from the government, but certainly there are from various ruling coalitions, including the academic coalition. In the United States there are in addition other complications, which are intradepartmental. Departments of psychiatry have become huge organizations with many branches. Often the chairman, consciously or unconsciously, imitates the prevailing methods of the corporate state. The chief of the department is generally an administrator concerned only with the smooth organization and with producing as many finished products as possible. He must deliver so many well-trained doctors and psychiatrists. Thus the school maintains the function of providing professional men, but not that of establishing a climate propitious to academic freedom. In many cases the chief of department becomes increasingly skillful in administrative practices and more and more stale in clinical, teaching, and research activities. Since he must retain some academic prestige, in some instances he persuades other people to do academic work for him. Thus he asks people to write articles or even books in which the name of the chief appears as the senior author, although he may have done little or none of the work. For these services he will reward his collaborators with academic titles, such as professor or assistant professor, just as kings of old used to appoint devoted subjects as dukes, counts, barons, and so on.

In most cases economics does not enter into the picture, only prestige and power. The atmosphere is thus different from that prevailing in other institutions of learning, such as colleges and nonmedical universities, where economics plays a role and makes the situation even worse. Obviously I do not imply that this method is the only one by which promotions are made. Merit still remains the main qualification in many departments.

In order to maintain top efficiency some chairmen do not want to grant autonomy to the different sections of the department. Such autonomy would stimulate self-determination and all the prerogatives which go with academic freedom. On the contrary, some chairmen want to retain the controlling power by appointing the new members and the chiefs of the various sections.

It is easy to determine what is wrong with such organization of hospitals and departments of psychiatry. The directors of the hospitals and the chairmen of the departments cannot be properly checked and balanced by the subordinate members of the staff. The sections should have as much autonomy as necessary to create a climate of academic freedom. A rotating system of chairmanship of departments and sections should be in operation. Fortunately this is the case now in an increasing number of departments. With the rotating system some efficiency would undoubtedly be lost, but the values gained in a climate of academic freedom would in the long run show telling results. Theoretically members of hospital staffs or of departments who feel manipulated within the system of hierarchy could complain to the commissioner of mental health or to the dean of the school. This is seldom the case, as the climate of courage for such steps rarely exists. And courage is necessary, because commissioners and deans are generally on the side of the recognized authorities, on whose benevolence they themselves depend. The would-be protesters might be labeled queer or paranoid.

In order to avoid these situations many psychoanalytic schools have organized and developed independent institutions. Alas! We may avoid Scylla and veer toward Charybdis. In a brilliant article published in 1958 in the *Saturday Review*, Erich Fromm exposed the intrigues which had taken place in the psychoanalytic association in its early history. By interviewing and quoting witnesses, Fromm documented the historical truth of these power manipulations. We would be extremely naïve to think that these maneuvers go on only among the orthodox Freudians. When the founding fathers of a school retire or die, new coalitions are formed. As in Roman, Napoleonic, or recent Russian history, at first dyarchies or triumvirates are formed, but eventually only one chief emerges. The chief will maintain the ideas of the founding chiefs (now part of the ideology of the establishment) and will keep at the periphery dissenting or not totally compliant members of the faculty.

In other cases, a conspiracy against a chief occurs; he is finally ousted and he founds another group. Often these splittings are purported to occur because of the different ideologies held by the members of the group. Actually the difference in ideology is only a pretext or a manifest motivation, just as it was in the religious wars of the past. Scientific organizations should welcome differences in ideology which certainly would add to the spirit of inquiry.

In conclusion, power as a force which tends to deflect, restrict, or eliminate the will of the individual is indeed more powerful than many other psychological factors that psychoanalysis has for a long time dealt with. Only if the individual becomes fully conscious of this power, and fully conscious of his will, may his self flourish, grow, and reach autonomy. At times he may have to pay the big price of standing alone, but he will be more of himself. And by being more of himself, he will be able to give more of himself to others. He must become aware that although it is true that he is partially made of biological components, whether we call them instinctual drives or genetic codes, and although it is true that he is also partially made of interpersonal and sociocultural influences, he is also made by the choices that he himself has made in life. Yet, not totally, but in his most significantly human part, he is made of what he himself has voluntarily chosen. But again, his choices are not entirely free. As analysts, we must do whatever we can to remove or weaken any power, external or internal, which restricts his free and constructive choices.

REFERENCES

1. ADLER, A.: A study of organ inferiority and its psychical compensation. *Nerv. Ment. Dis. Monogr.*, No. 24, 1917.
2. ADLER, A.: Understanding human nature. New York: Greenbreg, 1927.
3. ARIETI, S.: Volition and value: A study based on catatonic schizophrenia. *Compr. Psychiat.*, 2:74-82, 1961.
4. ARIETI, S.: The intrapsychic self: Feeling, cognition and creativity in health and mental illness. New York: Basic Books, 1967.
5. ARIETI, S.: The psychodynamics of schizophrenia: A reconsideration. *Amer. J. Psychother.*, 22:366-381, 1968.
6. ARIETI, S.: The structural and psychodynamic role of cognition in the human psyche. In: S. Arieti (Ed.), *The World Biennial of Psychiatry and Psychotherapy*, Vol. 1. New York: Basic Books, 1970.
7. ARIETI, S.: *The Will to Be Human*. New York: Quadrangle, 1972.
8. FARBER, L.: The ways of the will: Essays toward a psychology of the will. New York: Basic Books, 1966.
9. FROMM, E.: Debate with Jacob Arlow on psychoanalysis. *Saturday Rev.*, June 14, 1958.
10. GOULDNER, A. W.: The coming crisis of western civilization. New York: Basic Books, 1970.
11. HORNEY, K.: Our inner conflicts. New York: W. W. Norton, 1945.
12. LORENZ, K.: On aggression. New York: Harcourt, Brace and World, 1963.
13. MAY, R.: Love and will. New York: W. W. Norton, 1969.
14. RACAMIER, P. C.: Psychoanalytic therapy of the psychoses. In: S. Nacht (Ed.), *Psychoanalysis of Today*. New York: Grune & Stratton, 1959.
15. SALZMAN, L.: Personal communication, 1971.

31

Vico and Modern Psychiatry

There is today a revival of interest in the eighteenth-century philosopher Giambattista Vico. His ideas have been reevaluated in reference to modern psychiatry. This paper, read at a symposium on Vico held in 1976, illustrates the relations between Freud's and Jung's theories and Vico's. It also illustrates the influence of Vico on my psychiatric research.

THIS SYMPOSIUM reveals again the magnitude of Giambattista Vico's impact on contemporary thought. Since psychiatry, especially in its psychodynamic and psychoanalytic branches, plays such an important role in twentieth-century thinking, it is appropriate to inquire whether connections can be found between Vico and this discipline. In my opinion connections are not difficult to find, but generally they have been overlooked. To the best of my knowledge, I was the first psychiatrist to point out the connections between my field and Giambattista Vico. I did so in articles published in 1950 and 1952, and in the first edition of my book, *Interpretation of Schizophrenia,* published in 1955. Dr. Blasi and Dr. Mora have made my task easier with their discussions, respectively, of Vico and developmental psychology and Vico and Piaget. I shall first discuss Vico as precursor of Freud and Jung. Then I shall describe how Vico's conceptions helped me to interpret schizophrenia.

VICO AND FREUD

Both Vico and Freud engaged in a search for a deep psychological meaning in the apparently irrational myths, habits, and ways of thinking of ancient people. Vico was actually the first to describe some mental mechanisms, for instance, projection; but Freud was the one to present them in obvious psychologic terms, to include them in the framework of a Darwinian biology, and to make them available to people living in a cultural climate much more receptive to these ideas. Was Freud influenced by Vico? I don't know whether we can answer this question. The great German psychologist Wilhelm Wundt knew Vico's work, to which he referred in his book *Völkerpsychologie;* and it could be that Freud was influenced by Vico through Wundt, but I am not in a position to prove this possibility.

What Vico studied concerning the mind of ancient people may be connected with what Freud called the primary process. In Chapter 7 of his main book, *The Interpretation of Dreams,* Freud advanced the hypothesis that there are two fundamentally different kinds of mental processes, which he termed primary and secondary (1). According to Jones, "Freud's revolutionary contribution to psychology was not so much his demonstrating the existence of an unconscious, and perhaps not even his exploration of its content, as his proposition that there are these two kinds of mental processes" (2).

Freud gave the first description of the two processes and tried to differentiate the particular laws or principles that rule the primary process only. He called the primary process "primary" because, according to him, it occurs earlier in the ontogenetic development and not because it is more important than the secondary. Later Freud postulated that the primary process occurs earlier phylogenetically, too. The secondary process is the process of the normal adult who is awake; it is the process that follows the rules of thought of ordinary logic.

Now if we want to find correlates in the field of philosophy, we can say that Vico is the philosopher of the primary process and Descartes, with his "clear and distinct ideas," is the philosopher of the secondary process. It was much easier, of course, for Descartes to be understood by the intellectual masses, already educated in secondary process matter from the time of Plato and Aristotle. Vico, as a striking innovator, encountered more difficulty in making his ideas understood.

It is difficult to compare Freud's views on the primary process with Vico's views, for several reasons. Some of these reasons are connected with the different purposes of the two authors; other have to do with recent developments that have occurred in the psychoanalytic school. At first it seemed that in the study of the primary process classic psychoanalysis focused on the cognitive or symbolic processes that belong to the unconscious. When Freud later divided the psyche into three agencies (id, ego, superego), the unconscious did not correspond exactly to the id. The id was seen predominantly as a reservoir of psychic energy (or libido), not as a type of cognition but as a way of dealing with psychic energy. It is obvious, however, that any comparison between Vichian and Freudian conceptions must be made in the field of cognition.

At this point I will outline the major points of agreement between Freud's conceptions and Vico's:

1) Both Vico and Freud give great importance to the nature and origin of mental processes. Both authors believe that things cannot be understood from the ways they are at the time they are considered but from the ways they came to be. Vico writes: "The nature of things is nothing but their coming into being at certain times and in certain special ways. These times and ways being as they are and not otherwise, things come to be as they are and not otherwise" (3). Vico applies this point of view not only psychologically but also, as Auerbach put it, as a form of justification of historical relativism as well as an affirmation that history is subject to law and order (4). Freud applies this basic idea predominantly at a psychological level; what occurs in the adult psyche has its foundation in early childhood. As revolutionary as Vico's affirmation was for sociology and history, so was Freud's affirmation, at a time when psychological phenomena and psychiatric conditions were studied in cross country section, that is, in their present aspect, not in a longitudinal section or unfolding in time. There is no doubt that to know the origin of things is a gigantic step toward the understanding of their nature.

2) Both Vico and Freud compare primitive or ancient people to children of modern time. The underlying presupposition, which could not be formulated in this way by Vico, is that ontogeny recapitulates phylogeny. Vico speaks of the ancient or primitive world as *primo mondo fanciullo* (first childlike world) (5). The comparison between the primitive world and childhood is made all through the *Scienza nuova*.

3) Both Vico and Freud see the development of the human mind as a progressive succession of stages, from the most primitive to the most complex. According to both Vico and Freud, society and history mirror the development of the individual, and the development of the modern individual recapitulates the development of society. The relationship between all these points of view is obvious. As I have already mentioned, Freud had the benefit of Darwin's contributions. Vico did not have such benefit and could not draw his conclusions from biological data, only from historical and literary sources.

A comparison between the mental stages described by Vico and those described by Freud is not easy because of their different terminologies and approaches. Vico speaks of the *bestioni* (big, beastlike humans) and of civilized men; he also refers to the ages of Gods, Heroes, and Men. Freud gives the following various classifications: (2) unconscious, preconscious, conscious; (b) id, ego, superego; (c) oral, anal, genital stages of libido. Again we could stress that Vico's levels are predominantly phylogenetic and Freud's predominantly ontogenetic. However, Freud's oral stage, characterized by a feeling of omnipotence, narcissistic traits, godlike attitudes, and an impelling tendency to satisfy wishes, has many points in common with Vico's primitive stages.

4) Both Vico and Freud reach the conclusion that man projects his own beliefs and feelings into the world and tries to interpret the world through this projection. According to Vico, man in his ignorance makes himself the ruler of the cosmos and makes an entire world out of himself:

> When men do not know the natural causes which produce things and cannot even give analogical explanation, they attribute to things their own nature. For instance, uneducated people say that the magnet loves the iron. . . . The human mind, because of its indefinite nature, wherever it wanders in ignorance, makes itself the ruler of the universe concerning whatever it does not know (6).

Vico could not use the word "projection," which was coined by Freud in 1896, and formulated the concept that man attributes his own nature to the world.

5) Both Vico and Freud believe in a mental language common to all nations; that is, they both believe in the symbolic function of the human mind and in the existence of universal symbols.

Psychoanalysis studies symbols that are private and individualistic and those that are universal or recur among a large number of people everywhere. Whereas psychoanalysis studies symbols as they appear in dreams and in symptoms of psychopathologic conditions, Vico studies symbols as they appear in myths. The universal symbols in some respects correspond to Vico's "fantastic universals." In psychoanalytic theory, the symbol is conscious, the symbolized idea is unconscious (7). Although Vico could not express himself in these words, it is obvious in reading the *Scienza nuova* that he felt that ancient people were not fully aware of the meaning implicit in their myths.

6) Both Vico and Freud believe that incest is forbidden by man, not by nature, contrary to what Socrates thought (8).

At this point, it may be important to underline some basic differences between Vico's and Freud's basic concepts:

1) Both thinkers are very much concerned with primitive mentality, but their emphases are different. Freud wants to interpret and clarify

the irrationality of the mental processes that follow the primary process. He stresses that these mental processes are irrational, primitive, and inferior to normal activities of the psyche. They are so inferior that the normal person is ashamed of them, feels guilty because of them, and therefore represses them. Psychoanalysis will uncover them ("Where id was, ego must be"), so that the person can discard them altogether. Vico, too, realizes that the mentality of what he calls *bestioni* was a lower form, but in this apparent irrationality he sees some rationality, some truth that appears in symbolic universals, expressed in disguised, poetical forms, especially in the medium of myth.

2) Whereas Freud relies mostly on the study of dreams for an understanding of the archaic mind, Vico relies mostly on the study of myths and poetry. Myths and poetry are to Vico what dreams and symptoms are to Freud. They occupy approximately an equal role in the two systems. Fantasies and imagination in the waking state are as important in Vico's system as dreams are in Freud's.

3) Both Vico and Freud deal with what in today's psychological terminology we call cognition and motivation. However, whereas Freud stresses motivation by far, Vico stresses cognition.

VICO AND JUNG

Jung's work also deserves special consideration in a study of the relation between Vico and modern psychiatry.

1) The main point in common between Vico and Jung is the paramount role that archaic thinking plays in their systems. What in the Freudian system is included in the primary process becomes the collective unconscious in Jung's theoretical framework. Whereas Freud embraced Darwin's major concepts in evolution and applied them to his new psychoanalytic science, Jung followed Lamarck; that is, he believed in the inheritability of characteristics acquired from the environment. The collective unconscious would contain deposits of constantly repeated experiences of humanity (9). For instance, one of the commonest experiences is the apparent daily movement of the sun. This experience reappears in numerous modifications in the myth of the sun-hero among various peoples.

Although modern biology has disproved the validity of the concept of the inheritance of acquired characteristics, Jung's scholarly search for similarities in the customs, beliefs, and ways of thinking of ancient people has led to important psychological conceptions. I have no evidence that Jung derived his major concepts from Vico, but certainly both authors' search for similarities in ancient people must be considered an important common characteristic. Vico, of course, did not attempt any biological interpretation of the recurrence of myths.

2) For Jung, the archetype is the unity of psychological deposits, originated from the environment. The archetype is, by definition, an innate state of readiness to produce again and again similar or identical mythical or primitive ideas. These components of the collective unconscious are called by Jung not simply archetypes but various names: primordial images, mythological images, and behavior problems. To some extent they correspond to a mixture of Vico's fantastic universals and Vico's recurring common principles of human beings. Like Vico's fantastic universals, the archetypes tend to repeat archaic forms of cognition. The three common principles of Vico are divination, marriage, and burial, which give origin respectively to religion, morality, and belief in immortality. Although there is no exact parallel between Vico's fundamental principles and Jung's archetypes, the similarities are conspicuous.

The theory of recurrence, as formulated by Vico, may be more simply reformulated as the recurrence at various historical periods of various expressions of archaic mentality. Although the expressions of archaic mentality are part of the potential repertory of the human mind at any time, they may be elicited in clusters or in large numbers by particular historico-cultural and geographical factors.

3) Unlike Freud, who saw predominantly pathology and irrationality in the recurrence of the forms of archaic mentality, Jung stressed that myths as well as the other archaic mental processes may be rational or irrational. They may be either symptoms of disease or constructive symbols. Jung is thus in this respect closer to Vico, who saw in the ancient myths the wisdom of past ages.

VICO'S INFLUENCE ON MY WORK

When I started my research on schizophrenia, approximately thirty-five years ago, I found myself in an advantageous position on account of two factors. One of them was the discovery made shortly after my arrival in America of a book by Heinz Werner, which opened to my understanding the vast vistas of a comparative developmental approach. But the other advantageous position was my knowledge of Giambattista Vico, which I had acquired during my premedical studies in Italy, at the Liceo Galileo in Pisa. As a matter of fact, I soon discovered the great parallel between Vico's and Werner's approaches.

In my early studies of schizophrenia I became particularly interested in the modalities of thinking of the schizophrenic patient. I soon realized that the schizophrenic patient, when he thinks in a typically schizophrenic way, adopts a type of cognition that corresponds not only to Freud's primary process thinking but also to Vico's archaic mentality. As a matter of fact, I called the special "logic" of the schizophrenic "paleologic," or archaic logic. I wrote that what seem schizophrenic forms of irrationality are instead reemerging archaic forms of rationality.

Paleologic is founded mainly on Von Domarus's principle, which, in a slightly modified form, is as follows: "Whereas the normal person accepts identity only upon the basis of identical subjects, the paleologician accepts identity based upon identical predicates" (10). For instance a patient thought that she was the Virgin Mary. Her delusional thought process was the following: "The Virgin Mary was a virgin; I am a virgin; therefore, I am the Virgin Mary." The delusional conclusion was reached because the identity of the predicate of the two premises (the state of being virgin) made the patient accept the identity of the two subjects (the Virgin Mary and the patient). In order to remove her feeling of utter inadequacy, the patient needed to identify with the Virgin Mary, who was her ideal of feminine perfection. She also felt extreme closeness and spiritual kinship to the Virgin Mary. Nevertheless, she would not have been able to implement this identification had she not regressed to an archaic modality of thinking.

In primitive societies the same paleologic mode of thought prevails. For instance, Lévy-Bruhl reported a Congo native saying to a European that an evil man, a crocodile, and a wildcat were one and the same person because all of them had an evil spirit (11). The common characteristics or predicate (having an evil spirit) led to the identification. Books of anthropology are replete with similar examples. The paleologician does not respect Aristotle's three laws of thought. Vico advanced similar ideas about the origin of mythological figures such as satyrs and centaurs. He wrote that the ancients, being unable to abstract the same property from two different bodies, united the bodies in their minds. Vico explained mythological metamorphoses in a similar way; if a subject acquires a new property that is more characteristic of a second subject, the first is transformed into the second. For instance, if a woman who used to travel or to change in many ways finally stopped at a certain place, and no further change occurred in her life, in the myth she might appear as transformed into a plant. In logical language we could say that the paleologician has difficulty separating predicates from subjects and tends to identify with subjects that have one or more predicates in common.

Another characteristic that I described in the schizophrenic is the concretization of the concept. What in a normal person is conceived of in an abstract way assumes a concrete, perceptual, or quasi-perceptual representation in schizophrenic thinking. Vico described similar processes in ancient people. He gave numerous examples of how the idea is replaced by an image; how a concept becomes a fantastic universal. The immediate, the particular, and the concrete replace a concept that can be applied to a whole class. For instance, Jupiter becomes a vast animate and sensitive body that replaces the concept of supreme heroism and power; Hercules becomes the concrete embodiment of the abstract concept of strength. Thus concepts become personified, anthropomorphized. In some mentally ill patients, particularly the schizophrenic, the abstract idea is translated into a perception, in the form of a hallucination, fantasy, or delusion which is mediated by images.

Vico gave great importance to visual images. According to him, the fables of the ancients, before they were expressed in words, consisted chiefly of visual images. Language, or poetry, subsequently transcribed what was at first predominantly "imaged" in the visual field.

In the last fifty years images have lost the important position they held in the older books of psychology. The loss of interest in images in American psychology and psychiatry was possible because their most important functions had not been recognized and also because they did not lend themselves to objective or behavioristic investigations.

An image is a memory trace that assumes the form of a representation. It is an internal quasi-reproduction of a perception that, in order to be experienced, does not require the corresponding external stimulus. Although we cannot deny that at least rudimentary images occur in subhuman animals, there seems to be no doubt that they are predominantly a human characteristic. In fact, we can affirm that images are among the earliest and most important foundations of human symbolism. If we use the term "symbol" to mean something that stands for something else which is not present, the image must be considered one of the first symbols. For instance, I close my eyes and visualize my mother. She may not be present, but her image is with me; it stands for her. The image is obviously based on the memory traces of previous perceptions of my mother. My mother then acquires a psychic reality that is not tied to her physical presence.

Image formation is actually the basis for all high mental processes. It introduces us into the inner world that I have called fantasmic (12). It enables the human being not only to reevoke what is not present but also to retain an affective disposition for the absent object. For instance, the image of my mother may evoke the love I feel for her. Primitive forms of cognition, which do not make use of language, are mediated predominantly by images.

In dreams, too, concepts are transformed into images predominantly visual in type. Psychoanalysis has given a great deal of attention to the images of dreams but not enough to the other types. Under the influence of Vico, I have called attention to the importance of the fantasmic stage of development. This is a stage in which images prevail over other cognitive constructs. This stage cannot be found in pure form either ontogenetically or phylogenetically, but there cannot be any doubt about its existence, as I have described elsewhere (13).

The fantasmic stage represents an important intermediary form of organization that the evolving mind goes through while on its way toward an ultimate level, where universals, or concepts, or Descartes' clear and distinct ideas are possible. The fantasmic stage reappears in various stages of schizophrenia in the form of hallucinations, or in thoughts that rely more on images than on abstract concepts.

There is an additional point that I have derived from Vico, and which I think has influenced my psychotherapeutic approach toward all categories of patients. First of all, I must state that modern psychiatry has advanced different concepts and hypotheses about the goal of human mental health. At first, for many psychiatrists the goal seemed to be adjustment; that is, a state of psychological harmony with the environment, a concept that is a derivation of biological adaptational theories. Later, many psychologists and psychiatrists—for instance, Fromm, Horney, and Maslow—came to feel that adjustment cannot possibly be considered man's ultimate goal. Adjustment may actually stultify or limit the individuality of man, especially if it is adjustment to an unhealthy society. These authors believe that self-realization or self-actualization is man's goal. Although this point of view constitutes a certain progress over the concept of adjustment, in my opinion it also fails to explain the human condition. For instance, Horney refers to self-realization as the fulfillment of one's potentialities, just as an oak tree is the fulfilled potentiality of an acorn. This example of the acorn, first found in Aristotle's writings, cannot be appropriately applied to man. The unfolding of man's psychological development is not necessarily inherent in a potentiality. Inasmuch as the human symbolic functions are susceptible of infinite combinations, man is forever an unending product, capable of unpredictable growth. We should not confuse potentiality with possibility.

According to Caponigri, the first principle of the modification of the human mind is to be found in the definition of man that Vico advances in the *Diritto universale*, namely, *posse, nosse, velle, finitum quod tendit ad infinitum*, a finite principle of possibility, of knowing, and of willing that tends to the infinite (14). The *posse* of this definition, according to Caponigri, indicates Vico's insight into man's "indefinite nature." "This is the insight that the being of man cannot be enclosed within a determinate structure of possibilities, such, for example, as might be fixed by any law of cause and effect, but that it moves, rather, among *indeterminable alternatives*, and even further, by its own movement, generates these alternatives" (15).

The existentialist Italian philosopher Abbagnano has further elaborated the concept of possibility as differentiated from that of potentiality (16). Also the French author Lapassade describes man as always *inachevé* (17).

I have gradually come to see the goal of mental health not as self-realization or actualization of alleged potentialities but as self-expansion. The self of man evolves indefinitely along certain alternatives, which it generates. As I wrote elsewhere:

> This is not to say that man is infinite; he is indeed finite, but in his own finitude he is always unfinished. Biological growth stops at a certain stage of development, but psychological growth may continue as long as life does. By psychological growth we mean the expansion of feelings, understandings, and possibilities of choices and actions with agreeable and often unforeseeable effects. Man thus cannot aim at self-realization but at an unknown, undetermined, and undeterminable self-expansion. The quality and extent of this expansion will depend on what he can make of his inner experiences, conceptual life, interpersonal relations, work, and actions (12).

I believe that these words portray an indirect but very strong Vichian influence.

REFERENCES

1. FREUD, S.: *The Interpretation of Dreams*. New York: Basic Books, 1960.
2. JONES, E.: *The Life and Work of Sigmund Freud*, Vol. 1. New York: Basic Books, 1953.
3. *The New Science of Giambattista Vico* (hereinafter *NS*), translated by Thomas G. Bergin and Max H. Fisch. Ithaca: Cornell University Press, 1968, par. 147.

4. AUERBACH, E.: *Literary Language and Its Public in Late Latin Antiquity and in the Middle Ages*. New York: Pantheon Books, 1965.
5. *NS*, par. 69.
6. *NS*, par. 180.
7. FENICHEL, O.: *The Psychoanalytic Theory of Neurosis*. New York: Norton, 1945.
8. *NS*, par. 336.
9. JUNG, C. G.: *Two Essays on Analytical Psychology*. New York: Pantheon Books, 1953.
10. DOMARUS, E. VON: The specific laws of logic in schizophrenia. In: J. S. Kasanin (Ed.), *Language and Thought in Schizophrenia*. Berkeley: University of California Press, 1944.
11. LÉVY-BRUHL, L.: *Les fonctions mentales dans les sociétés inférieures*. Paris: Alcan, 1910.
12. ARIETI, S.: *The Intrapsychic Self: Feeling, Cognition, and Creativity in Health and Mental Illness*. New York: Basic Books, 1967.
13. ARIETI, S.: *Interpretation of Schizophrenia*, 2nd ed. New York: Basic Books, 1974.
14. CAPONIGRI, A. R.: *Time and Idea: The Theory of History in Giambattista Vico*. Chicago: Regnery, 1953.
15. *Ibid.*, my italics.
16. ABBAGNANO, N.: *Possibilità e libertà*. Turin: Taylor, 1956.
17. LAPASSADE, G.: *L'entrée dans la vie*. Paris: Éditions de Minuit, 1963.

Some Memories and Personal Views

FROM THAT COLD NIGHT of January 11, 1939, when I kissed my mother and father goodbye and escaped from Mussolini's hordes, to today, few if any have been the moments in my life equal in significance to the one, just passed, in which I received from the President of the American Academy of Psychoanalysis the Frieda Fromm-Reichmann Award.

This award has a deep meaning for me, first of all because it is linked with the name of the great teacher from whom I learned much, and whom I much revered. It is important for me, as it was for the others who preceded me in receiving this honor, to point out that those paths that Frieda Fromm-Reichmann so bravely opened up have been pursued by her pupils and probably one day will be followed and extended by her pupils' pupils. In an era when many thought that psychoanalytic treatment for the schizophrenic patient was hopeless, Frieda Fromm-Reichmann with her devotion and the originality and clarity of her teaching showed to us that her treatment was not in vain, and we gathered around her to learn and to be inspired.

It would be excessive modesty, however, not to mention that this award gives me pleasure because it is a recognition of my work. And in the few minutes at my disposal and in the most general way, I shall make an attempt to tell you what I have tried to do with my work, what I have tried to say.

More than all the other training to which I have been exposed, the preparatory work that I did at the William Alanson White Institute of New York made me understand that one becomes a person by virtue of relations with other human beings and not of inborn instinctual

The Frieda Fromm-Reichmann Award, honoring persons who have made significant contributions to knowledge of the etiology, nature, or therapy of schizophrenia, has been conferred on Dr. Arieti by the American Academy of Psychoanalysis. This statement was made at the annual meeting of the American Academy of Psychoanalysis in Boston on May 11, 1968 following the presentation of the Frieda Fromm-Reichmann Award.

drives. The countless ways, the infinite nuances with which people love or hate, help or hurt one another, in no other conditions can be better observed than in the study of the schizophrenic disorder.

Soon it appeared to me that this approach had to be applied in conjunction with others. The numberless messages of hate and love go through numbered doors, and the ever-expanding universe of people and symbols return to the uniqueness of the sentient self, to the individuality of the intrapsychic. What I am trying to say is that the sequence of the external influences is integrated by intrapsychic mechanisms so that it becomes personal history and the autonomous way of meeting the world becomes the personality.

In referring specifically to the schizophrenic patient, I mean that he makes his own contribution to his own condition. The environmental forces, as influential as they are, do not mold him entirely. The schizophrenic disorder is not simply a reaction; and, incidentally, I am delighted to see that finally the American Psychiatric Association has abolished the label "schizophrenic reaction" in the official nomenclature. The irrationality of the patient is not something that has been passively or directly transmitted by the parents as a language is. The environmental irrationality is a very powerful psychodynamic factor in schizophrenia, inasmuch as it leads to emotional states that trigger off special forms of abnormal cognition. In its turn, abnormal cognition expands enormously, transforming to often unpredictable consequences the original irrationality and adding new ones.

Since 1948 I have tried to illustrate the mechanisms of this special cognition. I have also attempted to show how late experiences in life, mediated by formally normal conceptual cognition, rekindle the old conflicts and evoke primary process mechanisms. I have also tried to show that when interpersonal relatedness is established in the treatment of the schizophrenic, the patient can become more aware of the active role he plays in his illness; how at times he can actually choose between the realm of psychosis and the realm of reality; how even in such apparently immutable processes as hallucinations and delusions, he can recognize that it is up to him to resist the seduction of the abnormal mechanisms and to accept the anxiety and suffering of a meaning that is not masked by psychotic media. The patient will be able to do so if he feels that the therapist is there to share the anxiety and suffering of his conflict. In other words, the patient is not expected to passively absorb interpretation, freely offered to him. The analyst only gives him tools with which he himself must fight his own illness.

I have found that it is difficult for some psychiatrists, even those prominent and creative in their specific fields, to appreciate this battle against reductionisms of all sorts and to accept an expansionist or pluralistic approach. It is difficult, I repeat, but it is not impossible if one of the advocators of this pluralistic approach can eventually get the Frieda Fromm-Reichmann Award.

As to Frieda Fromm-Reichmann herself, she too was a pluralist. She was influenced by four teachers with different orientations, the four teachers to whom she dedicated her book: Sigmund Freud, Kurt Goldstein, Georg Groddeck, and Harry Stack Sullivan.

I believe that it is appropriate to conclude these few remarks with one of the memories of Frieda Fromm-Reichmann that is dear to me. It is the memory of a meaningful little event that some of you in the audience may have actually witnessed with me. In January 1957, she gave a speech to the graduating class of the William Alanson White Institute. I was one of the many people listening to her, and I was very much impressed by the many things she said about her experiences in Chestnut Lodge and Palo Alto. But what has remained vivid in my mind was her mimicking of a female schizophrenic patient who always walked with a thumb extended and the other fingers flexed over the palm of her hand. Frieda did not interpret this gesture as others would have. For her, the extended thumb was not a phallic symbol, nor did it indicate penis envy. It meant, "I am one: alone, alone, alone!"

What does the cry of loneliness mean to the schizophrenic patient or, for that matter, to any human being? It means that one has been abandoned by the interpersonal world or is very much in need of intimacy with the interpersonal world. But the pain of aloneness and loneliness is felt inside, of what the lonely thumb stood for, in the depth of the intrapsychic.

Acceptance of the National Book Award

The following is the acceptance speech made by Dr. Arieti on his receiving the 1975 National Book Award for his book, *Interpretations of Schizophrenia*.

In accepting this award I have all the excitement, the joy, the trepidation, the rebirth experience of people whose work has been recognized. This work of mine with schizophrenic patients, work to which I have devoted more than a third of a century, approximately thirty-four years, has been and continues to be not just part of my profession, but of my blood, my soul, the meaning of my life.

This personal involvement and recognition fortunately does not limit my understanding of what is implied in the selection of my book for this Award. This Award is much more than an appreciation of my work. First of all, it is a tribute to psychiatry, especially to psychodynamic psychiatry. To the best of my knowledge this is the first time that the National Book Award in the field of science has been given to a psychiatric book. In selecting this book, the judges honored many previous psychiatrists, without whose contributions this book could not have been written. I do not think only of Sigmund Freud, but also of Harry Stack Sullivan, Frieda Fromm-Reichmann, and many others, whose pioneer work led to a psychodynamic understanding and treatment of schizophrenia.

Secondly, in choosing this book the judges recognized the importance of schizophrenia as a mental illness and as a significant social fact. In spite of the progress made, the number of people suffering from this condition is increasing, and more hospital beds are occupied by schizophrenics than by patients affected by any other disease. In my book I insist that the doors of the hospitals can be opened for a large number of treated patients and I show how, step by step, they can be helped to resume their peace and their role in society.

Thirdly, the judges must have accepted my message that it is possible for the therapist to help the patient "to experience the human tie more intensely than any fear, more strongly than any need for distance." As I described in my book, we therapists are able to learn and practice ways

473

of bringing trust to the distrustful, clarity to the bewildered, speech to the mute, creativity to the chaotic, confident expectation to the hopeless, and companionship to the lonely. And in so doing we can suggest a larger vista for the human horizon, a larger use for the human bond, and optimism for the solution of those other conditions in health or illness that, although difficult, are not so obscure, so hard to approach, so desperate, so far from the usual reach of man's words and care.

In other words, the judges have understood that the study of schizophrenia transcends schizophrenia. No other condition in human pathology permits us to delve so deeply into what is specific to human nature. Although the main objective of the therapist of the schizophrenic is to relieve suffering, he will have to deal with a panorama of the human condition, which includes the problems of truth and illusion, bizarreness and creativity, grandiosity and self-abnegation, loneliness and capacity for communion, interminable suspiciousness and absolute faith, motivated self-destruction and unmotivated crime, blaming and self-accusation, surrender to love and hate and imperviousness to these feelings.

In this field of psychiatry the rigid borders between neurology and psychology, biology and social science become blurred and confused. What emerges with greater clarity are the ways to understand each other and care for each other.

Bibliography of Silvano Arieti, M.D.

BOOKS:

Interpretation of Schizophrenia. First Edition, 1955. Translated into several languages. 12 American printings.

The Intrapsychic Self: Feeling, Cognition and Creativity in Health and Mental Illness, 1967.

The Will to Be Human, 1972.

Interpretation of Schizophrenia. Second Edition, 1974. Completely revised and expanded.

Creativity: The Magic Synthesis, 1976.

American Handbook of Psychiatry. First Edition (Editor), 1959 and 1966.

The World Biennial of Psychiatry. (Editor-in-Chief), Vol. 1, 1971; Vol. 2, 1973.

American Handbook of Psychiatry. Second Edition. Completely revised and expanded. (Editor-in-Chief), 1974 and 1975.

New Dimensions in Psychiatry. (Co-edited with Gerard Chrzanowski) Vol. I, 1975; Vol. II, 1977.

Love Can Be Found (with James Arieti), 1977.

PAPERS:

1. Histopathological Changes in Experimental Metrazol Convulsions in Monkeys. *American Journal of Psychiatry,* 98, 1941, 70-76.
2. The Vascularization of Cerebral Neoplasms Studied with the Fuchsian Staining Method of Eros. *Journal of Neuropathology and Experimental Neurology,* 1, 1942, 375-393.
3. Frontal Lobe Tumor Expanding into the Ventricle—Clinicopathologic Report. *The Psychiatric Quarterly* 17, 1943, 227-240.

4. Progressive Multiform Angiosis (with E. W. Gray). *Archives of Neurology and Psychiatry*, 51, 1944, 182-189.
5. The "Placing-into-Mouth" and Coprophagic Habits. *The Journal of Nervous and Mental Disease*, 99, 1944, 959-964.
6. Multiple Meningioma and Meningiomas Associated with Other Brain Tumors. *Journal of Neuropathology and Experimental Neurology*, III, 1944, 255-270.
7. An Interpretation of the Divergent Outcome of Schizophrenia in Identical Twins. *The Psychiatric Quarterly*, 1944, 18, 587-599.
8. Primitive Habits and Perceptual Alterations in the Terminal Stage of Schizophrenia. *Archives of Neurology and Psychiatry*, 1945, 53, 378-384.
9. General Paresis in Senility. *American Journal of Psychiatry*, 101, 1945, 585-593.
10. Primitive Habits in the Preterminal Stage of Schizophrenia. *The Journal of Nervous and Mental Disease*, 102, 1945, 367-375.
11. Cerebral Changes in the Course of Pernicious Anemia and Their Relationship to Psychic Symptoms. (With A. Ferraro and W. H. English) *Journal of Neuropathology and Experimental Neurology*, IV, 1945, 217-239.
12. The Effects of Sex Hormones on the Copulatory Behavior of Senile White Rats. (With R. S. Minnick and C. J. Warden) *Science*, 103, 749-750.
13. Histopathologic Changes in Cerebral Malaria and Their Relation to Psychotic Sequels. *Archives of Neurology and Psychiatry*, 1946, 56, 79-104.
14. The Processes of Expectation and Anticipation. *The Journal of Nervous and Mental Disease*, 106, 1947.
15. Special Logic of Schizophrenic and Other Types of Autistic Thought. *Psychiatry*, 11, 1948, 325-338.
16. Primitive Intellectual Mechanisms in Psychopathological Conditions. *American Journal of Psychotherapy*, IV, 1950, 4-15.
17. New Views on the Psychology and Psychopathology of Wit and of the Comic. *Psychiatry*, 13, 1950, 43-62.
18. Autistic Thought: Its Formal Mechanisms and Its Relationship to Schizophrenia. *The Journal of Nervous and Mental Disease*, III, 1950, 288-303.
19. Anti-Psychoanalytic Cultural Forces in the Development of Western Civilization. *American Journal of Psychotherapy*, VI, 1952, 63-78.
20. The Pineal Gland in Old Age. *Journal of Neuropathology and Experimental Neurology*, XIII, 1954, 482-491.
21. Some Aspects of Language in Schizophrenia. In H. Werner (Ed.),

On Expressive Language. Worcester, Mass.: Clark University Press, 1955.

23. Some Basic Problems Common to Anthropology and Modern Psychiatry. *American Anthropologist,* 58, 1956, 26-39.

24. The Possibility of Psychosomatic Involvement of the Central Nervous System in Schizophrenia. *The Journal of Nervous and Mental Disease,* 123, 1956, 324-333.

25. What Is Effective in the Therapeutic Process? *The American Journal of Psychoanalysis,* XVI, 1957, 30-33.

26. The Double Methodology in the Study of Personality and Its Disorders. *American Journal of Psychotherapy,* XI, 1957, 532-547.

27. The Two Aspects of Schizophrenia. *The Psychiatric Quarterly,* 31, 1957, 403-416.

28. Some Socio-Cultural Aspects of Manic-Depressive Psychosis and Schizophrenia. *Progress in Psychotherapy,* IV, 1959, 140-152.

29. The Triple Aspect of the Psychopathology of Schizophrenia. *Congress Report of the 2nd International Congress for Psychiatry,* Zurich, 1957, 209-213.

30. Schizophrenic Thought. *American Journal of Psychotherapy,* XIII, 1959, 537-552.

31. Manic-Depressive Psychosis. In S. Arieti (Ed.), *American Handbook of Psychiatry.* New York: Basic Books, 1959.

32. Schizophrenia: The Manifest Symptomatology, the Psychodynamic and Formal Mechanisms. In S. Arieti (Ed.), *American Handbook of Psychiatry.* New York: Basic Books, 1959.

33. Schizophrenia: Other Aspects; Psychotherapy. In S. Arieti (Ed.), *American Handbook of Psychiatry.* New York: Basic Books, 1959.

34. Rare, Unclassifiable, Collective, and Exotic Psychotic Syndromes. (With J. M. Meth) In S. Arieti (Ed.), *American Handbook of Psychiatry.* New York: Basic Books, 1959.

35. Recent Conceptions and Misconceptions of Schizophrenia. *American Journal of Psychotherapy,* XIV, 1960, 3-29.

36. Schizophrenia. *Encyclopaedia Britannica,* 1960.

37. The Experience of Inner Status. In *Perspectives in Psychological Theory,* 1960.

38. Etiological Considerations of Schizophrenia. In *The Out-patient Treatment of Schizophrenia.* New York: Grune & Stratton, 1960.

39. Aspects of Psychoanalytically Oriented Treatment of Schizophrenia. In *The Out-patient Treatment of Schizophrenia.* New York: Grune & Stratton, 1960.

40. Volition and Value: A Study Based on Catatonic Schizophrenia. *Comprehensive Psychiatry,* 2, 1961, 74-82.

41. A Re-examination of the Phobic Symptom and of Symbolism in

Psychopathology. *The American Journal of Psychiatry*, 118, 1961, 106-110.

42. The Loss of Reality. *Psychoanalysis and the Psychoanalytic Review*, 48, 1961, 3-23.

43. Introductory Notes on the Psychoanalytic Therapy of Schizophrenics. In *Psychotherapy of the Psychoses*. New York: Basic Books, 1961.

44. Hallucinations, Delusions, and Ideas of Reference Treated with Psychotherapy. *American Journal of Psychotherapy*, XVI, 1962, 52-60.

45. Psychotherapy of Schizophrenia. *Archives of General Psychiatry*, 6, 1962, 112-122.

46. The Microgeny of Thought and Perception. *Archives of General Psychiatry*, 6, 1962, 454-468.

47. The Psychotherapeutic Approach to Depression. *American Journal of Psychotherapy*, XVI, 1962, 397-406.

48. Studies of Thought Processes in Contemporary Psychiatry. *The American Journal of Psychiatry*, 120, 1963, 58-64.

49. Psychopathic Personality: Some Views on Its Psychopathology and Psychodynamics. *Comprehensive Psychiatry*, 4, 1963, 301-312.

50. The Psychotherapy of Schizophrenia in Theory and Practice. In *Psychiatric Research Report 17*, American Psychiatric Association, 1963.

51. The Rise of Creativity: From Primary to Tertiary Process. *Contemporary Psychoanalysis*, 1, 1964, 51-68.

52. The Schizophrenic Patient in Office Treatment. *Psychotherapy of Schizophrenia, 3rd International Symposium*, Lausanne, 1964, 7-23.

53. Conceptual and Cognitive Psychiatry. *The American Journal of Psychiatry*, 122, 1965, 361-366.

54. Contributions to Cognition from Psychoanalytic Theory. In *Science and Psychoanalysis*, Vol. III. New York: Grune & Stratton, 1965.

55. Schizophrenic Cognition. In *Psychopathology of Schizophrenia*. New York: Grune & Stratton, 1966.

56. Creativity and Its Cultivation. In S. Arieti (Ed.), *American Handbook of Psychiatry*, 3, 1966, 722-741.

57. Transferência e Contra-Transferência no Tratamento do Paciente Esquizofrênico. *Jornal Brasileiro de Psiquiatria*, 15, 1966, 163-174.

58. The Psychoanalytic Approach to the Psychoses. *The American Journal of Psychoanalysis*, XXVI, 1966, 63-65.

59. Emphasis on the Healthy Aspects of the Patient during Psychoanalytic Therapy. *The American Journal of Psychoanalysis*, XXVI, 1966, 63-65.

60. Rapida Rassegna degli Studi del Pensiero Schizofrenico da Bleuler

ai Giorni Nostri. *Archivio di Psicologia Neurologia e Psichiatria,* III-IV, 1967, 237-254.

61. Il Processo Secondario nella Psicodinamica della Schizofrenia. *Archivo di Psicologia Neurologia e Psichiatria,* III-IV, 1967, 255-269.

62. New Views on the Psychodynamics of Schizophrenia. *American Journal of Psychiatry,* 124, 1967, 453-458.

63. Some Elements of Cognitive Psychiatry. *American Journal of Psychotherapy,* XXI, 1967, 723-736.

64. Depressive Disorders. In *International Encyclopedia of the Social Sciences.* New York: The Macmillan Company & The Free Press, 1968.

65. The Creative Process, as Intrepreted by a Psychiatrist. *Journal for the Study of Consciousness,* Vol. 1, 3-15, 1968.

66. The Present Status of Psychiatric Theory. *American Journal of Psychiatry,* 124, 1968, 1630-1639.

67. Some Memories and Personal Views. *Contemporary Psychoanalysis,* 5, 1968, 85-89.

68. The Psychodynamics of Schizophrenia: A Reconsideration. *American Journal of Psychotherapy,* XXII, 1968, 366-381.

69. Toward a Unifying Theory of Cognition. *General Systems,* 10:109-115, 1965.

70. The Meeting of the Inner and the External World: In Schizophrenia, Everyday Life and Creativity. *The American Journal of Psychoanalysis,* XXIX, 1968, 115-130.

71. Current Ideas on the Problem of Psychosis. *Excerpta Medica International Congress Series No. 194, Problems of Psychosis.* International Colloquium on Psychosis, Montreal, 5-8 November, 1969, 3-21.

72. Cognition and Feeling. In M. Arnold (Ed.), *Feelings and Emotions.* New York: Academic Press, 1970.

73. The Role of Cognition in the Development of Inner Reality. In J. Hellmuth (Ed.), *Cognitive Studies,* Vol. 1. New York: Brunner/Mazel, 1970.

74. The Concept of Schizophrenia. In R. Cancro (Ed.), *The Schizophrenic Reactions: A Critique of the Concept, Hospital Treatment, and Current Research.* New York: Brunner/Mazel, 1970.

75. The Structural and Psychodynamic Role of Cognition in the Human Psyche. In S. Arieti (Ed.), *The World Biennial of Psychiatry and Psychotherapy.* New York: Basic Books, 1970.

76. The Origins and Development of the Psychopathology of Schizophrenia. In M. Bleuler and J. Angst (Eds.), *Die Entstehung der*

Schizophrenie (The Origin of Schizophrenia). Bern: Verlag Hans Huber, 1971.

77. Psychodynamic Search of Common Values with the Schizophrenic. *International Congress Series No. 259, Psychotherapy of Schizophrenia.* Proceedings of the IVth International Symposium, Turku, Finland, August 4-7, 1971. Amsterdam: Excerpta Medica.

78. The Origin and Effect of Power. In J. H. Masserman (Ed.), *Science and Psychoanalysis, Vol. XX: The Dynamics of Power.* New York: Grune & Stratton, 1972.

79. The Therapeutic Assistant in Treating the Psychotic. (With S. Lorraine) *International Journal of Psychiatry*, 10, 1972, 7-22.

80. Causality, Awareness, and Psychological Events. In *Festschrift for Ludwig von Bertalanffy.* London, 1972.

81. Anxiety and Beyond in Schizophrenia and Psychotic Depression. *American Journal of Psychotherapy*, XVII, 1973, 338-345.

82. Critical Evaluations: Concepts of Schizophrenia. I. An Abnormal Way of Dealing with an Abnormal Situation. *Canadian Psychiatric Association Journal*, 18, 1973, 253-256.

83. Schizophrenic Art and Its Relationship to Modern Art. *Journal of the American Academy of Psychoanalysis*, 1, 1973, 333-365.

84. Volition and Value: A Study Based on Catatonic Schizophrenia. In S. C. Post (Ed.), *Moral Values and the Superego Concept in Psychoanalysis.* New York: International Universities Press, 1973.

85. An Overview of Schizophrenia from a Predominantly Psychological Approach. *American Journal of Psychiatry*, 131, 1974, 241-249.

86. The Cognitive-Volition School. In S. Arieti (Ed.), *American Handbook of Psychiatry*, Vol. 1. New York: Basic Books, 1974.

87. Affective Disorders: Manic-Depressive Psychosis and Psychotic Depression: Manifest Symptomatology, Psychodynamics, Sociological Factors, and Psychotherapy. In S. Arieti (Ed.), *American Handbook of Psychiatry*, Vol. III. New York: Basic Books, 1974.

88. Schizophrenia: The Psychodynamic Mechanisms and the Psychostructural Forms. In S. Arieti (Ed.), *American Handbook of Psychiatry, Vol. III.* New York: Basic Books, 1974.

89. Individual Psychotherapy of Schizophrenia. In S. Arieti (Ed.), *American Handbook of Psychiatry*, Vol. III. New York: Basic Books, 1974.

90. Rare, Unclassifiable and Collective Psychiatric Syndromes. (With J. R. Bemporad) In S. Arieti (Ed.), *American Handbook of Psychiatry*, Vol. III. New York: Basic Books, 1974.

91. Psychosis. In *Encyclopaedia Britannica*, 1974.

92. Acting Out and Unusual Behavior in Schizophrenia. *American Journal of Psychotherapy*, XXVIII, 1974, 333-342.

93. Psychiatric Controversy: Man's Ethical Dimension. *The American Journal of Psychiatry,* 132, 1975, 39-42.
94. Sexual Problems of the Schizophrenic and Preschizophrenics. In M. Sandler and G. L. Gessa (Eds.), *Sexual Behavior: Pharmacology and Biochemistry.* New York: Raven Press, 1975.
95. La schizofrenia e l'approccio psicoterapeutico. *Revista Sperimentale di Freniatria e Medicina Legale delle Alienazioni Mentali,* Istituti Ospedalieri Neuropsichiatrici S. Lazzaro, Vol. 1C, Fasc. VI, 1975.
96. The Psychotherapeutic Approach to Schizophrenia. In D. Kemali, G. Bartholini, and D. Richter (Eds.), *Schizophrenia Today.* Oxford, Eng.: Pergamon Press, 1976.
97. Acceptance Speech, 1975 National Book Award in the field of sciences for *Interpretation of Schizophrenia,* Second Edition.
98. Psychoanalysis of Severe Depression: Theory and Therapy. *Journal of the American Academy of Psychoanalysis,* 4, 1976, 327-345.
99. Psychotherapy of Schizophrenia. In L. J. West and D. E. Flinn (Eds.), *Treatment of Schizophrenia: Progress and Prospects.* New York: Grune & Stratton, 1976.
100. Cognitive Components in Human Conflict and Unconscious Motivation. *Journal of the American Academy of Psychoanalysis,* 5, 1977, 5-16.
101. Vico and Modern Psychiatry. *Social Research,* 43, 1976, 739-752.
102. The Parents of the Schizophrenic: A Reconsideration. *Journal of the American Academy of Psychoanalysis,* 5, 1977, 347-358.
103. Psychotherapy of Severe Depression. *American Journal of Psychiatry,* 134, 1977, 864-868.
104. The Irrational in Psychoanalysis—Theoretical and Clinical Aspects. Papers presented at the IVth International Forum, New York, 1972. *Weiterentwicklung der Psychoanalyse und ihrer Anwendungen.* Gottingen and Zurich: Verlag fur Medizinische Psychologie im Verlag Vandenhoeck & Ruprecht.
105. A Psychotherapeutic Approach to Severely Depressed Patients. *American Journal of Psychotherapy,* 1978.
106. New Views on the Psychodynamics of Phobias. *American Journal of Psychotherapy,* 1978.

Acknowledgments

CHAPTER 1: Reprinted from AMERICAN JOURNAL OF PSYCHIATRY, 131:3, March 1974, pp. 241-249. © Copyright 1974 American Psychiatric Association. Reprinted by permission.

CHAPTER 2: Copyright © 1948 (renewed 1976), by The William Alanson White Psychiatric Foundation, Inc. Reprinted by special permission of the William Alanson White Psychiatric Foundation, Inc. from PSYCHIATRY (1948) 11:325-328.

CHAPTER 3: Reprinted from AMERICAN JOURNAL OF PSYCHOTHERAPY, Vol. XVI, No. 1, pages 52-60. January, 1962.

CHAPTER 4: Reprinted from PSYCHOTHER. SCHIZOPHRENIA, 3rd International Symposium, Lausanne 1964, pp. 7-23. Copyright © by Karger (Basel/New York) 1965.

CHAPTER 5: Reprinted from AMERICAN JOURNAL OF PSYCHOTHERAPY, Vol. XVII, No. 3, pages 338-345, July 1973. Presented at the Thirteenth Emil A. Gutheil Memorial Conference of the Association for the Advancement of Psychotherapy, New York City, Nov. 5, 1972.

CHAPTER 6: Reprinted from JOURNAL OF AMERICAN ACADEMY OF PSYCHOANALYSIS, Vol. 5, No. 3, pp. 347-358. Copyright © 1977 by John Wiley & Sons, Inc.

CHAPTER 7: Reprinted from AMERICAN JOURNAL OF PSYCHOTHERAPY, Vol. XIV, No. 1, pages 3-29. January, 1960. Read before the Association for the Advancement of Psychotherapy on October 24, 1958, in New York City.

CHAPTER 8: Reprinted from COMPREHENSIVE PSYCHIATRY, Vol. 2, No. 2, April, 1961, pp. 74-82. Read at the mid-winter meeting of the Academy of Psychoanalysis, New York, December 11, 1960.

CHAPTER 9: Reprinted from THE JOURNAL OF NERVOUS AND MENTAL DISEASE, Vol. 99, No. 6, June 1944, pp. 959-964.

CHAPTER 10: Reprinted from the ARCHIVES OF NEUROLOGY AND PSYCHIATRY, May 1945, Vol. 53, pp. 378-384. Copyright © 1945, by American Medical Association.

CHAPTER 11: Reprinted from THE JOURNAL OF NERVOUS AND MENTAL DISEASE, Vol. 123, No. 4, April, 1956, pp. 324-333.

CHAPTER 12: Reprinted from AMERICAN JOURNAL OF PSYCHIATRY, 124:12, June 1968, pp. 52-61. Copyright ©, 1968, American Psychiatric Association. Reprinted by permission.

CHAPTER 13: Reprinted from THE AMERICAN JOURNAL OF PSYCHIATRY, Vol. 118, No. 2, August, 1961, pp. 106-110. Copyright © 1961, The American Psychiatric Association. Reprinted by permission.

CHAPTER 14: Presented at the Eighteenth Emil A. Gutheil Memorial Conference of the Association for the Advancement of Psychotherapy, New York City,, October 23, 1977.

CHAPTER 15: COMPREHENSIVE PSYCHIATRY, Vol. 4, No. 5, October, 1963, pp. 301-312.

CHAPTER 16: Reprinted from AMERICAN JOURNAL OF PSYCHOTHERAPY, Vol. XVI, No.

3, pages 397-406. July, 1962. Presented at the Second Emil A. Gutheil Memorial Conference of the Association for the Advancement of Psychotherapy, New York, Oct. 29, 1961.

CHAPTER 17: Reprinted from JOURNAL OF THE AMERICAN ACADEMY OF PSYCHOANALYSIS, Vol. 4, No. 3, July-September 1976, pp. 327-345. Copyright © 1976 by John Wiley & Sons, Inc.

CHAPTER 18: Reprinted from THE AMERICAN JOURNAL OF PSYCHIATRY, Vol. 134, No. 8, August, 1977, pp. 864-868. Reprinted by permission.

CHAPTER 19: Reprinted from AMERICAN JOURNAL OF PSYCHIATRY, 132:1, January 1975, pp. 39-42. Copyright © 1975, American Psychiatric Association. Reprinted by permission.

CHAPTER 20: Reprinted from THE JOURNAL OF NERVOUS AND MENTAL DISEASE, Vol. 106, No. 4, Oct. 1947, pp. 471-481.

CHAPTER 21: Reprinted from the ARCHIVES OF GENERAL PSYCHIATRY, June 1962, Vol. 6, pp. 454-468. Copyright 1962, by American Medical Association.

CHAPTER 22: Reprinted from GENERAL SYSTEMS, Vol. 10, 1965, pp. 109-115.

CHAPTER 23: Reprinted from FEELINGS AND EMOTIONS. © 1970 Academic Press Inc., New York.

CHAPTER 24: Reprinted from THE WORLD BIENNIAL OF PSYCHIATRY AND PSYCHOTHERAPY, Vol. 1, pp. 3-33. © 1970 by Basic Books, Inc. Reprinted by permission.

CHAPTER 25: Reprinted from THE JOURNAL OF THE AMERICAN ACADEMY OF PSYCHOANALYSIS, Vol. 5, No. 1, January 1977, pp. 5-16. Copyright © 1977 by John Wiley & Sons, Inc.

CHAPTER 26: Copyright © 1950 by The William Alanson White Psychiatric Foundation, Inc. Reprinted by special permission of The William Alanson White Psychiatric Foundation, Inc., from PSYCHIATRY (1950), 13:43-62.

CHAPTER 27: CONTEMPORARY PSYCHOANALYSIS, Vol. 1, No. 1, Fall 1964, pp. 51-68. Presidential address to the William Alanson White Psychoanalytic Society, May 27, 1964 (revised version).

CHAPTER 28: Reprinted from AMERICAN JOURNAL OF PSYCHOTHERAPY, Vol. VI, No. 1, pages 63-78. January, 1952.

CHAPTER 29: Copyright © 1948 (renewed 1976) by The William Alanson White Psychiatric Foundation, Inc. Reprinted from AMERICAN JOURNAL OF PSYCHOTHERAPY, Vol. XI, No. 3, pages 532-547. July, 1957. Read before the William Alanson White Psychoanalytic Society, New York City, Jan. 25, 1957.

CHAPTER 30: Reprinted from SCIENCE AND PSYCHOANALYSIS, Vol. XX; *The Dynamics of Power*, pp. 16-32. J. H. Masserman, M.D., editor. © 1972 by Grune & Stratton, Inc.

CHAPTER 31: Reprinted from SOCIAL RESEARCH, Volume 43, Number 4, Winter 1976, pp. 739-752.

Index

On schizophrenia,
phobias
depression,
psychotherapy, and
the farther shores
of psychiatry

DATE			
MR 20 '80	MR 19 '86		
DE 4 '80	AP 8 '86		
AP 27 '82	MY 1 '88		
SE 24 '84	MY 4 '92		
OC 17 '84	MY 05 '93		
DE 13 '84			
MR 4 '85			
MR 25 '85			
NO 12 '85			
DE 3 '85			
MR 18 '86			